THE NORMAL CHILD

THE NORMAL CHILD

Some Problems of the Early Years and their Treatment

by

RONALD S. ILLINGWORTH

M.D. (Leeds), F.R.C.P. (Lond.), D.P.H., D.C.H.

Professor of Child Health, The University of Sheffield.
Honorary Physician to the Children's Hospital Unit
and Honorary Pædiatrician to The Jessop Hospital for Women,
The United Sheffield Hospitals

FIFTH EDITION

With 52 Illustrations

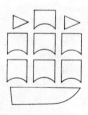

The Williams & Wilkins Company

Baltimore

SANS TACHE

First Edition	.	.	.	.	. 1953
Reprinted	.	.	.	.	. 1954
Second Edition	.	.	.	.	. 1957
Reprinted	.	.	.	.	. 1959
Third Edition	.	.	.	.	. 1964
Fourth Edition	.	.	.	.	. 1968
Reprinted	.	.	.	.	. 1971
Fifth Edition	.	.	.	.	. 1972

Translated into Greek (Third and Fourth Editions)
,,   ,,   Spanish
,,   ,,   Japanese

ISBN 0 443 00862 0

© Longman Group Limited 1972

*Any correspondence relating to this volume should
be directed to the publishers at 104 Gloucester Place,
London, W1H 4AE*

Printed in Great Britain at The Pitman Press, Bath

PREFACE TO THE FIFTH EDITION

In preparing this volume I read several times through the previous edition, reading every word, so that I could bring the book fully up to date. The continuing interest in the normal child is reflected in the fact that 191 new references have been added—rather more than were added when I prepared the fourth edition. However 125 old references have been removed, so that those to papers before 1960 are retained only when they are of particular interest or importance.

I have made extensive revisions to the sections on breast feeding and artificial feeding, largely rewriting the latter, and paying special attention to the prevention of obesity and other problems, in the light of recently acquired knowledge about possible errors of feeding methods in early infancy. I have largely rewritten the chapters on immunization and on twins, and made extensive revisions to the sections on crying, discipline, obesity, pica, breath-holding attacks and the ill child, and many other sections. I have introduced a new chapter entitled "The Young School Child," with sections on bringing the best out of a child, the mentally superior child, the backward intelligent child, dislike of school, bullying, delinquency, smoking and solvent sniffing. I have done my best to bring the book thoroughly up to date to the middle of 1971.

In case further editions of this book are required, I should be most grateful for any criticisms or comments, and in particular suggestions for deletions or additions.

Sheffield, 1972   R. S. ILLINGWORTH

PREFACE TO THE FIRST EDITION

It has long been recognized that a knowledge of anatomy and physiology is a necessary basis for the study of medicine and every medical student accordingly has to learn about the structure of the human body and how it works. It is notable, however, as Ryle pointed out some years ago, that while one would have thought that the study of health would seem to be the proper preliminary to the study of disease, health has no special place in the curriculum. Ryle said "It is surely an omission that so little attention has been paid by the students of disease and their teachers to that state from which deviation or departure must occur before the existence of disease is recognized." In the case of Pædiatrics, it certainly cannot be said that a knowledge of the normal child, of his growth, mind and development, is regarded, in England at least, as an essential basis for the study of the sick and diseased child. Yet it would seem obvious that a knowledge of the normal should precede the knowledge of the abnormal. Individual variations in the anatomical, physical, mental and biochemical make-up of the normal healthy child are so great, that a thorough grounding in the normal and in the normal variations which occur, is an essential preliminary to the fuller study of disease.

In some teaching schools, there is too much emphasis on the rare and the "interesting," and too little emphasis on the common conditions which form the large bulk of family practice. In the case of children, many of these common conditions consist of variations from the normal which hardly amount to disease, but which cause a great deal of anxiety and concern to the parents. The doctor may leave the medical school ill-equipped to deal with them. He learns a great deal from his own children, but lacking that knowledge of the normal and of normal variations which he should have learnt as a student, he is liable to read far too much into his experience with his own family and to make unwarranted generalizations which will prove harmful when applied to his patients.

It is the reponsibility of the teacher to interest the student in the common rather than the unusual, the important rather than the rare, in persons and people rather than in cases, in health as well as in disease, in prevention as well as in cure. He must instil in him a thorough knowledge of the normal, as an essential basis for the study of the abnormal.

It is because I felt that this knowledge of the normal is not easy to acquire from the available textbooks that this one was planned.

This book is intended to describe the problems other than disease which arise in the normal child in his first three years. It is not intended to be a handbook of child management, to give a description of the normal child, or to discuss biochemical and other laboratory investigations. The variations in the normal biochemistry of childhood are so great and the interpretation of the findings so difficult that, if properly covered, such a discussion would fill a book in itself. Questions of physiology, embryology, nutrition and general medicine, are omitted except only in so far as they are strictly relevant to the subjects under discussion. A knowledge of those is assumed. The book does set out to describe the normal variations in the normal child, variations which cause a great deal of worry to the parents, and which, if improperly managed, may cause a great deal of suffering to children. It sets out to give the doctor as much help as possible in trying to decide whether an individual child is normal or abnormal: it sets out to give him as much guidance as possible in the management of simple behaviour problems, such as any doctor concerned with the care of children ought to be able to deal with himself. The range of topics discussed includes behaviour problems, feeding problems, problems of physical and mental development, and certain problems of preventive pædiatrics. It is intended for all doctors who are concerned with the care of children, especially family doctors and doctors in the Child Welfare Service. It is hoped too that it will help them with their own children.

In planning the book I was constantly faced with the difficulty of deciding what is normal and what is abnormal, and what, therefore, should be included in the book and what excluded. It is almost impossible to define the normal. It is certainly not synonymous with the average. A child may differ very widely from the average child in physical and mental development and yet be perfectly normal. An attempt has been made to include the extreme range of normal variations which may occur. This was a matter of great difficulty, for so little has been written about the subject, and differences of opinion are wide. The preparation of the book has certainly taught me how much we do *not* know about the normal child, and how much awaits investigation.

Behaviour problems are included in the book because every normal child has them. I feel that a child with no behaviour problems would be highly abnormal. The book may well be criticized for including topics which are on the borderline between health and disease, such as cyclical vomiting and motion sickness. They are, however, extremely common, and are unrelated to any known organic disease, and accordingly it was felt that they should find a place in this book. Infections are not discussed, but a section is devoted to the prevention of infection and so to the preservation of health.

Another difficulty experienced was that of repetition. So many different subjects have been discussed in this book that any attempt to give a reasonably comprehensive account of each individual problem has inevitably led to minor repetitions. I felt that this was preferable to an excess of cross references, which are so often irksome to the reader. Many of the repetitions are simply due to the fact that numerous different problems arise from the same basic causes.

It is difficult in a book of this nature to give full credit to all papers which have been read in its preparation. It was felt undesirable to list all the hundreds of articles read. Instead an effort has been made to include at the end of the book only those references which the reader will find of value. Specially recommended reading is printed in heavy type. A few references to articles which are particularly worth reading, but which are not specifically referred to in the text, are given at the end of this list. References to articles which are not otherwise relevant to the subject under discussion are referred to by asterisk, and the reference is given at the foot of the page. Any references which I was unable to read personally are denoted by the words "quoted by," referring to the author who referred to that work in his paper or book. I have made every effort to include in the references those papers which do not accord with my opinion, so that both sides of the question can be read.

In conclusion, I wish to express my gratitude to Professor Wilfred Vining of Leeds, who taught me so much when I was a student, and to Dr. Arnold Gesell, of New Haven, who taught me so much about the normal child while I was in his Department. The section on Developmental Problems is inevitably based largely on Gesell's works—on knowledge which I acquired from him and his staff, and from his numerous books and papers. In the section on Behaviour Problems I have frequently referred to an excellent series of articles in the *Journal of Pediatrics* by Dr. Harry Bakwin, and I wish to thank the Editor for permission to do so.

Professor Vining (Leeds), Professor Capon (Liverpool), Dr. Donald Court (Newcastle-upon-Tyne) and Dr. Doxiadis (Sheffield) have read and criticized the entire script. Dr. Harold Waller (Tunbridge Wells), Dr. John Emery (Sheffield), Dr. John Lorber (Sheffield) and Mr. Robert Zachary, F.R.C.S. (Sheffield) have read parts of it. To all these friends I wish to express my thanks. The opinions expressed in the book, however, are my own, and they do not necessarily accord with those of my friends. This could not be, for many of the subjects are highly controversial, and in the present state of our knowledge, purely matters of opinion, so that on some of the topics there was no agreement between my critics. Readers of the book will probably differ still more, and I should like it to be known that I should welcome their criticisms and suggestions.

R. S. ILLINGWORTH.

CONTENTS

CHAPTER I

NORMAL BREAST FEEDING

If lactation is properly managed, over 90 per cent of mothers can fully breast feed their babies.[25]

Many studies have indicated that in developed countries, there is more breast feeding in the upper classes than in the lower ones.[27]

The Advantages of Breast Feeding

The Incidence of Infection

By far the most important advantage of breast feeding is the fact that it is the safest method of feeding the baby. Where the standard of hygiene is good, the difference between the incidence of infections in breast- and bottle-fed babies is probably small. In places where hygiene is poor, and especially in tropical countries, the difference is great. In fact Jelliffe,[16] in an excellent paper which should be read in full by anyone interested in the subject, wrote that in the tropics "It is no exaggeration to say that breast feeding for at least six months is necessary for very survival itself." He added: "The feeding bottle can be regarded without exaggeration as a lethal weapon in the hands of the majority of tropical mothers."

The danger of artificial feeding is gastroenteritis. This is partly due to contamination of the feeds and feeding utensils by careless handling and storage. The fact that it does not occur in fully breast-fed babies may be due partly to the fact that the more acid stools of the fully breast-fed baby discourage growth of pathogenic *Esch. coli*.

There is some evidence that fully breast-fed babies acquire fewer respiratory infections, not only during the period of full breast feeding but for some months afterwards. Joenson[17] in his 445-page monograph on breast feeding in the Faroe Islands, found that fully breast-fed babies had fewer colds and attacks of bronchitis or pneumonia than artificially-fed babies, and when they did get a cold they were less likely to develop bronchitis after it: 1·87 per cent. of those who were artificially fed from birth developed pneumonia, as compared with 0·15 per cent. of those fully breast fed for 6 months. Similar observations were made in Sweden.[23]

It is interesting to note that human milk inhibits intestinal infection by the poliomyelitis virus. In studies of the Sabin vaccine,[29] the poliomyelitis virus was found in the fæces of 65 per cent. of artificially-fed babies and only 44 per cent. of breast-fed ones. The difference, based on a study of 483 infants, was highly significant. It is known to be due to the effect of neutralizing antibodies in human milk. Significant amounts of hæmagglutinating antibody to pathogenic *E. coli*, and of neutralizing antibodies to poliomyelitis, have been demonstrated in the stools of young breast-fed infants.[19]

It is a fallacy to suppose that human breast milk is sterile. In one study it was found that 93 per cent. of newborn babies were drinking staphylococci in their mother's milk.

Convenience

There can be little doubt that in most ways breast feeding is far easier for the mother. There is no equipment to sterilize and there are no feeds to mix and measure. When the mother visits friends or travels, it is much easier for her to feed the baby on the breast than to take all the necessary equipment for artificial feeds. When the baby demands feeds at night, as he usually does in the first 10 weeks, it is easier for her to feed the baby on the breast than to prepare an artificial feed. Not all mothers have a refrigerator in which to keep the day's feeds ready made up. In my opinion too many mothers with organic diseases, such as rheumatic carditis, are advised to bottle feed their babies on the grounds that it will be easier for them. In fact, artificial feeding causes much more work than breast feeding.

Psychological Factors

Numerous workers have tried to determine whether there is any relationship between the duration of breast feeding and subsequent behaviour. Many have suggested that there is such a relationship, and that babies acquire psychological advantages from feeding at the breast. There is no scientific evidence to this effect, and it is obvious that it would be exceedingly difficult to produce such evidence. The mother who prefers to breast feed her baby may be different in other attitudes from the mother who wishes to feed her baby on the bottle. There are differences in the social background of breast-fed and bottle-fed babies. It would be virtually impossible to control the variables in a study of this nature. The fully breast-fed baby may gain from closeness to one woman only, his mother. A mother may feel satisfaction at being able fully to breast feed her baby, and this may indirectly help her child. He may gain from the effect which breast feeding has on her. It may increase the bond of love between the two. The bottle-fed baby may be given his feeds by various people, and is not constantly close to one woman.

Psychiatrists claim that rapid weaning from the breast causes psychological trauma to the baby, and may be responsible for behaviour problems years later. They may be right, but they have not provided evidence for this view.

Chemical Differences and Digestibility

There are numerous differences between human and cow's milk. In cow's milk there is more protein, more volatile long chain fatty acids, more thiamin and riboflavin, four times more calcium, more sodium, less iron and less vitamin C. There are differences in the amino-acid content, in the nature and degree of absorption of carbohydrates, and in many other features.

Breast fed babies are less likely to develop tetany and it may be that owing to the lower sodium content of human milk they are less likely to develop hypernatraemic dehydration with infections.

Other Advantages

Breast fed babies are less likely than artificially fed babies to become fat. Perianal soreness is less common. It is said that they are less liable to develop ulcerative colitis. Sudden unexplained deaths (cot deaths) are less common in breast fed babies. There is evidence, not accepted by all, that women who breast feed are less likely to develop carcinoma of the breast.[24]

A recently described problem in newborn babies is intestinal obstruction due to inspirated milk curds (lactobezoar), sometimes leading to perforation. It is confined to artificially fed babies.[4,11,21]

There is much more fluoride in cow's milk, especially when it is dried, than in human milk, but it is not harmful.[6] There is more strontium in human milk.

Disadvantages

There are certain disadvantages of breast feeding.

The mother who is fully breast feeding has less freedom than a mother who feeds her baby on a bottle. She alone can feed her baby. It is less easy for her to get her shopping done, she cannot return to work and she cannot have short breaks away from the child.

Some mothers object to breast feeding because they say that it spoils the figure. This can be partly prevented by providing adequate breast supports during lactation.

The loose stools of the fully breast-fed baby provide more work for the mother than the much firmer stools of the baby fed on cow's milk. It is much easier to clean the baby up if he is bottle fed.

There can be no doubt that a fully breast-fed baby is more likely to be underfed than a bottle-fed baby. It is sometimes an advantage that an anxious mother does not know how much milk the baby is obtaining from the breast at each feed. Mothers who are feeding their babies on the bottle are apt to be worried when the baby takes less than the usual quantity. On the other hand, the mother who is fully breast feeding may think that she is providing enough milk when she is not doing so. The difficulty is avoided by regular weighing.

Painful overdistension of the breast, soreness of the nipple, mastitis and breast abscess are disadvantages of breast feeding. Lactorrhœa is a trivial but annoying accompaniment of lactation in many women.

Some mothers worry about breast feeding. They are anxious because they fear that they may not have enough milk. They are certainly worried if they have any of the breast complications described above. This may explain in part the repeated statement that breast feeding causes fatigue. It is difficult to see why it should do, if the mother is taking an adequate diet. On the other hand, a woman who is feeding her baby on the bottle has extra work to do in the way of cleaning and sterilizing bottles and teats, and preparing feeds, unless someone else does it for her.

In an overcrowded home, a mother may feel embarrassed about feeding her baby on the breast. It is said that there is some association between hæmorrhagic disease of the newborn and breast feeding.[28] It was found that breast fed babies not given additional Vitamin K were more liable to bleed than artificially fed babies. It has been shown[18] that the prothrombin time tends to be lower in newborn breast fed babies than in those receiving cow's milk.

Preparations for Breast Feeding and the Establishment of Lactation

The expression of colostrum in the latter weeks of pregnancy[15] and the use of Waller plastic nipple shells for retracted nipples are of doubtful value.[12]

When Should the Baby be put to the Breast?

There is no rule about this. If the mother would like to put her newly born baby to the breast as soon as he is delivered, there is nothing against it, as long as the baby is fit. It will help to contract the uterus, for when the baby sucks, the oxytocin liberated by the pituitary causes uterine contractions ("after pains"). Some mothers feel the urge to put the baby to the breast as soon as he is born. This may be analogous to the licking of the newborn by sheep and other animals. If the mother is tired, no harm will be done if the baby is kept off the breast for 12 to 24 hours. In general, the full-term baby is likely to be put to the breast 6 to 12 hours after delivery.

Piglets start sucking before the last of the litter is born.

How the Baby gets the Milk

The baby obtains the milk by four mechanisms. He expresses it, he sucks it, and the breast expels the milk, partly through the myo-epithelial cells of the breast and partly through the draught reflex. By a cine-radiographic technique,[1] the mother's nipple being coated by a barium paste, it was shown that the baby expresses the milk from the ducts into the nipple by the movement of his jaws. He then presses the nipple with his tongue against his palate, and expresses the milk. He obtains the milk from a feeding bottle in the same way. The role of suction is doubtful, though suction does occur. When the baby brings his lips tightly round the nipple and areola, he seems to adhere to the breast, because he has created a vacuum, and in order to get him away from the breast without causing pain, the mother inserts her little finger into the angle of his mouth in order to release the vacuum. In the same way babies suck air out of the feeding bottles, with the result that the teat becomes flat and they can get no more milk until the teat is withdrawn from their mouth in order that air can enter the bottle.

The draught reflex, termed in animals the "let-down" reflex, is an essential part of breast feeding. When the baby begins to suck, the stimulus causes the liberation of oxytocin from the pituitary. This passes into the blood stream and causes the milk to pass from the cells of the breast into the ducts, so that it is available for the baby. In the first few days after delivery, the oxytocin causes the uterus to contract, and the mother may therefore feel cramps in the lower part of the abdomen. The reflex is accompanied by an anti-diuretic effect. When the reflex occurs, the mother feels the breast become tight and almost uncomfortable. If one watches the baby when he is put to the breast, one can see that he takes a few sucks and then appears to stop and wait. In about 30 seconds, when the reflex has occurred, he begins to suck vigorously. One may also notice milk leaking out of the opposite breast. A conditioned reflex may become established, whereby the flow of milk begins when the breast is being prepared for a feed, or even when the baby begins to cry. The reflex can be induced artificially by pituitrin snuff or oxytocin spray into the nose. It can be inhibited by adrenaline. It is important to note that it is inhibited by fear or emotion. This is of great clinical importance, because the mother can readily be worried by tactless remarks about the baby's face or head, or about the likelihood that there will not be sufficient milk. The slightest suggestion that the baby is abnormal may be quite enough to reduce the milk supply. A good mother may be worried if her baby is separated from her by being placed in a nursery. She may worry about her child's appearance, grunting respirations, nævoid staining on the forehead or back of the neck, or other features. She may be anxious because the baby is drowsy or irritable. She may be worried by undue interference on the part of the nurse who is trying to help her to establish breast feeding. She may be upset by test feeds, and she may suffer pain from a sore nipple or overdistended breast. Embarrassment at breast feeding in a ward with others present may be sufficient to inhibit the flow of milk. Frequent weighings may also lead to anxiety. The mother is in an emotional state in the puerperium, and every effort should be made to avoid causing her unnecessary anxiety, because of its effect on the milk supply—partly through the mechanism of the draught reflex. The reflex is inhibited in cows if they take a dislike to a new farmhand. A farmer told me that his cows let the milk down better if milking is carried out to a musical accompaniment. It has in fact been shown scientifically that music at milking time produced a 6 per cent. increase in the milk yield of the cow and goat. There have not to my knowledge been studies of the effect of different types of music.

The Feeding Schedule

The obvious and natural way to feed a baby in his first few weeks is to feed him more or less when he wants it—and most intelligent mothers will do this, whether instructed otherwise or not. I am against a rigid schedule, and I am against a strict self-demand schedule. One can be too rigid either way. I suggest that the baby should be fed more or less when he wants it. That does not mean that he should never be awakened for a feed if the mother wishes to go out shopping, or if domestic arrangements make it desirable to get the baby fed. It does not mean that the moment that the baby cries, everything should be dropped to feed him. It does mean feeding him in the night when he demands it, as most babies do in their first 10 weeks or so; it does mean that he should not be deliberately left crying for a prolonged period because the alarm clock has not announced that it is now time for the baby to feel hungry.

A reasonable self-demand schedule is the common-sense schedule. It allows for the fact that all babies are different, some becoming hungry sooner than others; it allows a child to catch up if he has been underfed earlier, for under an elastic schedule a baby can demand more frequent feeds until he has caught up to the average weight; it does allow the mother to satisfy his basic needs, which include particularly food, love and comfort. Though a rigid schedule may satisfy some babies, if it happens to coincide with their stomach emptying time, it will certainly not satisfy others. It will lead to a prolonged crying, which in turn disturbs the parents (and perhaps the neighbours), and which tires the baby and causes him to take his feed less well. It leads to air swallowing, which in turn makes him take less, or makes him vomit. Psychiatrists claim that it is harmful for the baby's psychological development to be left crying for prolonged periods. It is difficult to prove this, but it does seem reasonable to satisfy the child's need for food.

It is nonsense to claim that a self-demand schedule leads to bad habit formation. Within a month or so babies fed on an elastic schedule get into a rhythm of quite regular feeds. Babies who are fed when they demand it at night spontaneously drop the night feed at 10 to 12 weeks or so of age.

In discussing the feeding schedule with parents it is essential to bear in mind the possible difficulties. These are as follows:

(1) Babies cry for reasons other than hunger. If the baby stops crying when he is picked up, he is not seriously hungry. If he continues to cry when picked up, he is either hungry or uncomfortable or both. He may be uncomfortable because of evening colic. One should never allow a mother to believe that she should feed the baby every time he cries. She should feed him when he is hungry. If she is of low intelligence and unable to understand this, I would instruct her to feed the baby on a fairly rigid schedule—of about 3-hourly feeds in the case of a small baby, or about 4-hourly feeds in the case of a larger baby.

(2) The baby who is cold, drowsy, premature, ill or mentally subnormal cannot be relied upon to demand feeds. He should be fed on a rigid schedule.

(3) Some babies, between the fifth and the tenth day, demand very frequent feeds—up to 12 in the 24 hours. This is a nuisance for the mother, but good for her breasts.[14] It does not mean that there is insufficiency of milk.

(4) Some babies demand feeds so infrequently that insufficient stimulus is given to the breasts and lactation fails. I have seen several babies who from the age of a week or two only demanded three feeds in the 24 hours. They should be encouraged to take more frequent feeds.

(5) A mother may find it difficult to feed a baby at rather irregular periods. If she prefers to use a rigid schedule, she should.

It has been argued that a rigid schedule is essential in a maternity hospital. All babies at the Jessop Hospital, Sheffield, are fed on a self-demand schedule, and we have experienced no difficulty at all.[10] Each mother has her baby at her bedside, and picks him up as soon as he cries for food, and feeds him. The ward sister finds that the self-demand schedule enables her to supervise feeds, where necessary. On a rigid schedule such supervision would be impossible. Many visitors have remarked about the quietness of the hospital. Babies are never left to cry. In my opinion, they shouldn't be.

There is no place for self-demand feeding after the age of 2 or 3 months. Babies develop a fairly rigid schedule of their own, and the mother will guide this to coincide with her own convenience.

Prelacteal Feeds

There is no rule as to whether a baby should be given fluids in the first 2 or 3 days before lactation becomes established. If the weather is hot, and the child appears to be thirsty, I would give him boiled water in the first 2 or 3 days. Failure to do so may cause him to become dehydrated and acidotic, and to lose weight excessively. I have smelt acetone in the breath of such babies. The so-called dehydration fever may occur—a rapid rise of temperature, promptly settling when fluid is given.

When there is no evidence of thirst, fever or dehydration, I would prefer to withhold extra fluids. It must always be remembered that infection can readily be introduced by giving prelacteal feeds. Where hygiene is poor, the safest feed for the baby is breast milk only.

Forced Fluids for the Mother

It is unnecessary and undesirable to try to cause the lactating mother to drink large quantities of fluid. The best regulator of the mother's fluid needs is thirst. If she satisfies that, there is no need for her to take more fluid. It will do nothing to increase the milk supply.

At the Jessop Hospital, Sheffield, we carried out a controlled study on 210 mothers.[14] Those who were caused to drink a large quantity (average 3 litres per day) produced if anything rather less milk than those who were left to drink only what they wanted (average daily intake 1·9 litres). There is no evidence that cows produce more milk when given extra water to drink. It was suggested by Gunther[10] that the flooding of the body with water may antagonize the draught reflex on account of its association with the antidiuretic hormone.

The Mother's Diet

The mother's diet is reflected in the chemical composition of the milk. There is a significant relationship between the quantity of dietary protein and milk protein, and between the dietary fat and the milk fat. There is no evidence however, that a high protein intake increases milk secretion, although carbohydrates may. Fat in large amounts may reduce the milk supply.[10]

There is some evidence that proteins may pass through into the breast milk and even cause allergic manifestations in the baby. Rhesus antibodies pass into the milk, but do no harm. No special food preparations and no drugs increase the amount of milk produced.

It is customary to advise mothers not to eat onions and pickles when lactating, but it is uncertain whether this restriction is necessary. It is known that if cows eat garlic, a member of the onion family, the milk tastes unpleasant on account of the allyl sulphide in it. It has also been said that if a mother eats large quantities of oranges, the baby may have colic, but I doubt this.

Drugs and Breast Milk

Many drugs are excreted in milk.[20] The following are of importance, in that they may affect the baby: thioracil, radioactive iodine,[3] iodides, bromides, lithium,[30] alcohol, phenobarbitone, anticoagulants[5] and possibly penicillin. Ergot, senna, rhubarb, cascara and aloes might theoretically affect the baby. Organochlorine compounds including dicophane (D.D.T.)[22] pass into the milk in considerable quantities, much more than the maximum acceptable amount, and this has caused anxiety in Sweden, Australia and elsewhere, because of the possibility that it could lead to tumour formation. The danger of radioactive iodine taken by the mother is that it may lead to carcinoma of the thyroid in the child.

Many fatalities occurred in Turkish babies because breast feeding mothers had eaten the seed of wheat treated by hexachlorobenzene; the babies developed rashes, diarrhœa and vomiting.

Numerous other drugs pass into the breast milk without harming the baby. They include carbimazole, isoniazid, pyrimethamine, quinine, antihistamines, sulphonamides, chloramphenicol, novobiocin, mandelic acid and caffein. Norethynodrel (contraceptive pill, enovid) passes through in fairly large quantities.

Breast milk Jaundice

This is rare, and is due to the presence of 3 alpha 20 beta diol in the mother's milk. The baby is jaundiced while breast fed, but the jaundice disappears promptly when the baby is taken off the breast.[2]

The Duration of the Feed

It would be irrational to suggest that each feed should be restricted to a set time, because this would imply that all babies are the same in the speed of sucking, and that all nipples and breasts are the same. Yet one constantly hears that mothers have been told to feed their baby for "10 minutes on each side." Some babies suck much more rapidly than others. Older babies are likely to suck more quickly than younger ones. Milk comes slowly out of some breasts and almost pours out of others. Some nipples are difficult for the baby to suck. Many babies are difficult for the first few days, and withdraw and cry, so that only a small part of the duration of the feed is spent in actual sucking.

We know from serial test feeds that most babies obtain nearly all the milk in the first 4 or 5 minutes. I would certainly say that no baby needs more than about 15 minutes' actual sucking on each side. Beyond that time he is merely using the nipple as a pacifier, and is likely to swallow air. If he is not allowed long enough, he will not obtain enough milk. If he is given too long, he will swallow air and so have "wind". In addition he may make the nipple sore. If a mother tries to make him go on sucking on the first breast after he has obtained the milk, he is likely to become tired and then suck badly on the second breast, going to sleep before he has got enough.

I recommend that the baby should be fed on the first breast until he suddenly slows down in his sucking, and fed on the second breast until he goes to sleep or stops sucking.

Many advocate severe restriction of the duration of the feed in the first 2 or 3 days, on the grounds that more prolonged sucking will cause soreness of the nipple. I am uncertain whether this is true. In parts of Africa, mothers sleep on the floor of the hut with the baby sucking at the breast. Soreness of the nipple in these women is very rare.

Emptying the Breast

The amount of milk produced depends in large part on the emptying of the breast. Any farmer knows that if a cow is not milked fully, she will produce less milk.

I feel that there is much to be said for regular manual expression of milk after every feed for the first 10 days, in order to ensure full emptying. This stimulates the breast to produce more milk. This step is not essential, but it is a step which is likely to ensure the success of lactation. Where possible, the expressed milk is given to the baby by a sterile spoon (provided that the milk has been expressed into a sterile basin).

Because of the importance of emptying the breast, both breasts should be given at each feed. I do not think that it matters whether there is alternation in the use of the breasts at successive feeds or not.

The technique of manual expression is as follows. Expression of milk is achieved by two movements. The first is compression of the whole breast between the two hands, starting at the margin of the breast tissue and continuing down as far as the areola. Firm pressure is maintained throughout the movement, which is repeated ten or twelve times. The aim of this movement is to impel milk from the smaller into the larger ducts and lacteal sinuses. The second movement is designed to empty the sinuses. The breast tissue just behind the areola is pinched sharply and repeatedly between the thumb and forefinger of one hand while the breast is held firmly fixed by the other. The direction of this force is backward towards the centre of the breast rather than towards the base of the nipple. A common mistake is to move the finger and thumb over the surface of the skin, thus rubbing the skin. The finger and thumb remain over the same piece of skin and should not move over it. The other common mistake is to move the skin over the breast tissue instead of compressing the sinuses. It should be possible to make the milk squirt out when the movement is properly performed. Unless overdistension is severe it causes no discomfort to the mother.

A woman had persistent trouble with sore nipples, and so fed her baby entirely on expressed breast milk. She was so efficient in expression that in two lactation periods she sold a surplus of 750 litres of milk for 3,717 dollars. Another woman sold 570 litres in one lactation period for 2,020 dollars. A wet nurse is known to have produced 5,770 ml of milk in one day, and was able to maintain seven babies at a time with the quantity produced.

There have been reports from many parts of the world concerning breast feeding by grandmothers and even women who had never been pregnant.[8,9,26] David Livingstone described several examples of grandmothers nursing a child.[31] Wieschoff wrote that in Java it is the custom for babies to be nursed by their grandmothers if their own mothers are too busy. He quoted examples of the same practice in the Maoris, North American Indians, Africans and South Americans. Folley[7] wrote: "It has now been proved that it is possible by suitable experimental treatment to bring into lactation not only castrated (ovariectomized) virgin lactating animals, but males as well."

The Feeding of Twins

The easiest and the quickest way to feed twins on the breast is to feed them simultaneously, one on each breast (*Fig. 1*). The babies' legs are behind the mother, and each head is supported by the mother's hands with the help of a pillow or cushion. If one twin feeds on the right breast at one feed he feeds on the left at the other. Some mothers are reluctant to do this, for it is not very comfortable, but it does save time and it avoids the difficulty of keeping one baby crying for food while the other is being fed. It is not possible if the twins demand feeds at different times and refuse to suck when they are both put to the breast at the same time. A self-demand schedule is obviously difficult with twins, because they are apt to want feeding at different times. I would advise a more or less rigid schedule, allowing such elasticity as is convenient.

Every effort should be made to enable the mother to produce sufficient milk for both. It would seem desirable to practise manual expression as a routine after feeds from the third day until lactation is well established in order to stimulate the supply of sufficient milk.

When to Wean

There is no rule as to when the baby should be weaned from the breast. On the one hand he should not be weaned too late, in countries where the hygiene is good, because he is apt to become anæmic and to be difficult about taking different foods. On the other hand, he should not be weaned unnecessarily early if there is abundance of breast milk.

The following are my suggestions with regard to weaning:

(1) Weaning should begin not later than 4 or 5 months, because he is apt to become difficult about weaning later. This applies only to countries in which hygiene is good. In others breast feeding should be continued for at least 9 months.

(2) He should be weaned if he reaches about 16 lb (7 kg), because at that weight he would probably be taking 40 oz (1·1 litres) of milk from the mother (150 ml/kg), and at that stage it is better for him to have a mixed diet.

(3) He should be weaned on to thickened feeds if he is taking 200 to 225 ml at a feed, whatever his weight or age, because that would probably mean that he is taking 1·1 litres of milk per day.

(4) He should be weaned if after 1 or 2 months the milk supply is not adequate. There is no need to go to the trouble and expense of buying bottles and teats and preparing these for feeds. He can be given thickened feeds from a spoon or cup.

(5) He should be weaned in the case of illness in the mother, each on its merits. He should be taken off the breast if the mother develops a breast abscess.

Weaning is normally completed by the age of 8 or 9 months, but it does not matter if the baby has odd breast feeds for the remainder of the first year. Babies often demand a breast feed in the late evening before their night's sleep, and seem to be reluctant to part with this feed.

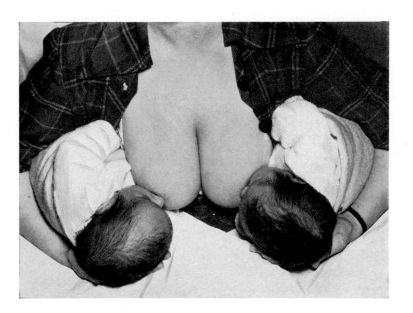

FIG. 1. Twins being fed simultaneously on breast.

To face p. 12

The choice of the particular feeds at which thickened foods should be introduced is purely a matter for the mother's convenience.

Amongst primitive people, in whom weaning is delayed, many different means are used to make the baby part with the breast. Some apply bitter sap to the nipples. Others wrap the nipples in human hair, or apply tobacco, soot, aloes, garlic, ginger, red pepper, or goat dung.

References

1. Ardran, G. M., Kemp, F. H., Lind, J. (1958). "Cine-radiographic Study of Breast Feeding." *Brit. J. Radiol.*, **31**, 156.
2. Arias, I. M., Gartner, L. M. (1970). "Breast Milk Jaundice." *Brit. Med. J.*, **4**, 177.
3. Bland, E. P., Docker, M., Crawford, J. S., Farr, R. F. (1969). "Radioactive Iodine Uptake by the Thyroid of Breast Fed Infants After Maternal Blood Volume Measurements." *Lancet*, **2**, 1039.
4. Cook, R. C. M., Rickham, P. P. (1969). "Neonatal Obstruction Due to Milk Curds." *J. Pediat. Surgery*, **4**, 599.
5. Eckstein, H. B., Jack, B. (1970). "Breast Feeding and Anticoagulant Therapy." *Lancet*, **1**, 672.
6. Ericsson, V., Ribelius, U. (1970). "Increased Fluoride Ingestion by Bottle Fed Infants and its Effect." *Acta Paed. Scand.*, **59**, 424.
7. Folley, S. J. (1956). *The Physiology and Biochemistry of Lactation.* Edinburgh. Oliver and Boyd.
8. Foss, G. L., Short, D. (1951). "Abnormal Lactation." *J. Obst. and Gynæc. Brit. Emp.*, **58**, 35.
9. Greenway, P. J. (1937). "Artificially Induced Lactation in Humans." *E. African Med. J.*, **13**, 346.
10. Gunther, M. (1953). "Too Little Milk." *Univ. Coll. Hosp. Mag., London*, **38**, 82.
11. Howat, J. M., Wilkinson, A. W. (1970). "Intestinal Obstruction in the Neonate." *Arch. Dis. Childh.*, **45**, 800.
12. Hytten, F. E., Baird, D. (1958). "The Development of the Nipple in Pregnancy." *Lancet*, **1**, 1201.
13. Illingworth, R. S., Stone, D. (1952). "Self-Demand Feeding in a Maternity Unit." *Lancet*, **1**, 683.
14. Illingworth, R. S., Kilpatrick, B. (1953). "Lactation and Fluid Intake." *Lancet*, **2**, 1175.
15. Ingelman-Sundeberg, A. (1958). "The Value of Antenatal Massage of Nipples and Expression of Colostrum." *J. Obst. and Gynæc. Brit. Emp.*, **65**, 448.
16. Jelliffe, J. B. (1962). "Culture, Social Change and Infant Feeding." *Am. J. Clin. Nutrition*, **10**, 19.
17. Joensen, H. D. (1954). "Studier over Brysternaeringens Udbredelse og Betydning." *Ann. Soc. Scient. Faeroensis Torshavn.*
18. Keenan, W. J., Jewett, T., Glueck, H. I. (1971). "Role of Feeding and Vitamin K in Hypoprothrombinemia of the Newborn." *Am. J. Dis. Child.*, **121**, 271.
19. Kenny, J. F., Boesman, M. I., Michaels, R. H. (1967). "Bacterial and Viral Coproantibodies in Breast Fed Infants." *Pediatrics*, **39**, 202.
20. Knowles, J. A. (1965). "Excretion of Drugs in Milk." A Review *J. Pediat.*, **66**, 1068.
21. Levkoff, A. H., Gadsden, R. H., Hennigar, G. R., Webb, C. M. (1970). "Lactobezoar and Gastric Perforation in a Neonate." *J. Pediat.*, **77**, 875.
22. Lofroth, G. (1968) "Pesticides and Catastrophe." *New Scientist*, **40**, 567.
23. Mellander, O., Vahlquist, B., Mellbin, T. (1959). "Breast Feeding and Artificial Feeding." *Acta Pædiat. Uppsala*, Suppl. 116.
24. Schaefer, O. (1969). "Cancer of the Breast and Lactation." *Can. Med. Ass. J.*, **100**, 625.

25. SEDGWICK, J. P. (1921). "A Preliminary Report of the Study of Breast Feeding in Minneapolis." *Am. J. Dis. Child.*, **21**, 455.
26. SLOME, C. (1956). "Non-Puerperal Lactation in Grandmothers." *J. Pediat.*, **49**, 550.
27. SMITH, D. V. (1969). "Attitudes to Breast Feeding." *Brit. Med. J.*, **2**, 695.
28. SUTHERLAND, J. M., GLUECK, H. I., GLESER, G. (1967). "Hemorrhagic Disease of the Newborn. Breast Feeding as a Necessary Factor in the Pathogenesis." *Am. J. Dis. Child.*, **113**, 524.
29. WARREN, R. J., LEPOW, M. L., BARTSCH, C. T. E., ROBBINS, F. C. (1961). "Influence of Breast Milk on Intestinal Infection with Sabin Type 1 Poliovirus Vaccine." *Am. J. Dis. Child.*, **102**, 685.
30. WEINSTEIN, M., GOLDFIELD, M. (1969). "Lithium Carbonate Treatment During Pregnancy." *Dis. N. System*, **30**, 828.
31. WIESCHOFF, H. A. (1940). "Artificial Stimulation of Lactation in Primitive Cultures." *Bull. Hist. Med.*, **8**, 1403.

CHAPTER 2

DIFFICULTIES IN BREAST FEEDING

Difficulties in the Mother

Overdistension of the Breast

Some degree of overdistension of the breast is quite common in the first few days after delivery. In mild forms there is some discomfort which is relieved when the baby sucks. In moderate forms the pain is relieved when the baby sucks, but the breast rapidly refills, so that half an hour or so after a feed the breast is uncomfortable again. In more severe forms the baby cannot get the milk, partly because he cannot get his jaws far enough behind the nipple, and partly because of obstruction in the breast. In the most severe forms pain is severe and the breast is œdematous. It is thought that inelasticity of the skin is an important factor. It is also caused by inadequate emptying of the breast either because the baby is not allowed to suck, or because he is drowsy or sucks badly.

Overdistension of the breast causes pain, insomnia and worry. If the baby is allowed to suck when distension is fairly severe, he will suck the nipple and make it sore, because he cannot get his jaws far enough behind the nipple. The greater danger is the failure of lactation because the breast is not being emptied.

Overdistension can often be anticipated and so prevented. When the breast fills up unusually rapidly—in the case of a primipara at the end of the first or early in the second day—stilbœstrol should be given (10 mg six-hourly) in order to slow down the coming in of the milk. It is stopped as soon as the danger is over. Routine expression is a help. The baby should be encouraged, if necessary, to take frequent feeds.

If the breast fills rapidly after feeds, it is essential to give stilbœstrol until the danger is over. The baby should not be allowed to suck if distension is moderately severe. If manual expression is painful, the electric "Humalactor" may be used successfully. The breast should be adequately supported and sedatives may be needed. In severe cases, expression will have to be avoided because it causes too much pain.

In all cases, as soon as the overdistension has subsided, the breast must be expressed at every feed time in order to stimulate milk production, until lactation is firmly established.

Local overdistension is fairly common. A segment of the breast is painful and distended, the rest of the breast tissue being unaffected. It may be due to the mother lying in a particular position, or to an abnormal opening in the duct, or to a badly fitting support. The absence of fever and malaise distinguishes it from mastitis. It is readily relieved by massage and expression of the affected segment.

Soreness of Nipple

Soreness of the nipple is common. It is experienced by about 20 per cent. of women at some stage. It may be due to the baby biting the nipple. It may be due to suction, the baby creating a vacuum around the nipple when he is sucking. Mavis Gunther[6] wrote this form can be recognized by a dark band across the nipple with petechial hæmorrhages. She ascribed it to the mother's posture making it difficult to get the nipple far enough into his mouth, so that he has to suck too hard. The mother should not lean back against a pillow when feeding the baby, but instead should lean forward or lie on her side. A bland cream, such as Cetavlex, will ease the soreness. It may be partly due to irritation by clothes.

Soreness may be due to dermatitis, arising from the use of detergents; it clears if 0·5 per cent. hydrocortisone ointment is applied for two days. The regular use of soap and water after feeds may predispose to soreness. The trouble may be due to defective protraction of the nipple. Such a nipple lies during suckling in the front of the baby's mouth instead of well back against the palate, and suction falls on its surface instead of on the areola. It has already been explained that if a baby sucks on an overdistended breast, he is apt to make the nipple sore. Some feel that if the baby sucks too long in the first 2 or 3 days, soreness of the nipple may result, but I doubt this. It does seem reasonable to suppose that if the baby is allowed to stay on the breast after obtaining the milk, using the nipple as a pacifier, he may make it sore. In our controlled study of self-demand feeding at the Jessop Hospital, Sheffield, we showed that a self-demand schedule reduced the incidence of soreness of the nipple.[10] Poor hygiene may be an important factor. It should be remembered that many mothers are genuinely afraid of being hurt when the baby sucks, and that when they complain of pain there is no abnormality of the nipple to be seen.

The dangers of soreness of the nipple are several. It is painful for the mother, and pain can reduce supply of milk—partly by inhibiting the draught reflex. In addition it causes worry and insomnia, and both have an adverse effect on lactation. If the baby is wrongly allowed to continue to suck after soreness has developeed, the pain increases and failure of lactation is likely to result. Many babies are taken off the breast on account of improperly treated soreness of the nipples, the mother having felt that she "could not carry on any longer" with breast feeding because it was so painful. There is a danger that the staphylococcus, which has probably gained entry at the site of the abrasion on the nipple, will cause mastitis and abscess. Sometimes the nipple bleeds when the baby sucks, and the baby is then found to have melæna.

As soon as any soreness develops and any lesion can be seen, the baby should be taken off the affected breast. The milk is expressed at the usual feed intervals and given to the baby. An antibiotic cream is applied to the nipple four times a day, and as soon as the nipple has healed the baby is returned to the breast.

Too Large a Nipple

One occasionally sees nipples which are so large that the baby cannot get his jaw back sufficiently to obtain the milk. In such cases the milk has to be expressed by hand and given to the baby in a bottle.

Blood in the Milk

When a nipple is deeply cracked, blood may be found in the milk. Occasionally, however, one sees blood in the milk when there is no visible crack or fissure. This may be due to a duct papilloma, and the woman should be carefully studied and followed up by the gynæcologist on that account. There is no doubt that in some mothers there is no discoverable cause for the bleeding, but one presumes that there must be an anatomical cause. For psychological reasons it may be better to take the baby off the breast and suppress lactation by stilbœstrol (10 mg four-hourly for 10 days or so).

Lactorrhœa

Milk may leak out of one breast when the baby is sucking at the other breast. It may leak out of both breasts when the draught reflex occurs, as a result of conditioning, before the baby begins to suck. It may also occur at night when the breast remains unemptied for a long period. It is a nuisance for the mother, though it is harmless. She has to wear a pad of cotton wool to avoid soiling of the clothes. It does not mean that there is a large amount of milk, though mothers usually believe that this is the case.

Lactorrhœa occurs in various pathological conditions,[3] including pineal tumours, encephalitis, acromegaly, adrenal tumours, and chorionepithelioma. It is related to depression of œstrogen activity and to secretion of prolactin. It is sometimes caused by drugs of the reserpine and phenothiazine group,[6] chlordiazepoxide and thioridazine. It may follow withdrawal of the contraceptive pill.[21]

The Axillary Tail

Swellings in the region of the axilla are likely to be due to the "axillary tail" of breast tissue rather than to accessary breasts.

Insufficiency of Milk

Ætiology. The main reasons for insufficiency of milk are inadequate emptying of the breast, genetic factors, worry and fatigue.

Inadequate emptying of the breast may be due to overdistension; a retracted nipple making suckling difficult; failure to put the baby to the breast; inadequate frequency of feeds; poor suckling by the baby—because he is drowsy, irritable or premature, or because he has been given complementary feeds. If a baby is given complementary feeds in the first 3 or 4 days, lactation is extremely likely to fail *unless there is full manual expression of the breast.* If a baby is given a supplementary feed and a complete bottle feed in between breast feeds, the breast will remain unemptied for a long period.

Worry and anxiety have a profound effect on the milk supply. Fatigue also has a considerable effect. The contraceptive pill is said to reduce the milk supply.[21] Smoking has a similar effect. The ready availability of tins of artificial food must be regarded as one of the main reasons for the insufficiency of milk. Artificial feeds are given too readily, so that the baby empties the breast less well, and lactation fails.

The Diagnosis of Insufficiency. The diagnosis is made on the basis of symptoms, the appearance of the child and the result of test feeds. *When the deficiency is only slight there may be no sign other than defective weight gain. The child seems to be contented, sleeps well and the stools are normal.* When the insufficiency is of moderate degree the baby cries excessively. He is likely to demand frequent feeds—long after the new-born period, in which frequent demands for food by normal babies are common. He may refuse the breast or suck at the breast for 2 or 3 minutes and then withdraw and cry. He may suck at the breast for a normal time and go to sleep, only to waken up half an hour later and cry. The crying is not stopped by picking him up. He may suffer from flatulence and colic as a result of sucking at an empty breast, with consequent air swallowing. Excessive air swallowing may cause vomiting. Weight gain is defective. He is likely to be constipated. If the deficiency is marked, the stools become green and contain mucus without fæcal matter. After a time the child looks undernourished, with a loss of tissue turgor. When severe deficiency of milk continues, the child may lose his appetite and become too languid and exhausted to cry for food at all.

If there is doubt about the diagnosis of underfeeding it should be confirmed by test feeds. When a test feed is done the baby is weighed before and after every feed for a whole day, so that the total weight gain can be calculated. It is essential that he should be weighed before and after every feed, for the amount of milk produced varies considerably from hour to hour. In general, the most productive feed is the first in the morning. The late afternoon or early evening feed tends to be the most deficient. If complementary feeds are needed, it is important to know which feed is most deficient, for after these feeds the complements should be given.

It must be admitted that in a busy baby clinic one can often fairly safely assess the amount of milk which the baby is obtaining from the mother by means of the weight gain. Knowing that an average baby after the first 10 days requires approximately $2\frac{1}{2}$ oz. per pound (150 ml/kg) per day, a weight gain of less than half the minimum "normal" weight gain of 6 oz. (19 g) per week would suggest that the baby is receiving less than half the required quantity of milk from the mother—provided that there is no other cause for the defective weight.

The limitations and fallacies of test feeds must be thoroughly understood. It is particularly important to remember the normal rate at which milk comes in. By the fifth day the child is not likely to obtain more than 1 oz. (28 ml) per pound in the day, and by the seventh day he is not likely to obtain more than $1\frac{3}{4}$ oz. per pound (110 ml/kg). I have seen a child taken off the breast on the second day of life on the grounds that there was not sufficient milk for him. It must be remembered that there are individual variations in the amount of milk needed to satisfy a baby and to give an average weight gain. A test feed may show that the baby is receiving $2\frac{1}{2}$ oz. per pound (150 ml/kg) per day but that does not prove that the baby would not like to have more. His crying in spite of an intake which is enough for average babies may be due to hunger. The child at all the feeds must be weighed on the same scales, for scales are frequently inaccurate. He must be weighed without clothes. The passage of urine or fæces after a feed just before weighing will affect the figures for that feed. I have already mentioned the fact that the test feed shows not the amount of milk which the mother is producing but merely the quantity which the child has obtained from the breast. A child who is drowsy, perhaps as a result of being overclothed, will not suck well and test feeds may give an entirely fictitious idea of the amount of milk available. It is obvious that test feeds are much more significant if the breast is fully emptied after every feed, the quantity of milk expressed being added to the quantity taken by the baby. This method alone gives an adequate picture of the quantity of milk produced by the mother.

Treatment

Historical. Recommended prescriptions for insufficiency of milk used to include powdered earthworms, and the dried udder of a goat. Platt and Gin[17] described a variety of galactagogues in use in China. They include cuttle-fish soups, shrimps' heads cooked in wine, cooked sea slugs, powdered dead silk worms in old wine, and sweet wine made from glutinous rice with the larvæ of blow-flies collected from fæces. Barats[1] recommended breast milk enemas. Zlocisti[22] advised that the husband should stimulate the breast by sucking it himself. An interesting Slavonic recipe consisted of instructing the mother to tickle a trout in the nearby stream, force its jaws open, express some milk into its mouth and then let it free. She then produced more milk.

Treatment Recommended. In the puerperium, if the baby is continuing to lose weight on the fifth day, or has not begun to gain weight, a complementary feed should be given after the breast feed. It is absolutely essential, however, that in addition the mother's breast should be expressed after each feed and the milk given to the baby. The baby must be given the breast before the complementary feed. Before the fifth day, nothing but boiled water should be given to the baby.

There is often a temporary falling off of the milk supply when the mother gets up and returns to work. Test feeds will show in which feeds the supply of milk is inadequate, and appropriate complements are then given. In addition, the breasts must be expressed after every feed, and the expressed milk is given to the baby. One must see that the feeds are sufficiently frequent (i.e. not merely three per day) and that the baby is being given long enough on each breast. As soon as possible the complementary feed is dropped.

A good idea of the quantity of breast milk available when a baby is receiving complementary feeds can be obtained by observing how much the baby takes from the bottle. An average baby requires approximately $2\frac{1}{2}$ oz. (150 ml) of milk per kg per day. Supposing that a 10-lb. (4·5 kg) baby is being given a complementary feed after each breast feed, and the mother says that he is taking 18 oz. (510 ml) of properly constituted cow's milk in the 24 hours, it is clear that the baby is probably taking not more than 7 oz. (200 ml) of milk per day from the mother—provided that his weight gain is an average one. (A baby's weight gain may be a great deal more than 6 oz. (170 g) a week. If so, he may be receiving more than the calculated average requirement of $2\frac{1}{2}$ oz. per pound (150 ml/kg per day).) It is most unlikely that there will ever be a sufficient supply of breast milk in such a case, and he should probably be put fully on to the bottle. In general, if it is shown that the mother is not producing as much as half the calculated requirements, in spite of proper emptying of the breast, it is usually wiser to put the baby fully on to artificial feeds. This is an individual matter, and if the mother is anxious to continue partially breast feeding her baby it is her affair, and she should not be discouraged from doing so. It takes a long time to feed the baby on the breast at each feed, then to express the breast, and then to give a complementary feed.

When a mother comes to the doctor after the first 2 weeks, and the baby's weight gain is inadequate, the decision as to what to do will depend on how much the baby has gained, provided that there is no other cause for defective weight gain, such as vomiting or an infection. If he is gaining 4 oz. (113 g) or 5 oz. (142 g) a week, the introduction of manual expression of the breast after every feed, together with attention to the frequency of the feeds, and to the time on the breast, can usually be relied upon to increase the weight gain to 7 oz. (198 g) or 8 oz. (227 g) a week, without giving complementary feeds. The expressed milk is given to the baby. If the weight gain has been less than 113 g a week, in my experience one cannot usually increase the weight gain to the required figure without giving a complementary feed. If the weight gain has been a mere 1 or 2 oz. (28 or 57 g) in the week, one might as well put the baby on to the bottle right away. It should be noted that if a baby has not been seen for 2 or 3 weeks, the weight gain may be deceptive. The fact that he has gained, say 21 oz. (600 g) in the last 3 weeks does not by any means prove that the milk supply is adequate: he might have gained 18 oz. (510 g) in the first 2 weeks and only 3 oz. (90 g) in the last week.

As for the nature of the complementary feed, it matters little, as long as it is properly constituted. In a hospital, if expressed milk from another mother is available, it should be given (after it has been boiled or pasteurized). Otherwise a dried milk or ordinary cow's milk is given diluted, with added sugar if necessary. As for the quantity, enough is given to satisfy the baby, and it should not be restricted. If test feeds have shown that the breast milk supply is only defective in one or two feeds in the 24 hours, the complement is given after these feeds only. A supplementary feed, that is a complete feed of cow's milk, is never given except in the weaning period, for if it is given it will mean that the breast will remain unemptied for a prolonged period. If the baby has been breast fed up to 6 or 8 weeks or so, and is then found to be obtaining insufficient milk from the mother, I would not advocate the use of complementary feeds at all. I would wean the baby on to thickened feeds—feeding him by spoon and cup. There would then be no need to buy bottles, teats and the other equipment for artificial feeding, and one would avoid the time taken in cleaning and sterilizing the bottles and other equipment. Every effort must be made to avoid worrying the mother, and she should be given as much rest as possible.

Failure of Lactation

Unwillingness of the Mother to Breast Feed her Child

This may be a matter of necessity. The early return to work in industry or elsewhere makes artificial feeding almost inevitable. More often, failure is due to a lack of desire to feed the baby on the breast. This may be due to the feeling that breast feeding is too tying. The mother wants to be free to go out to places of entertainment, and to shop without feeling bound to return by a given time to feed her baby. She may have no idea of the importance or value of breast feeding. A friend of mine visited a magnificently equipped American maternity unit and, on seeing a woman feeding her baby on the bottle, asked her why she was not feeding him on the breast. The mother laughed and said, "Well, it never struck me!"

Some mothers (and fathers) regard breast feeding as an unpleasant or disgusting procedure. There are presumably deep-seated psychological reasons for this attitude. I think that it is wrong to make determined efforts to persuade such a mother to breast feed her baby. Others do not wish to breast feed their baby because they have had a previous painful experience with sore nipples or breast abscess.

Other Reasons

By far the commonest cause of failure is a mere lack of desire to breast feed. The mother thinks that it does not matter whether the baby is breast fed or not, and if the slightest difficulty arises or the slightest symptoms develop in the baby she takes him right off the breast without consulting any doctor or nurse. She may consult her own mother or her neighbours, and the advice then given is almost invariably that the baby should be put on to the bottle. If the mother has failed to breast feed a previous child, she will be all the more ready to feed her second baby on cow's milk. Another major cause of the failure of lactation is the lack of enthusiasm of the doctor and nurse. They have little interest in maintaining lactation and recommend artificial feeding for no good reason at all.

Jelliffe,[11] writing about infant feeding in the tropics, declared: "For failure, the main ingredients are lack of certainty, anxiety and the alternative pursuits of modern women, all ultimately interfering with the key psychosomatic let down or milk ejection reflex, and a subsequent vicious circle of inadequate milk flow, a dissatisfied hungry baby, and a worried traumatized mother, with ultimate failure of lactation." He wrote that the feeding bottle in the tropics is becoming a status symbol, the more wealthy mothers feeding the baby on the bottle. It is an interesting paradox that in developing countries the bottle should become a status symbol, while in this country the incidence of breast feeding is much higher in the upper social classes than in the lower ones.

Other common reasons for unnecessary abandonment of breast feeding include the following:

(1) The idea that the breast milk is not suiting the baby. Except in the case of beriberi, breast-milk jaundice, galactosæmia, phenyl-ketonuria, or lactose intolerance, this diagnosis is always wrong. The symptoms are always due to something else. I have seen countless babies taken off the breast on account of this idea, when in fact the vomiting was due to congenital pyloric stenosis.

(2) The idea that the breast milk is too watery. This idea is always wrong. It is true that the first part of the milk appears watery. The last part of the milk from the breast is the richest in fat. Analysis of the total milk output would reveal a normal fat quantity, provided that the mother's diet is adequate.

(3) The idea that the breast milk is too strong. I have once seen a baby have bulky stools because the mother was drinking 5 pints (2·8 litres) of milk a day and the cream of a further 3 pints (1·7 litres). Otherwise I have never seen symptoms arising from the mother's diet or abnormality in the breast milk. For practical purposes the diagnosis is always wrong.

(4) Mismanagement of the sore nipple or overdistension. The correct management of feeding problems in the baby will be described in the section to follow. Mismanagement of these commonly leads to the abandonment of breast feeding.

(5) Mismanagement of the normal falling off of milk supply when the mother returns to work. The commonest time at which babies are weaned is about the end of the second week, when the mother returns to work. This may be due to a combination of factors, partial involution of the breast as a result of inadequately treated overdistension, or fatigue and worry about her ability to manage the child. If the baby is tided over 2 or 3 days of insufficiency of milk by judicious comple-mentary feeds and milk is expressed by hand, in the majority of cases the milk increases in quantity and the baby can be fully breast fed.

It is now known that oral contraceptives may reduce lactation. This is of importance in tropical countries, in which breast feeding is necessary for the child's survival.

Suppression of Lactation

Lactation has to be suppressed if the mother develops a breast abscess or other acute illness. It is wrong to suggest that there is no need to give any medicine, on the grounds that if the baby does not suck, the

the milk supply will cease; the mother is likely to suffer painful distension before this happens.[4,15] Stilboestrol, 5 mg three times a day
for 12 days, is the cheapest drug for the purpose, and it is satisfactory.
It is said that there may be withdrawal bleeding from the vagina when
the drug is discontinued. Some say that the dosage should be tapered off
after 10 days, or else lactation may restart. It has been argued that
stilboestrol may increase the risk of thromboembolism; but if the
woman is under 25 to 30 years of age, delivery was not by Cæsarian
section, the blood group is O, there are no varicose veins and no history
of previous thromboses, it is safe to use the drug. Other preparations
are much more expensive.[4] They include one intramuscular injection
of 15 mg of hexoestrol, or an androgen and oestrogen combination. In
my opinion stilboestrol is the drug of choice.

It should be noted that suppression is said to be less effective once
lactation has started.

Difficulties in the Baby

Irritability in the New-born Period

Irritability when the breast is offered is a common condition in
the new-born period and is a common reason for taking the baby off
the breast and putting him on to the bottle. It distresses the mother and
takes much of the nurse's time. It is surprising that so little is written
about it.

The baby, a full-term one, who has had a normal delivery, behaves
normally between feeds. He shows no sign of cerebral irritability and
there is no suggestion of birth injury. When taken to the breast, as
soon as he touches the nipple he screams violently and may refuse to
suck, or else he may suck for a few seconds and withdraw to scream
and fight. He may snarl at the breast and bite it hard, making the
mother withdraw instantly in pain, so making the baby more annoyed.
The more nervous and anxious the mother, the worse he becomes; the
calmer she is, the sooner he settles down. The whole feed is apt to
become a fight and a thoroughly unpleasant and exhausting experience
for the mother. The natural response of the nurse is to try to force
the baby to take the breast, holding his head and binding his limbs
down so that he cannot fight. Any attempt to discipline the child
aggravates matters. A child knows where the breast is without being
forced to it. When his cheek is touched the rooting reflex is initiated
and he roots for milk. The holding of the child's head by the cheeks
only annoys him further. Rough handling of any kind, even before the
feed, makes him worse. A depressed nipple, which he finds difficulty
in sucking from, increases his irritability. His irritability is also apt

to be increased by excessive clothing, which makes him too hot, and a rigid feeding schedule, which keeps him crying for food.

The irritability is apt to arouse the suspicion that there is not enough milk for him. This seems to be confirmed by his defective weight gain. If a test feed is carried out, the suspicions of the unwary are again apt to be confirmed, for it is likely to show that he has obtained only a small amount of milk from the mother. Many babies are taken off the breast for this reason or on the grounds that the breast milk is "not suiting" him, causing him to cry and to be irritable. This diagnosis, of course, is always wrong.

Gunther[5,6] thought that the irritability is usually due to the baby finding it difficult to breathe, either because his nose is embedded in the breast, or because the upturned upper lip is obstructing the nostrils. She wrote that an adequately shaped breast, presenting a nipple as a knob, with yielding tissues beneath, acts as a stimulus to the baby to suck. Without it the baby may be apathetic or irritable.

The treatment is not entirely satisfactory. One should certainly see that the baby can breathe, by ensuring that the nose is not obstructed. A self-demand schedule is a rational approach to the problem, because it is likely that a child who is not kept waiting for a long time for his feed will be less irritable. It is certainly not the whole answer, however, for babies fed on this schedule may still show extreme irritability at feed times. It is reasonable to suppose that it would help to have the baby constantly by the side of the mother rather than in a nursery, when his cries are apt to go unheeded. He should be picked up and cuddled by his mother as much as she wishes. It is particularly desirable that he should be cuddled for a fairly long time before a feed. He is more likely to approach the breast calmly in this case than if he is merely brought into the mother's room from the nursery and put to the breast immediately. He should be handled with the utmost gentleness and taken to the breast gently and without any forcing. The room should be quiet and interruptions should not be allowed. It is then purely a matter of patience. The less the nurse interferes the better. The nature of the problem should be fully explained and discussed with the mother. She must then fight her own battle. It is very difficult to stop the nurse interfering in an attempt to help the mother, but interference is undesirable. The mother has to get used to the baby, and the baby to the mother. The nurse should be present at first to give moral support, but no more. As soon as possible she leaves the room. The child should not be stopped from licking the breast, and he should not be hurried. The whole feed may take almost an hour, though only a small part of that time is spent by the baby in actual sucking. The essential thing is to reassure and encourage the mother. She must know that there is nothing wrong with her, her breast or the baby, and that it is purely a temporary phase which, though very troublesome as long as it lasts, will resolve itself in a few days if only patience and tolerance are shown. If overdistension of the breast develops as a result of the poor sucking by the baby it should be treated by manual expression. By the age of 10 or 14 days, if not sooner, the child becomes reasonable and well behaved.

Inertia and Drowsiness

In my experience inertia and drowsiness can be more worrying for the doctor than irritability, but it is less worrying for the mother. The baby does not seem to want feeding. He has no interest in it. If left on a self-demand schedule he does not demand feeds. Everyone is conversant with this behaviour in a small premature baby, but we are here concerned with the well full-term baby who, like the irritable baby, shows no evidence of birth injury. Gunther[6] ascribed it to inadequate protractility of the nipple. The presence of the normal nipple far back in the baby's mouth initiates sucking; if it does not protract this stimulus to sucking is lost. Marked physiological jaundice may be a factor in some. In others underclothing or overclothing is responsible. A mentally defective child is particularly liable to be disinterested in feeds in the new-born period, but it would be a serious mistake to suppose that most babies with such inertia are mentally defective. Inertia may result from cerebral trauma, but most of the babies show no other signs of cerebral trauma and grow up to be normal children. They are frequently children of a particularly placid disposition.

A fairly rigid schedule is necessary until the child begins to be more alert and to demand feeds. Only patience and gentle coaxing without undue forcing will enable the child to suck adequately. As with the irritable child, the problem nearly always resolves itself by 10–14 days of age. Only occasionally the baby continues to be disinterested in food and the maintenance of nutrition is not easy. It is always necessary to be sure that there is no infection.

Inertia in the baby is apt to lead to defective emptying of the breast. Unless manual expression is carried out during the period in which the baby is sucking badly, lactation may fail.

Sleepiness after the New-born Period

Many babies in the first 2 months or so fall asleep after they have sucked from one breast and before sucking from the second. Textbooks advise that they should be awakened by gentle slaps and other methods. Some apply pressure on the big toe in an attempt to awaken the baby.

It is often, however, impossible to awaken him. The mother should avoid rocking while feeding the baby, but rocking is not usually the cause of the trouble. It may be that the baby obtains all that he requires from one breast and so falls asleep. It is largely a matter of immaturity, and it rights itself as the baby gets older (usually by 8 weeks or so). It is particularly annoying if the baby, having fallen asleep in this way, awakens in about 2 hours, feeling hungry and cries.

The problem may be caused by efforts to make the child suck longer than he wants on the first breast, because of a rigid rule that the baby should suck 10 minutes on each breast. If he is forced to go on sucking after he has obtained the milk, he is liable to fall asleep on the second breast because he is tired, and so he does not obtain enough milk.

An older baby may obtain the food so quickly that after about 5 minutes on each breast he falls asleep. This may worry the mother, but a study of the child's weight gain immediately enables one to reassure the mother and explain that he is obtaining a perfectly adequate amount of milk unusually quickly.

Overclothing as a cause of drowsiness must always be remembered. It is common. At all times sleepiness of recent onset should arouse the suspicion of an infection.

Flatulence and Gastric Colic

Too many symptoms are ascribed to flatulence. It undoubtedly does occur in babies, but it is overdone. Crying for any reason—loneliness, desire to be cuddled, hunger—is ascribed to wind, and various medicines are given to bring it up. I have several times had older children (aged 1–2 years) referred to me on account of excessive wind. The excessive crying at night, which had been ascribed by the parents to wind, was simply a behaviour problem.

All wind which comes up from the stomach is wind which has been swallowed. The more immature the baby the greater the flatulence, because the greater is the amount of air which he swallows in sucking. The young baby in the first month or so is unable to approximate his lips closely to the areola of the breast, and milk consequently leaks out of the corner of his mouth as he sucks and air swallowing occurs. The older baby approximates his lips tightly to the areola, creating a vacuum in the process of sucking, and he swallows little air. Provided that none of the other causes mentioned below are found, the mother can be reassured and told that he will not be troubled with excessive wind in a few weeks, when he is older.

Flatulence may be caused by the baby gulping the milk down too quickly. It is usual to blame the baby for this, accusing him of being a greedy baby. He is then given chloral or boiled water before a feed in order to make him less hungry, or else the interval between feeds is increased. I feel that by far the commonest cause of this condition is an unduly rapid flow from the breast. It is easy to see that when a baby is suddenly disturbed while sucking at the breast and withdraws from it, the milk is squirting out of the breast. This is due to contractile myoepithelial cells between the secretory epithelium and the basement membrane. Many mothers interpret the cause of the gulping correctly and note that it occurs particularly when the breast is distended, at the first feed in the morning. Some writers, recognizing the cause of the trouble, have recommended that the breast should be constricted by the mother's fingers during the feed so that the baby cannot obtain the milk so quickly. It is difficult, however, for the mother to regulate the flow properly. Either she does not constrict it enough and the flow is unaffected, or else she constricts it too much so that the baby swallows air, because he does not get the milk sufficiently easily. The best method is for the mother to express a small quantity of milk say, 1 oz. (28 ml) when the breast is distended, and after that to allow the baby to suck. By regulation of the quantity expressed excessive flow when the baby sucks is prevented.

Flatulence may be due to a wrong position in feeding the baby. If he is fed while almost horizontal, air tends to accumulate anteriorly and therefore does not come up until there is considerable distension of the stomach. Milk is then apt to be brought up with it. If the child is held well propped up during a feed the air rises to the cardiac end of the stomach and therefore comes up more rapidly. If when he is laid down, he is placed on his left side, air in the stomach tends to pass into the intestine, and so may cause discomfort. It is better to lay him on the right side.

Excessive wind is also due to the baby being allowed to suck on an overdistended breast. He is unable to obtain the milk and so he swallows air. Probably the commonest cause is sucking from the breast after all the milk available has been obtained. If there is an inadequate supply of milk the baby may obtain all the milk there is in much less than the 10 minutes commonly allowed for sucking and swallow air in the remaining time. The supply may be adequate, but the baby, who has obtained all the milk in about 3 minutes on each breast, may be kept on the breast because the mother has been instructed to feed the baby for 10 minutes on each side. Sometimes a mother feeds a baby for much longer than 10 minutes on each breast. This is nearly always wrong after the new-born period, for the baby merely swallows air and so suffers from flatulence and colic.

A baby of any age who is left to cry for a long time swallows air in the process, and may even vomit as a result. This is one of the reasons why a rigid feeding schedule may lead to feeding difficulties.

Three Months' Colic, or Evening Colic

The term "three months' colic" is intended to imply that the colic disappears after about three months from birth. It is not a good term, and causes confusion. I prefer the term "evening colic" because the pain is almost confined to the evening.[9] For unknown reasons, I see less of it now in my Baby Clinic than I did in the past.

The typical story is as follows. A few days after birth, though sometimes only on return from the Maternity Hospital, the baby, having been perfectly good during the day, has attacks of crying in the evening, mostly between 6 p.m. and 10 p.m.

In an attack his face suddenly becomes red, he frowns, draws his legs up and emits piercing screams, quite unlike the cry of hunger or loneliness. They are likely to continue for 2 to 20 minutes, even though he is picked up. The attack usually ends suddenly, but sobbing is apt to continue for several minutes. He is just about to fall asleep, obviously tired out, when a further attack occurs. Attacks continue at regular intervals till about 10 p.m., when he lapses into sleep. During the attack one may hear loud borborygmi, and much flatus is passed per rectum, giving temporary relief. No unusual amount of wind is brought up by mouth. Gentle pressure or massage of the abdomen, or placing him in the prone position, gives some relief, and he obtains relief by sucking, though an additional feed does not give more than temporary relief. The attacks recur nightly, but almost always cease by the end of the third month.

There are all degrees of severity of these attacks, and the description above applies to the severe one. In milder forms the baby is just mildly irritable in the evening, without definite screaming attacks. In mild forms the attacks cease by about the eighth week, while in the severest forms the baby may not be entirely happy in the evenings till the fourth month. The average duration in a series of 50 cases was 9½ weeks: 54 per cent. had lost the attacks by 2 months of age, 85 per cent. by 3 months and 100 per cent. by 4 months.

Many have stated that the attacks do not begin in hospital. I think that the explanation of this idea lies in inaccurate observation in the maternity nursery. Thirty-six out of a series of 49 babies with colic observed by me had their first attack in hospital. Forty-four began in the first 15 days. True colic does not begin after 3 or at the most 4 weeks. It is said that the onset in premature babies is delayed for a period approximating the degree of prematurity. Forty-seven out of 50 babies in the series studied by me had their attacks after 5 p.m.

It appears to occur just as much in artificially-fed babies as in breast-fed ones.

The cause of the attacks is unknown. In my review of the literature I found an astonishing list of suggested causes. The suggestions include the following: overfeeding, underfeeding, too frequent feeds, too infrequent feeds, feeds too rich, feeds too weak, too hot or too cold; excess of fat, carbohydrate or protein; allergy, cod-liver oil, orange juice; congenital malformations of the alimentary tract, inguinal hernia, urethral colic, appendicitis, foreign bodies in the alimentary tract, lead poisoning, anal fissures, imperforate anus, peptic ulcer, disease of the gall bladder, respiratory tract or osseous system, volvulus, syphilis, intussusception, renal colic, nasopharyngitis, otitis, pyelitis and hyperacidity, tension developed *in utero* from a hypothetical uterine handicap or transmitted from a highly strung mother's system, exposure to cold, chilling of the extremities, abdominal binders, fatigue toxins from the mother, acidosis, introversion, and accumulation of acid in the kidneys. Others blame the mother for a "faulty feeding technique"—usually without defining the particular fault, though some say that the colic occurs because she fails to bring the baby's wind up. As we have shown that colic is not due to gastric flatulence, this explanation can be discarded—as it can by the simple method of feeding the baby and observing that in spite of "burping" him, the colic occurs as usual.

Some who ascribe colic to the mother's emotional problems give as evidence for this the statement that when affected babies are admitted to hospital, the colic subsides. Such babies should never be admitted to hospital, because of the risk of infection; but one obvious factor which would explain the observation, if it were true, would be the increasing age of the baby and possibly the fact that a busy nursery staff may not notice a baby's cries as much as a mother at home.

Several workers ascribe the colic to "hypertonicity" or "neuropathic constitution," whatever that means, claiming that these babies show a wide variety of signs such as vomiting, diarrhœa, constipation, abdominal distension, tetany and so on. There is no truth whatsoever in this. In my experience these babies are entirely normal apart from their colic. In my study of 50 babies with colic, whom I compared with 50 babies without colic, there was no difference with regard to their sex, birth weight, feeding history, their incidence of posseting, the number of stools or their weight gain. Their mothers differed in no way with regard to their age, parity or pregnancy history. Affected infants are certainly no more likely to show neurological signs of hypertonia than are other infants. I have not seen evening colic in association with diarrhœa. With regard to allergy, I have found no evidence of it.

In my series, there was no difference between affected and unaffected babies with regard to the family history of allergy, or the presence or development of other allergic manifestations.

It is customary to blame the parents for the colic. They are said to "pick the child up too much, and to bounce him too much after feeds." Psychiatrists in particular pin the responsibility for the baby's colic on to the mother's personality. Lakin[13] for instance, assessed the personality of 20 mothers of colicky babies, and 20 mothers of "well adjusted" infants. The mothers in the case of the colicky babies showed "poorer parent-child relationship, greater interpersonal conflict over role accepted, greater concern over their adequacy in the female role, less adequate marital adjustment, and less mothering love." A psychoanalyst described colic as a combination of congenital hypertonicity in the baby with primary anxious overpermissiveness in the mother.[19] Wessel et al.[20] blamed family tension for 22 out of 48 cases. They wrote: "Paroxysmal fussing is probably one of the earliest somatic responses to the presence of tension in the environment." The particular degree to which any infant reacts is probably determined by constitutional factors. In my opinion most of the so-called tension in parents of babies with colic is the result of the baby's colic, and not the cause of it. It is inevitable that severe colic in a baby will cause some degree of tension in a good mother. After careful observation of parents of these babies I do not believe that they are any different from parents of babies who have no colic. I do not see how family tension could produce these strictly rhythmical attacks of violent screaming with excessive borborygmi, attacks which should surely be due to pain from the nature of the scream and the fact that they continue unabated in the mother's arms. If the colic was due entirely to psychological tension, one would expect it to occur more often in the first born than in subsequent children but it does not. Furthermore, colic commonly occurs in only one of three or four babies in the family.

In the U.S.A. Paradise[16] carried out a useful study at Rochester Child Health Centre, investigating various possible factors in the background, and carrying out psychological tests on the mother, and on mothers who did not have colicky babies. He found that the incidence of colic was unrelated to the mother's age, social class, the baby's birth order, sex, weight gain, type of feeding, or family history of allergy. He could find no relation to emotional factors in the mother, but did find that there was a slightly higher incidence of colic in babies of mothers of superior intelligence—perhaps because they would report a baby's symptoms earlier than other mothers, or because they had a lower tolerance to the baby's cries. Mothers of affected babies were "stable, cheerful and feminine."

Jorup[12] in his careful study of these babies, showed that there is no excess of wind in the bowel (a finding which I can confirm), but thought that the colon showed "excessive propulsive activity"; when a barium enema was given it was expelled with unusual force. The attacks of pain coincided in time with violent colonic contractions. This would explain the excessive borborygmi which I have described.

Bruce[1] suggested that colicky babies are malingerers, for he wrote "I feel sure of one thing, infants are usually not in so much pain as they appear to be, or as their parents think they are." One feels that this would be difficult to prove.

At the Jessop Hospital, Sheffield, radiological studies of 20 infants during the actual attacks of colic in the evenings revealed no excess of gas in the stomach. The evidence all points to the colic being due to gas becoming blocked in loops of bowel. Why this should happen, we do not yet know. One can say with a fair degree of certainty, that colic is unrelated to "hypertonicity," "allergy," or "psychological factors in the mother." The role of immaturity of the nervous control of the alimentary tract, leading to obstruction of gas in loops of bowel, is a likely but unproven and certainly little understood cause.

Differential Diagnosis

Psychiatrists tend to apply the term "colic" to all babies who cry a great deal. To me the condition of evening colic is an entity of unknown ætiology, almost confined to the evenings, with characteristic rhythmical crying attacks. It is obvious to me that most of the psychological studies of so-called colic have included many conditions of quite different and obvious ætiology. For instance, some babies cry a great deal because of their personality. There are happy smiling babies and babies who are easily annoyed and upset. It would not be surprising if one had to find that the parents of such babies were different from the parents of placid babies.

It is easy to ascribe a baby's evening crying to "colic" when it is merely due to hunger. Mothers tend to produce less milk in the evenings, so that underfeeding in the evenings may readily occur. In this connection the apparent relief given to babies with colic by sucking is a real cause of confusion, and leads mothers to give frequent feeds all through the evening. In fact, if the baby is getting enough from the breast, although he likes to suck when he has colic, he will not take a bottle feed. If he does take some milk from the bottle, the colic remains unabated. In my experience these babies are in a good state of nutrition, and quite up to the average weight or above it. The condition is certainly not due to overfeeding. Efforts to reduce the feeds will only cause more crying.

Many babies cry merely because they want to be picked up, but such crying stops when the mother takes the baby into her arms. Not all babies who cry have colic. They cry because they are hungry, wet, cold, hot, bored, or because they suffer from gastric flatulence. Some babies cry when the light is put out, others cry when the light is put on.

Treatment

A wide variety of treatments have been given to babies with colic.

Jorup[12] recommended methyl scopolamine nitrate ('Skopyl'). In a controlled study at Sheffield it proved to be useless. In another controlled study[8] I showed that dicyclomine hydrochloride was a specific treatment for the condition. Given in a dose of 4 ml half an hour before the evening feed, it gives excellent relief. In fact, if it failed to give relief I would think that the diagnosis was wrong. The drug has an anti-cholinergic action. I have not tried other drugs with a similar pharmacological action.

It has been suggested that the colic is due to progesterone deficiency.[2] Fifteen non colicky babies showed appreciable urinary pregnanediol glucuronide excretion, while 15 colicky babies did not— and they improved when the hormone was given. It should be noted, however, that a much cheaper and safer preparation, dicyclomine hydrochloride (below) is highly effective—if the diagnosis is correct. Paradise[16] made a curious observation, namely that certain sounds (motors, vacuum cleaners, washing machines), or vibrations, seemed to give relief. He regarded the colic as an expression of immaturity of the central nervous system, and thought that "the improvement by sucking activity, vibrations or sounds, rocking or enemas, may be due to interruption or decrease in certain afferent proprioceptive stimuli."

Infantile Colic related to Menstruation

It has long been thought that some babies are irritable during the mother's menstrual period. Whether this is related to the mother's irritability at that time is not clear. It does seem that there is sometimes a falling off in the milk supply during the period, and this may be the reason for the irritability.

It has been suggested that there are some substances in the breast milk during menstruation which cause discomfort to the baby. This has not been proved.

Overfeeding

In my opinion overfeeding is so rare that it can be ignored. I have seen only one or two possible cases. When vomiting, crying, colic, diarrhœa or other symptoms are ascribed to overfeeding, the diagnosis is almost certainly wrong. The most common cause of symptoms ascribed by doctors to overfeeding is in fact underfeeding. I have frequently seen ravenously hungry underfed babies whose feeds had been restricted because it was thought that they were being overfed. Animals know when to stop when feeding from their mothers. It would be surprising if human babies behaved differently in this respect.

When a baby has been underfed in the early days, and is then given as much as he wants, he will have a compensatory increase of appetite, with resultant rapid weight gain, until he has caught up to the expected weight—when his intake falls off and his weight gain slows to the average. I have seen a baby gain 28 oz. (800 g) in a week under these circumstances. No anxiety should be known about an unusual weight gain in a previously starved infant.

It is legitimate to ascribe obesity in the older baby to overfeeding. I prefer to term it wrong feeding. Such babies should have been weaned on to a mixed diet, with restriction of the milk intake.

Posseting and Vomiting

I do not think that it is profitable to attempt to distinguish the above terms. All babies bring some milk up, but some do it more than others. It occurs especially in the highly active, wiry, alert baby, who exhibits rapid movements of the arms and legs. It is usually more troublesome in the first few weeks, but it may be a nuisance in the latter part of the year.

In most young babies some milk wells up into the mouth after a feed. In others milk shoots out when the baby belches, and the "projectile vomiting" leads the unwary to diagnose congenital pyloric stenosis. It worries mothers, and they are apt to exaggerate the quantity brought up. The doctor assesses the truth of the story by the weight gain. I have been told on innumerable occasions that the baby brings the whole of every feed up, and yet I find that his weight gain is normal.

The treatment of this sort of "vomiting" is the treatment of the cause. By far the commonest cause of excessive flatulence in the breast-fed baby is sucking after the milk has been obtained. This is due either to insufficiency of milk or to allowing the baby to suck longer than the time usually recommended.

Babies frequently pass urine or a stool after a feed, and the napkin has to be changed. It is easy in changing the napkin to tilt the child so far back that milk is brought up. This is due to the relative incompetence of the cardio-œsophical sphincter in early infancy. After a feed the baby should be placed on his right side, with the head slightly higher than the rest of the body.

The chief condition from which normal posseting or vomiting has to be distinguished is congenital pyloric stenosis. This occurs in 1 in 150 males and 1 in 775 females. It commonly begins between the fourth and sixth week, and is characterized by one big vomit immediately after or during a feed. On palpation during a feed the pyloric tumour can be felt.

Whenever a baby vomits repeatedly, one should always ask whether there is blood in the vomitus. This would suggest chalasia of the œsophagus or hiatus hernia. The presence of bile in the vomitus would suggest intestinal obstruction.

Rumination

Rumination is a habit acquired by babies usually after the age of 3 months. The diagnosis can sometimes be made on the history alone, but it is usually made by observation of the child. The baby is usually a wide-awake alert one. It is equally common in the two sexes. Examination shows that the baby hollows his tongue, champs the jaws, strains, arches the back, keeping the mouth open, and holds the head back. He contracts the abdominal muscles and may make sucking movements of the tongue, bringing milk up. Some of the milk dribbles out, while the rest is swallowed. The child shows satisfaction at his achievement, obviously enjoying it. The loss of milk may be considerable, so that the weight gain is unsatisfactory, and he may even lose weight.

It is now thought that rumination is a sign of emotional deprivation,[14,18] and that the treatment consists of satisfying the baby's need for love. This may usually be true, but it is not necessarily always so; the cause may be difficult to determine. It is wise if in doubt to ask for a barium swallow x-ray examination to exclude a hiatus hernia.[7]

The problem is usually treated successfully by thickening the feeds. The head of the cot may be raised, or the child is placed in a chalasia chair, so that it is less easy for him to ruminate. The prone position may be tried if this fails, for it is difficult for a child to ruminate when prone.

The Baby's Stools

The great majority of babies pass the first stool during the first day of life; 69 per cent. of 500 full-term babies passed the first stool in 12 hours, and 94 per cent. within 24 hours of birth.

All who are responsible for the care of babies should be conversant with the normal changes in their stools. The first stool passed by the new-born baby may be the so-called meconium plug, which has a greyish-white or yellow appearance. Thereafter for the next 2 or 3 days he passes the typical meconium stool, which is dark green-black, tenacious, sticky and almost odourless. After 2 or 3 days this gradually changes to a less intense green-black and then to a green-brown greasy stool. There is then a gradual transition to the normal orange-yellow loose homogeneous stool of the fully breast-fed baby. This transition stage may take up to almost 3 weeks, and in this stage the stools contain mucus, are often explosive and may be frequent (up to twelve per day). They may be a bright green colour and they contain solid yellow soap plaques. A normal breast-fed baby may at times pass bright green stools for the first 6 weeks or so. An erroneous diagnosis of diarrhœa is readily made, but the child is well and thriving.

The stools of the fully breast-fed baby remain loose but change in character immediately after other foods are given. Even a small amount of cow's milk makes them much firmer. It should be borne in mind that when mixed feeds are given, the stools readily show notable changes in colour. Certain fruits, such as bilberries, given to older babies, cause remarkable coloration of the stools.

Striking colours may appear in the napkin of a baby receiving phenolphthalein in teething powders. The stool is surrounded by a salmon pink discoloration which turns a deep bright mauve when hot water is poured on to it. The alkalinity of the napkins causes the colour to change when the phenolphthalein is washed out of the stool.

Constipation

The majority of breast-fed babies who are said by their mothers to be constipated are merely having infrequent normal motions. There is a great deal of unnecessary anxiety about this. I was once asked to see a baby who had been given an enema by the doctor at the age of 24 hours on account of constipation. It is a strange fact that breast-fed babies often have periods in which they have infrequent motions. At one time they have five or six motions a day. A few weeks later they are having one motion every 5 or 6 days. Such infrequency is extremely common. Hardly a day passes in a welfare clinic without a mother complaining about her child's "constipation." I have frequently seen babies who only had a motion every 5 days. Such marked infrequency does not seem to occur in the first 2 or 3 weeks of life. It is exceptional to see a baby who has a motion as infrequently as every 10 or 12 days, but I have seen this, and it is certainly no cause for alarm. The baby rarely suffers any discomfort from infrequent bowel action, though occasionally he seems to be a little restless for a day or two before the stool is passed. There is little abdominal distension. Flatus is passed as usual. The child is in every way perfectly well. The old explanation of the phenomenon was spasm of the anal sphincter. There is no evidence for this, and any attempt to dilate the sphincter is unwarranted. No treatment of any kind is needed. Mothers who are worried should be reassured. They commonly try various kinds of purgatives, usually in an unavailing attempt to make the child have a motion. They give enemas and pass soap sticks into the rectum. All those treatments are wrong. The mothers should be told that there is nothing wrong with the child, that this infrequency is extremely common in normal breast-fed babies, and that instead of being anxious they should be pleased that they have fewer soiled napkins to wash.

The reason for the infrequency of the motions is unknown. The condition does not occur in artificially-fed babies, and this should be emphasized. It seems as if the loose stools of the breast-fed baby fail to supply a sufficient stimulus to the bowel to lead to emptying. The phases are not usually long lasting, and the baby who for a few weeks had infrequent motions gradually reverts to his former state of having two or three motions a day.

The starved child has the so-called "starvation stools"—small, often frequent, loose or semi-fluid stools containing mucus. They are often semi-transparent, dark green or green-brown, and have a faint old musty odour without any smell of fermentation or decomposition. In addition, the child shows defective weight gain and the appearance of an underfed baby.

The constipation of intestinal obstruction is diagnosed by the associated abdominal distension, illness of the child, absence of the passage of flatus and vomiting of material which is often green or fæcal. The diagnosis can be confirmed by a straight X-ray of the abdomen.

In Hirschsprung's disease the stools may be bulky and hard, even though the baby is fully breast-fed.

Diarrhœa

When mothers complain that their breast-fed child has diarrhœa, by far the commonest finding is that the baby has perfectly normal stools. The motions of a fully breast-fed baby are loose, and many mothers, not realizing this, think that he has diarrhœa. In the first 2 or 3 weeks of a baby's life there is often obvious mucus in the stools and the expulsion of a stool may be explosive. The stool at this stage shows soap plaques and curds and is often bright green in colour, thus adding to the suggestion that food is going through the baby improperly digested. In the first 6 or 8 weeks of life some breast-fed babies have frequent motions—up to 10 or 20 a day, or more. The unwary, diagnose gastro-enteritis, and I have known perfectly normal babies admitted to infectious disease hospitals on that account. True diarrhœa can occur in a fully breast-fed baby, but it is very rare, for gastro-enteritis is practically confined to artificially-fed babies. There have been outbreaks of mild diarrhœa in nurses and mothers in maternity units which have led to infection of the babies, but these are uncommon. True diarrhœa in a fully breast-fed baby is difficult to diagnose with certainty. It would hardly be diagnosed without coincident loss of weight, malaise and evidence of dehydration. It is unusual for stools to be green when freshly passed after about 10 to 12 weeks, and there should not be obvious mucus after that age, unless some purgative has been given. An important point in the diagnosis would be a sudden increase in the frequency of the stools.

The looseness of the stools sometimes met with as a result of substances passing through the mother's milk has already been mentioned. Orange juice sometimes upsets a baby and causes diarrhœa. It is extremely important to distinguish the loose green mucus stools of starvation. Such stools often lead to the erroneous diagnosis of diarrhœa. This is a tragedy, for the baby is then likely to be starved still further, whereas all that he needed was more food. I have seen a baby develop diarrhœa as a result of licking ointment of zinc and castor oil placed on the lips on account of soreness.

Defective Weight Gain

Though an average child after the first fortnight gains 6 or 7 oz. (170 or 200 g) a week, some normal children gain more and some less. I would consider that a weight gain of 5 oz. (140 g) a week was "normal" if the child were contented, had normal stools and looked well, and if the gain were maintained at that level.

The obvious cause of defective weight gain is insufficient food, and this diagnosis can readily be confirmed by test feeds. There are, however, other important causes which have to be considered. An important early cause is irritability, inertia or poor sucking. It is easy to make a mistaken diagnosis of underfeeding in those babies, being misled by defective weight gain and poor gain in test feeds. Expression of the breast after the baby has sucked shows that there is an adequate supply of milk, but the baby has not taken it.

Loneliness and separation of the baby from the mother may prevent a satisfactory weight gain. Prolonged crying due to a rigid schedule may prevent a satisfactory weight gain.

Defective weight gain may be due to excessive posseting or to vomiting. It is not uncommonly due to gross overclothing. In a baby whom I was asked to see because of failure to gain weight, a thorough search for infections had been made, with a negative result. Test feeds showed that the milk supply was adequate. The child was well but grossly overclothed, having fifteen layers of clothes in a room in which the temperature was 86°F (30°C). When this was dealt with the child gained weight normally. Overclothing may prevent a satisfactory weight gain not only by causing excessive perspiration but by making the baby drowsy, so that he sucks badly. It must always be remembered that any infections, however slight, may prevent a young baby gaining weight adequately.

References

1. Bruce, J. W. (1961). "Infantile Colic." *Ped. Clin. N. Am.*, **8**, 143.
2. Clark, R. L., Ganis, F. M., Bradford, W. L. (1963). "A Study of Possible Relationship of Progesterone to Colic." *Pediatrics*, **31**, 65.
3. Cope, E., (1968). "Galactorrhoea." *Practitioner*, **260**, 692.
4. *Drug and Therapeutics Bulletin* (1970). "Drugs that Inhibit Lactation." **8**, 1.
5. Gunther, M. (1955). "Instinct and the Nursing Couple." *Lancet*, **1**, 575.
6. Gunther, M. (1970). *Infant Feeding*. London, Methuen.
7. Herbst, J., Friedland, G. W., Zboralske, F. F. (1971). "Hiatal Hernia and 'Rumination' in Infants and Children." *J. Pediat.*, **78**, 261.
8. Illingworth, R. S. (1959). "Evening Colic in Infants. A Double Blind Trial of Dicyclomine Hydrochloride." *Lancet*, **2**, 1119.
9. Illingworth, R. S. (1954). "Three Months' Colic." *Arch. Dis. Childhood*, **29**, 165.
10. Illingworth, R. S., Stone, D. (1952). "Self-Demand Feeding in a Maternity Unit." *Lancet*, **1**, 683.
11. Jelliffe, J. B. (1962). "Culture, Social Change and Infant Feeding." *Am. J. Clin. Nutrition*, **10**, 19.
12. Jorup, S. (1952). "Colonic Hyperperistalsis in Neurolabile Infants." *Acta pæd. Uppsala*, **41**, Suppl. 85.
13. Lakin, M. (1957). "Personality Factors in Mothers of Excessively Crying (Colicky) Babies." Monograph of the Society for Research in Child Development, **22**, 7.
14. Menking, M., Wagnitz, J. G., Burton, J. J., Coddington, R. D., Sotos, J. F. (1969). "Rumination—Near Fatal Psychiatric Disease of Infancy." *New. Engl. J. Med.*, **280**, 802.
15. Millar, D. G., (1970) "Supression of Lactation." *Practitioner*, **205**, 251.
16. Paradise, J. L. (1966). "Maternal and Other Factors in the Etiology of Infantile Colic." Report of a prospective study of 146 infants. *J. Am. Med. Assoc.*, **197**, 191.
17. Platt, B. S., Gin, S. K. (1938). "Chinese Methods of Infant Feeding and Nursing." *Arch. Dis. Childhood*, **13**, 343.
18. Richmond, J. B., Eddy, E. J., Green, M. (1958). "Rumination, a Psychosomatic Syndrome of Infancy." *Pediatrics*, **22**, 49.
19. Spitz, R. A. (1951). *Psychoanal. Study Child.*, **6**, 255.
20. Wessell, M. A., Cobb, J. C., Jackson, E. B., Harris, G. S., Detwiler, A. C. (1954). "Paroxysmal Fussing in Infancy." *Pediatrics*, **14**, 421.
21. *World Medicine* (1969). "Does the Pill Affect Breast Feeding?" Leading Article. **4**, 39.
22. Zlocisti, quoted by Von Reuss, A. (1921). *Diseases of the Newborn*. London Bale and Danielsson.

CHAPTER 3

ARTIFICIAL FEEDING AND WEANING

Historical

The milk of many animals has been used for feeding babies. They include the goat, ass, camel, llama, caribou, bitch, mare, reindeer, sheep and water buffalo. In Paris in the nineteenth century, babies were fed direct from asses, which were kept in stables next door to the Maternity Hospital. In Malta babies were fed direct from goats.

Equipment Needed

This includes the following:

(1) Feeding bottles. These are of glass or plastic. Though the boat shaped bottle with a hole at each end is easy to clean through and through, the vertical kind with a hole at one end only is easier to boil in a pan, and is the type usually used.

(2) Teats. Rubber teats have an advantage over plastic ones in that if the hole is not large enough, one can readily enlarge it by inserting a needle into a cork, making the needle red hot, and inserting it into the hole until it is the appropriate size. The milk should almost pour out when the bottle is inverted. One should not need to shake the bottle, or still less to squeeze the teat between the forefinger and thumb. If on inverting the bottle one can count the drops, the hole is not big enough. If it is not big enough, the baby will find it difficult to get the milk, he will take too long over the feed, and so will swallow air. He will then have "wind," cry, and perhaps vomit. No feed should take more than ten or fifteen minutes. If it does, he will be likely to have "wind" as a result. It is absolutely essential to realize that the hole must be tested before every feed. One cannot rely on the maker's statement that the hole is a big one. We have seen numerous teats which were said to have a large hole, and in fact had no hole at all. The hole gets blocked by particles of milk and by the rubber swelling.

There is no such thing as an "anti-colic" teat. Some teats have a bulbous swelling in the middle. This is undesirable, because it is difficult to clean them properly. The danger of a flange to the edge of the teat is the difficulty in cleaning it.

(3) A funnel.

(4) A measuring glass in ounces or millilitres.

(5) A bottle brush—reserved for the purpose of cleaning the feeding bottle.

(6) A half or one pint mixing glass.

(7) Some one or two ounce medicine glasses which can be used for putting over the teat when the teat is on the bottle after the milk has been put in. This keeps the teat clean and uncontaminated until the baby wants the feed.

Preparation of the Bottle and Teat

It is absolutely essential that the bottle and teat should be sterile when given to the baby. Hence immediately after a feed the teat and bottle should be rinsed, because once the milk has dried on, it is more difficult to remove it. The bottle should then be scrubbed out with the special pan brush. The teat should be scrubbed and turned inside out, so that it can be thoroughly cleaned. Water is squeezed through the teat. The two are then washed out in a detergent such as Stergene, and then thoroughly rinsed. The day's bottles and teats are subsequently boiled, the bottles for ten minutes, leaving them in the pan afterwards with the lid off. The teats are boiled for three minutes and the water is poured off.

Instead of sterilizing the bottle and teat by boiling, they can be left completely submerged in 1 per cent. hypochlorite (Milton) $\frac{1}{2}$ oz. (14 ml) in 2 pints (1·1 litres) of water, for 3 hours before a feed. They should not be rinsed before use; the small amount of residual hypochlorite in the teat and bottle is harmless. The solution should be changed every 24 hours. Anderson and Gatherer[1] showed that the hypochlorite method was safer than boiling. In a study of 758 feeding bottles, 78 per cent. of the bottles and 70 per cent. of teats showed a satisfactory colony count when the hypochlorite method was used, as compared with 46 per cent. of bottles and 34 per cent. of teats when the boiling method was used for sterilization.

Carelessness in the preparation and sterilization of equipment, is one of the reasons for the prevalence of gastro-enteritis in artificially fed babies. In the first few months the feed must be sterile when given to the baby. The age at which some relaxation of this principle can be permitted is a matter of opinion. I would feel that by the age of 6 months fresh pasteurized milk may be given unboiled to a baby.

In a hospital all feeds are subjected to terminal sterilization either by autoclave or steam bath and stored in a refrigerator until wanted.

The Choice of Food

The choice lies between dried milk, fresh cow's milk and evaporated milk. There is nothing to choose between any of these except in price—though some prefer evaporated milk or fresh cow's milk because of the ease with which they are mixed. On the other hand, dried milk is easy to store and convenient to take on holiday or otherwise away from home. Trufood and S.M.A. are still more costly.

The chemical differences between the dried milks are so trivial, that it is quite inconceivable that a baby would have troublesome symptoms as a result of one preparation "not suiting him." In fact I have never yet had to change from one dried milk to another to find one which suits the baby—except in the case of the rare metabolic conditions, such as phenylketonuria, galactosæmia, disaccharide intolerance, hypercalcæmia and so on. On rare occasions one prescribes a soya bean preparation for a child allergic to cow's milk. Suitable preparations are Soyolk (Soya Food Ltd., 1½ oz. (42 g) made up with 1 pint (560 ml) of water), or Velactin (Wander; made from vegetable matter; 8 tablespoonsful to a half pint (280 ml) of water).

Evaporated milk is entirely satisfactory, provided that it is not kept in an open tin in a warm place. It must be stored in a refrigerator.

Fresh cow's milk is satisfactory and easy to use. It should be diluted with water, because of the high protein content. It should be boiled before use—at least up to about 6 months of age. It has been pointed out[2] that prolonged boiling causes a dangerous concentration of electrolytes which may result in hypernatræmia. When 227 ml of fat free milk were boiled for 15 minutes in a 6 inch pan the sodium content of the milk was doubled; when boiled for 12 minutes in a 9 inch pan it was trebled.

It is a common practice to change from one dried food to another because the child is vomiting, crying excessively or presenting other feeding problems. In the case of pyloric stenosis, it is extremely common to hear that the baby was taken off the breast on the grounds that the vomiting was due to the breast milk not suiting the baby, and then tried on one dried milk after another in an attempt to find one which would not cause vomiting. This should never be done. The diagnosis is bound to be wrong.

There is no need for a half-cream milk except for a premature baby, or one who on account of an infection has some looseness of the stools.

The Quantity of Food

The first step in calculating the amount of food to offer is to determine the expected weight, by adding 6 oz. (170 g) per week (in the first 3 months) to the birth weight. For instance, the expected weight of an 8 week old baby whose birth weight was 8 lb (3·6 kg) would be 8 lb + 6 × 8 oz. = 11 lb (5 kg).

If he is above the expected weight,

his feed will be calculated for his actual weight; if he is below it, his feed will be calculated for the expected weight.

The next step is to ensure that the fluid intake is adequate—$2\frac{1}{2}$ oz. per lb (150 ml/kg) per day. (In tropical countries the fluid intake will be higher.) The feeds are then calculated on the basis of the figures given in Table I. These feeds all give a calorie value of approximately 50 calories per pound.

TABLE I

Quantity of Food for Baby, per Pound of Expected Weight per Day

	Milk	Sugar	Water
Breast milk	$2\frac{1}{2}$ oz. (71 ml)	—	—
Cow's milk	$1\frac{3}{4}$ oz. (49 ml)	3·6 g	$\frac{3}{4}$ oz. (21 ml)
Full cream Cow & Gate . } Ostermilk No. 2 . . }	$1\frac{3}{4}$ measures	3·6 g	$2\frac{1}{2}$ oz. (71 ml)
Half cream Cow & Gate } Ostermilk No. 1 . . }	$2\frac{1}{2}$ measures	—	$2\frac{1}{2}$ oz. (71 ml)
Unsweetened Evaporated Milk	$1\frac{1}{2}$ oz. (42 ml)	1·8 g	$2\frac{1}{2}$ oz. (71 ml)

It is customary to add sugar to a feed, unless it is a sugar containing food. It is not really necessary, though some babies may become a little constipated without. It is quite unnecessary to use glucose instead of ordinary sugar; it is more expensive and in no way better.

Table II gives the average quantities likely to be taken by babies of four different weights.

These figures are approximate, but near enough provided that the baby is given more if he wants it. Having worked out the calculated requirements for the 24 hours, the total quantity is divided by the number of feeds he receives in that period, keeping to a convenient round figure. For instance, if a baby's expected weight is 12 lb and he is fed on cow's milk, the total quantity for the whole day would be

Milk . . 12 × $1\frac{3}{4}$ oz. = 21 oz. (588 ml)
Sugar . . 12 × 3·6 g = 43 g
Water . . 12 × $\frac{3}{4}$ oz. = 9 oz. (252 ml)

TABLE II

Average Quantities for Each of the Five Feeds

		Expected weight in pounds (or actual weight if greater)			
	oz.	6 (2·7 kg)	8 (3·6 kg)	10 (4·5 kg)	12 (5·4 kg)
Breast		3 (85 ml)	4 (113 ml)	5 (142 ml)	6 (170 ml)
Cow & Gate Full Cream Ostermilk No. 2	Milk (meas.)	2½	3½	4½	5
	Sugar (teaspoon)	1 (3·6 g)	1½ (5·4 g)	2 (7·2 g)	2½ (9·0 g)
	Water (oz.)	3 (85 ml)	4 (113 ml)	5 (142 ml)	6 (170 ml)
Cow & Gate Half cream Ostermilk No. 1	Milk (meas.)	3	4	5	6
	Sugar (teaspoon)	—	—	—	—
	Water (oz.)	3 (85 ml)	4 (113 ml)	5 (142 ml)	6 (170 ml)
Trufood	Milk (meas.)	2½	3½	5	6
	Sugar (teaspoon)	—	—	—	—
	Water (oz.)	3 (85 ml)	4 (113 ml)	5 (142 ml)	6 (170 ml)
S.M.A.	Milk (meas.)	3	4	5	6
	Sugar (teaspoon)	—	—	—	—
	Water (oz.)	3 (85 ml)	4 (113 ml)	5 (142 ml)	6 (170 ml)
Evaporated	Milk (oz.)	1 (28 ml)	1½ (42 ml)	1¾ (49 ml)	2 (57 ml)
	Sugar (teaspoon)	1 (3·6 g)	1½ (5·4 g)	2 (7·2 g)	2 (7·2 g)
	Water (oz.)	3 (85 ml)	4 (113 ml)	5 (142 ml)	6 (170 ml)
Fresh cow's milk	Milk (oz.)	2 (57 ml)	2½ (70 ml)	3½ (98 ml)	4½ (127 ml)
	Sugar (teaspoon)	1 (3·6 g)	1½ (5·4 g)	2 (7·2 g)	2 (7·2 g)
	Water (oz.)	1 (28 ml)	1½ (42 ml)	1½ (42 ml)	1½ (42 ml)

If he has 5 feeds a day, one would offer at each feed

Milk	.	.	.	4½ oz.	(128 ml)
Sugar	.	.	.	2 teaspoon	(7·0 g)
Water	.	.	.	1½ oz.	(42 ml).

There is no need to be more exact. The mother should be told that if the baby wants more he should be given more, but that he may want less than this, in which case a somewhat smaller quantity will be made up.

The formula described above for half-cream milk does not give quite the same calorie value as the other feeds in the quantities stated. Doxiadis and Paschos, however, showed that if babies on a weak formula are allowed to take what they want, they will compensate by increasing the volume taken. The danger of making the feeds considerably stronger (e.g. 9 measures in 6 oz. (170 ml) of water) is hyperelectrolytæmia.

The Danger of Overfeeding

In previous editions of this book I wrote that there is no danger of overfeeding a young baby. I argued that a baby knows when to stop and will not take too much. This may be true, but recent work in my Department at Sheffield has indicated that there is a real danger of wrong feeding. Eid[7] showed that babies who are gaining weight excessively even as young as 6 weeks of age are more likely than others to be overweight at the age of seven or eight.

Subsequently Taitz[17], in a study of 261 infants in the follow up clinic at the Jessop Maternity Hospital, Sheffield, found that 19·0 per cent. of breast fed babies had a weight gain velocity at 6 weeks above the 90th percentile, as compared with 59·6 per cent. of those artificially fed (74·6 per cent. of the boys, 46·0 per cent. of the girls). The reasons for this excessive weight gain were not altogether clear. Some mothers were using heaped measures of milk powder instead of flat ones. Some were adding too much sugar, but most were giving cereals and rusks.

It is most important that excessive weight gain in the early weeks should be avoided (see p. 265).

It is possible that an unwise diet in infancy has a bearing on the recent increase in cardiovascular disease in adults. It is well known that plaques are commonly found in the aorta of infants. Neufeld[15] examined the coronary arteries of children under 10 in different ethnic groups. Gross changes were found in male Ashkenazi children; Ashkenazi adults have a higher incidence of ischaemic heart disease than Bedouins and Yemenite Jews in Israel. We do not know whether overfeeding in infancy is related to cardiovascular disease in adults, but it may be. We do know that in experimental animals overfeeding in the early days shortens life.[3] Yudkin[22] has marshalled evidence that a high intake of refined sugar is a factor in the development of atherosclerosis. If it is true, it is important that mothers should not induce the sweet-eating habit in their children.

Taitz and Byers at Sheffield[18] have drawn attention to the excessive sodium load given by mothers to their babies. The mean sodium content of feeds taken from the milk kitchen at the Jessop Hospital, Sheffield, was 26 mEq per litre; 29 of 32 mothers in the follow-up clinic were giving feeds containing considerably more sodium; 15 were giving 31 to 35 mEq/l. and 2 were giving 36 to 40 mEq. Taitz and Byers noted that cow's milk contains over three times as much sodium as breast milk. This high sodium load may be a factor in the increasing incidence of hypertonic dehydration when infants suffer respiratory or alimentary infections. Guthrie[10] discussed the possibility that excessive salt intake is a factor in the development of hypertension. In experimental animals a salt intake similar to that taken by many babies causes hypertension and early death.

The Danger of Underfeeding

The dangers of underfeeding are several. Underfeeding often (but not always) leads to excessive crying. Malnutrition predisposes to infection and increases the risk of serious illness resulting from infection. It may also damage the developing brain. Dobbing in this country[5] and Winick[19,20,21] have shown that malnutrition during the period of maximum brain growth may cause permanent damage to the brain. Ten normal brains from well nourished Chilean children who died accidentally were compared with brains of nine infants who died of severe malnutrition during the first year of life. The brains of the latter were smaller in weight, protein content, RNA and DNA content and the number of cells. Undernutrition of the rat and pig in the early days caused a permanent reduction in brain weight. Infants who at 15 days weighed less than their birth weight were compared during their first year with infants matched for birth weight, length and gestational age; they continued to be smaller throughout their first year and to lag behind in total body growth, head circumference, chest circumference and skin fold thickness, but not in behavioural development.[4] Reference is made in the next chapter to the work of Eid[8] in this connection.

Making up the Feed

It is essential that the hands should be thoroughly washed and dried on a clean towel before the bottle and teats are handled. It is no use washing the hands thoroughly and then drying them on a dirty towel.

If dried milk is used, the quantity is measured out in the measure which should be kept in the tin. The powder is placed in the mixing glass, the lid is returned promptly to the tin and boiled water is added to the powder, which is then thoroughly mixed so that no lumps remain. It is a mistake to measure the milk powder with a teaspoon, because teaspoons vary so much in size. In the same way it is a mistake to measure the water in tablespoons, which are supposed to measure half an ounce, because tablespoons vary so much in size. The water should be measured in a measuring glass. After mixing, the milk is poured into the bottle, the teat is added, and the medicine glass is put over the teat. The bottle is then stored in a cool place.

Warming the Feed

It is the custom prior to giving the feed to the baby to warm it. If one does, one must see that it is not too hot, by pouring some onto the bare arm before giving it to the baby. In fact it is unnecessary to warm it at all before giving it to him.

There have been several trials of the use of cold milk for infants instead of warmed feeds. Gibson[9] gave 150 infants cold feeds from a refrigerator, and 89 per cent. accepted them without difficulty. Holt et al.[11] carried out a controlled study of the use of cold milk in feeding premature babies. They could find no difference in the sleep patterns, vocalizations, motility, food or fluid intake, weight gain or amount of regurgitation, as compared with babies fed on warmed feeds. They concluded that there is no advantage in heating the feeds. We tried a limited number of infants at the Children's Hospital, Sheffield, and found that most of them took it as well as warm feeds. In the case of roller dried milks (Cow and Gate), the fat tends to congeal if the feed is cold, and the milk may not come through the hole in the teat as well when cold as when warm. If one is in a hurry to obtain a feed for a baby (as when one is wanting to palpate an abdomen for a pyloric tumour), I would certainly use a cold feed if a warm one were not available.

If a baby requires feeds in the night, the milk should not be kept in a vacuum flask, for dangerous organisms may grow in it. Water may be kept warm in the flask and used for mixing the feed when required.

Method of Feeding

The baby should be partly or fully propped up, because it is difficult to swallow milk when lying down. The teat must be withdrawn from his mouth at intervals to allow air to bubble into the bottle, for otherwise he will suck all the air out of the bottle, creating a vacuum, leaving him unable to get the milk. The teat will be flat as a result of the vacuum.

After the feed, he should be allowed to bring the wind up, by patting him gently on his back in the sitting position.

It is essential to remember that the size of the hole in the teat must be tested *before every feed.* It readily gets blocked up.

Indications of Adequacy

The most important of all indications that he is getting enough is a good weight gain—of not less than 6 oz. (170 g) a week in the first three months.

Vitamins

Babies should be given additional Vitamin C from a month or two of age, and as soon as they are off dried milk they should be given additional Vitamin D, to prevent rickets. The British Welfare Clinic orange juice has now been discontinued. Vitamin D is added by manufacturers to the dried milks and to cereals such as Farex.

It was shown long ago[13,14] that vitamin D which has been added to milk is much more effective in preventing rickets than vitamin D in oil.

Weaning the Baby

There is no rule as to when to introduce thickened feeds. I frequently introduce them when a baby is 4 to 6 weeks of age. They can be introduced sooner if it is so desired. I normally introduce them when a child is a little over 10 lb (4·5 kg) in weight.

Weaning should be begun under the following circumstances:

(1) The child is 4 to 5 months old. If one waits longer, the baby is liable to resist the introduction of new foods.

(2) The child weighs 16 lb (7 kg). This would mean that he is taking 16 × 2½ oz. (70 ml) per day, which is 40 oz. (1·1 litres). I think that at that stage it is wise not to increase the quantity of milk further.

(3) He is taking 7–8 oz. (200 to 225 ml) feeds. It is inconvenient for the mother to prepare two bottles per feed. As stated above, it is wise to limit the quantity of milk which he is taking.

(4) He is constipated in spite of ensuring that the feeds are properly made up, and he is being given sufficient. The introduction of puréed fruit and other substances is likely to help.

(5) He is becoming too fat. The milk should be limited, and other foods should be introduced—avoiding excess of cereals. Puréed fruits,

as supplied by the manufacturers, have a high carbohydrate content. Other pureéd foods, such as meats and vegetables, have less carbohydrate added, but it would be better if possible to prepare the pureéd foods at home, so that they contain even less carbohydrate. Mothers should not think that all feeds given to babies need be sweet.

(6) There is insufficient breast milk, and the baby has been fed on the breast for a period such as 8 weeks or so. I would wean on to thickened feeds instead of advising the mother to buy bottles and teats and other equipment.

If after 2–3 weeks the mother cannot supply half the required quantity, it is doubtful whether it is justifiable to continue partly breast feeding and then giving complementary feeds. There is little value in part breast feeding unless the mother wishes to do this.

Before the baby can chew, he is given puréed meat, puréed vegetables, puréed fruit, soup, cereals, custard, potato mashed with gravy, banana mashed with milk and sugar, grated cheese or grated carrot. Some think that egg yolk should be avoided in the first 6 months because of the risk of allergy developing, but I am doubtful about this.

Babies normally begin to chew at about 7 months. They can then be given raw apple (without the skin and core), a biscuit, chocolate, toast and other solid foods.

The causes of food refusal when weaning is being attempted can be enumerated as follows:

(1) Dislike of the food offered—because of taste or appearance.

(2) The child is being forced to take it or is being rushed unduly.

(3) The food is too hot or the child remembers a previous similar food which was too hot and which burnt him.

(4) He wants a drink first.

(5) He is not hungry, perhaps because he is tired.

(6) He is uncomfortable because of a wet napkin or because of teething.

(7) The food is being offered in a cup or dish other than his favourite one.

(8) He is not allowed to help to feed himself.

(9) He prefers a cup to a spoon.

Weaning difficulties are intimately bound up with the development of food refusal in later years.

Looseness of the stools in the weaning period may be due to an excess of fruit in the diet, particularly rhubarb and pears.

Undue offensiveness of the stools may be due to excess of protein in the diet.

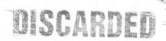

Flatulence and Colic

There are several causes of air swallowing in artificially-fed babies, most of them concerned with the teat of the bottle. Much the commonest is too small a hole in the teat. The hole should be tested for patency and adequacy before every feed. One often hears on questioning that the teat was tested when it was purchased, but not again. It is important to be conversant with the methods commonly used by mothers for testing the hole. A common and most undesirable practice is for the mother, having filled the bottle with milk and applied the teat, to suck it herself. She assumes that if she can suck milk the baby should be able to do likewise. Another method is to squeeze the teat when it is on the bottle, and still another is to fill the detached teat with water or milk and then to push a finger into it in order to determine whether milk can be expressed. These methods are wrong, because very considerable pressure is applied. Often the hole is tested when the bottle is filled with water. This is undesirable because water will flow more easily than milk. A common mistake it to test the hole when water or milk is in the bottle and then to fill the bottle with milk thickened with a cereal. I saw a 6-months-old child with extreme irritability, flatulence and loss of weight. Questioning showed that the mother had put the entire sago pudding into the bottle and expected the baby to suck it out. There is no need to shake the bottle in order to test the hole. When the bottle is inverted the milk should drop out at the rate of several drops per second without any shaking. The patency of the hole should be tested before every feed, because it readily becomes blocked up, particularly if dried milks are used.

It is common in the case of a baby suffering from excessive wind to find that the feed is taking 30 to 60 minutes. No feed should take more than 15 minutes if the hole in the teat is large enough.

Too large a hole in the teat is a rare cause of trouble. Some mothers enlarge the hole by cutting the teat with a pair of scissors, and the hole is then too large. If the hole is too large the baby is likely to gulp milk down and swallow air in the process.

If the bottle is not tilted so that the teat is kept full of milk, the baby will swallow air. If the mother fails to withdraw the teat from the baby's mouth at frequent intervals, and certainly when it becomes flat as a result of the creation of a vacuum in the bottle, the baby will be unable to obtain the milk and will swallow air in his efforts. (This difficulty is easily avoided by using a boat-shaped bottle with a teat on the sucking end only.) It is largely for these two reasons that it is always wrong to leave a baby to feed himself from a bottle which is propped on a pillow. An old teat, or one which has been repeatedly boiled, readily becomes flat when the baby sucks.

It will be seen that in investigating the cause of excessive flatulence in a bottle-fed baby a careful detailed history is essential. It is always necessary to see the bottle to test the patency of the teat oneself.

The use of a dummy or pacifier might conceivably lead to air swallowing, but it is not an important cause of flatulence.

As in the breast-fed baby, prolonged crying as a result of a rigid feeding schedule may cause air swallowing.

Posseting and Vomiting

Posseting occurs in a bottle-fed baby in the same way as it does in a breast-fed one. Excessive posseting or vomiting is often due to flatulence, which has been discussed above. If it still persists in spite of correction of the feeding technique, the feed can be thickened with cereal so that it does not come up so readily. Vomiting is only rarely due to the child taking too much food. In the case of an artificially-fed baby there is always the possibility that it is due to the child being given unsuitable food, such as undiluted cow's milk, or even less suitable articles of diet. The possibility of infections and of other organic disease must always be borne in mind.

Constipation

When a mother puts her child on to cow's milk after a period of breast feeding, she is apt to become worried about the much firmer consistency of the baby's stools and to think that he is constipated. The mother should be reassured.

True constipation in an artificially-fed baby is nearly always due to underfeeding. It may be due to making a feed up with too little water (i.e. giving less than $2\frac{1}{2}$ oz. (150 ml) of fluid per pound (kg) per day). It may be due to failure to add sugar to a dried milk of low carbohydrate content. If undiluted cow's milk is given, the baby is apt to have dry, hard, greasy, foul soap stools or bulky grey ones. Constipation may be due to overclothing or excessive perspiration as a result of a high external temperature. It may be due to excessive posseting or vomiting. Organic causes of constipation (such as megacolon and early hypothyroidism) have to be remembered just as much as in the breast-fed baby. True constipation may occur in spite of attending to all the above possible causes. The stools are hard and cause discomfort when they are being passed. It sometimes helps in these cases to change to a different carbohydrate, such as lactose or maltose. Brown sugar may be used instead of white. In the weaning period puréed prunes may be added to the diet. Purgatives are hardly ever required if attention to the above factors is given. If really necessary milk of magnesia is safe and non-irritating.

Diarrhœa

It is a great deal more significant when a mother complains that her bottle-fed baby has diarrhœa than when a breast-fed baby is brought up with that complaint. Gastro-enteritis is very rare in fully breast-fed babies, the disease being almost confined to bottle-fed ones.

Diarrhœa may be due to excess of sugar in the feeds or to the practice of giving glucose between feeds. A common mistake is to add sugar to dried foods which have a high carbohydrate content, such as half-cream Cow and Gate or Trufood. It may be due to disaccharide or fat intolerance. There are considerable individual variations in the tolerance of both fat and carbohydrate. Looseness of the stools due to fat intolerance is usually remedied by changing from a full-cream preparation to a half-cream one. Diarrhœa may be due to orange juice. This can be remedied by giving the Vitamin C in the form of ascorbic acid.

Diarrhœa is rarely due to overfeeding. The motions tend to be loose and frequent. There may be vomiting and the weight gain, which is sometimes excessive at first, falls off and weight may even be lost. It should be emphasized that underfeeding is infinitely commoner than overfeeding.

In the United States allergy to cow's milk is regarded as a common cause of intestinal disturbances in babies, and in particular of colic, vomiting and diarrhœa. In my experience it is rare.

Defective Weight Gain

The commonest cause of defective weight gain in an artificially-fed baby is underfeeding. This may arise in a variety of ways. It may arise simply from ignorance of the normal food requirements of a baby. It may arise from rigid ideas of the quantity of food which should be given. Many books about infant feeding give the impression that the quantities of food recommended at various ages must be strictly adhered to. This is wrong, for there are big eaters and little eaters. Some need more than the average amount of food to secure a satis-factory weight gain and to satisfy hunger. When advice is sought on account of excessive crying, the calculation that the food being given is adequate for an average child by no means implies that it is enough for the child in question. The child should have what he wants, whether it is more than the average or not. Rigid ideas of the quantity to be given are often based on totally unfounded fears of overfeeding the child.

Underfeeding may arise from feeding the baby by the actual weight rather than by the expected weight. Babies who have been underfed, perhaps as a result of defective lactation or for other reasons, have a compensatory increase of appetite which enables them to catch up to the expected weight. If extra food is not given to such children, excessive crying may result from hunger. It is for this reason, as well as on account of individual variations in appetite already discussed, that it is always wrong to feed babies by the instructions on the tin. Infant feeding should be much more individualized than that and the quantities given should be adjusted to the needs of the individual.

Defective weight gain may also be due to insufficient fluid in the feeds. In hot climates the quantity of fluid usually recommended in this country ($2\frac{1}{2}$ oz. per pound (150 ml/kg) per day) is inadequate. I saw several babies in the Middle East who were failing to thrive for this reason. Excessive clothing will prevent the usual weight gain on account of excessive perspiration.

In bottle-fed babies separation from the mother has always to be remembered as a sufficient cause for a child not gaining weight.

Defective weight gain may be due to excessive posseting, vomiting, diarrhœa or to any infection such as thrush.

One sees an occasional baby who, in spite of being given as much food as he wants, still gains weight unsatisfactorily. This can sometimes be remedied by adding a cereal to the feed.

Refusal to take the Calculated Requirements

Some babies who are otherwise perfectly well refuse almost from birth to take ordinary quantity of milk, and many are below the average weight as a result. It is impossible to find a reason for this behaviour. Such obvious causes as overclothing, coldness, too frequent feeds and infections are readily eliminated. They are not left crying excessively. They just do not take as much as they should. It seems to be an inherent characteristic of the child which is not due to any mismanagement, but food forcing is apt to result, and this aggravates the condition. It is rare and it is difficult to manage. I have often seen it in infants of small build who have an unusually small mother or father. The essential points in the management are patience, absence of forcing and absence of anxiety.

Refusal of the Bottle and Refusal to Part with the Bottle

It is not at all uncommon for a bottle-fed baby suddenly to refuse to have food from a bottle any longer. The refusal is usually easy to deal with as soon as it is recognized, for such children are nearly always willing to take food from a spoon or cup. There need be no anxiety about the child's ability to use a cup. It is surprising how often mothers feed children with a spoon when a cup would be much quicker and easier to use. Most children can approximate their lips adequately to a cup by about 5 months of age. They tend to manage thickened feeds from a cup sooner than ordinary liquids such as milk.

A baby may refuse milk yet be ready to take solids. I saw an 8-month child who had been on a mixed diet for 2 months, and who was put back on to the bottle by the doctor on account of a febrile illness. The baby refused to have anything to do with it and was brought up for a second opinion because of his marked loss of weight. He responded immediately to the return of a mixed diet.

A baby may refuse to part with the bottle. This is usually due to failure to offer the food by cup and spoon in place of the bottle. This should be done at the age of 5 or 6 months. Brennemann wrote that he had seen a girl of 18 years of age who could still only take milk from a bottle. No baby should have a bottle after the age of 12 months. It is better to discard it at about 6 months, before the baby has become too attached to it. It is quicker, furthermore, to feed the baby from a cup as soon as he can manage it.

References

1. ANDERSON, J. A. D., GATHERER. A. (1970). "Hygiene and Infant-feeding Utensils." *Brit. Med., J.* **2,** 20.
2. BERENBERG, W., MANDELL, F., FELLERS, F. (1969). "Hazards of skimmed Milk, Unboiled and Boiled." *Pediatrics,* **44,** 734.
3. BERG, B. N., SIMMS, H. S. (1965). "Nutrition, Onset of Disease and Longevity in the Rat." *Can. Med. Ass. J.,* **94,** 911.
4. DELICARDIE, E. R., VEGA, L., BIRCH, H. G., CRAVIOTO, J. (1971). "The Effect of Weight Loss from Birth to Fifteen Days on Growth and Development in the First Year." *Biol. Neonate,* **17,** 249.
5. DOBBING, J. (1970). "The Kinetics of Growth." *Lancet,* **2,** 1358.
6. DOXIADIS, S. A., PASCHOS, A. (1962). "Feeding Behaviour and Growth in the First Three Months of Life." *Mod. Problems in Pediatrics,* **7,** 202.
7. EID, E. E. (1970). "Follow up Study of Physical Growth of Children who had Excessive Weight Gain in the First Six Months of Life." *Brit Med. J.,* **2,** 74.
8. EID, E. E. (1971) "A Follow up Study of Physical Growth Following Failure to Thrive in the First Year of Life." *Acta Paediat. Scand.,* **60,** 39.
9. GIBSON, J. P. (1958). "Reaction of 150 Infants to Cold Formulas." *J. Pediat.,* **52,** 404.
10. GUTHRIE, H. A. (1968). "Infant Feeding Practices—a Predisposing Factor in Hypertension?" *Amer. J. Clin. Nutrition.* **21** 863.
11. HOLT, L. E., DAVIES, E. A., HASSELMEYER E. G., ADAMS, A. O. (1962). "A Study of Premature Infants Fed Cold Formulas." *J. Pediat.,* **61,** 556.
12. LEWIN, P. K., REID, M., REILLY B. J., SWYER, P. R., FRASER, D. (1971). "Iatrogenic Rickets in Low-Birth-Weight Infants." *J. Pediat.,* **78,** 207.
13. LEWIS, J. M. (1935). "Clinical Experience with Crystalline Vitamin D; the Influence of the Menstruum on the Effectiveness of the Antirachitic Factor." *J. Pediat.,* **6,** 362.
14. LEWIS, J. M. (1936). "Further Observations on the Comparative Antirachitic Value of Crystalline Vitamin D Administered in Milk, Corn Oil or in Propylene Glycol." *J. Pediat.,* **8,** 308.
15. NEUFELD, H. N. (1968). "Ischaemic Heart Disease in Children." *Lancet,* **1,** 408.
16. SELIG, M. (1970). "Are American Children still Getting an Excess of Vitamin D?" *Clinical Pediatrics,* **9,** 380.

17. TAITZ, L. S. (1971). "Infantile Overnutrition Among Artificially Fed Infants in the Sheffield Region." *Brit. Med. J.*, **1**, 315.
18. TAITZ, L. S., BYERS, H. D. (1971). "Excessive Sodium Concentration in Infant Feeds: A Possible Factor in the Pathogenesis of Hypertonic Dehydration Complicating Gastroenteritis." (*In Press*).
19. WINICK, M., ROSSO, P. (1969). "The Effect of Severe Early Malnutrition on Cellular Growth of Human Brain." *Pediatric Research*, **3**, 181.
20. WINICK, M. (1969). "Malnutrition and Brain Development." *J. Pediat.*, **74**, 667.
21. WINICK, M., ROSSO, P. (1969). "Head Circumference and Cellular Growth of the Brain in Normal and Marasmic Children. *J. Pediat.*, **74**, 774.
22. YUDKIN, J. (1971). "Nutrition and Atherosclerosis." *Brit. J. Hosp. Med.*, **5**, 665.

CHAPTER 4

WEIGHT AND HEIGHT

Birth Weight

The birth weight depends on genetic, racial, nutritional, uterine, placental and other factors. The mean birth weight is regarded as one of the indices of the health of a country; underdeveloped countries, in which malnutrition is common, have a lower mean birth weight than countries with a high standard of nutrition. The mean birth weight tends to be higher in the upper classes than in the lower classes, and amongst the more intelligent mothers. Nutrition in the third trimester of pregnancy[4,9,16,28] is of particular importance, malnutrition lowering the birth weight of the fœtus. In general, the greater the weight gain during pregnancy, the bigger is the fœtus likely to be.[5,18,28] There is also a positive relationship between a mother's prepregnancy weight and fœtal weight. Mothers of large babies tend to be taller and heavier than controls, to be older, and to have had more children, but there is little or no association between a large birth weight and the duration of pregnancy,[19] maternal hypertension or antepartum hæmorrhage. If the mother is over 24 years of age the birth weight rises with birth order and the mother's age.[23] Babies of diabetic or prediabetic mothers tend to be large, but some of their weight is due to œdema.[12]

It is said that there are seasonal factors; babies born in March, April and May tend to be larger; those born in June, July and August tend to be smaller.[23] There is a secular trend—the mean birth weight tending to decrease.

According to Ounsted,[19] the largest mean birth weight is in Lapland (3393 g), the Arctic (Russian Eskimos, 3481 g); and Portuguese Guinea (Africans, 3486 g). Rantakillio in North Finland[21] showed that the mean birth weight of the fœtus in the last weeks of pregnancy is relatively large; her figures and those of Babson et al.[3] are shown below.

Duration of Gestation (weeks)	Mean birth weight Rantakillio	Babson et al.
28	1230	1172
32	2250	1881
36	2900	2749
40	3460	3462

It is said that the largest live baby weighed 17 lb (7·7 kg) and the largest stillborn baby weighed 24 lb (10·8 kg).

The causes of a low birth weight were discussed in the well-known paper of Warkany et al.[28], under the heading of "Intrauterine Growth Retardation". They drew attention to the implications of a low birth weight in relation to the duration of gestation. The prognosis with regard to perinatal mortality, subsequent mental and physical growth and various abnormalities is worse than for the baby of comparable birth weight which corresponds to the duration of gestation.[15] Others have found that the mean intelligence of "small for dates" babies is less than that of babies of the same birth weight who were prematurely born. Churchill[7] found that the birth weight of 51 children with undifferentiated mental subnormality was significantly less than that of 51 children with an intelligence quotient over 110, when matched for age sex and neighbourhood.

The mean birth weight is below the average in mongols, and other chromosomal abnormalities, and children with the Prader-Willi, Seckel, Silver, De Lange and other syndromes, in children with the rubella syndrome or cytomegalovirus infection. It is smaller than usual when the placenta is small or infarcted, as in toxæmia. Many workers have shown[22] that smoking during pregnancy lowers the birth weight of the fœtus, and also increases the stillbirth and neonatal death rate. Eid[11] showed that boys born of mothers who smoked were significantly smaller at school age than those born of non-smokers.

McKeown[16a] and others have studied the birth weight in multiple pregnancy. That of twins is around 2395 g (mean duration of pregnancy 261 days), of triplets 1818 g (247 days) and quadruplets 1360 g (237 days). McKeown wrote that the retardation of growth of twins begins when the total weight is about 7 lb (3175 g), when it becomes difficult for the placenta to support the fœtus. The birth weight of twins is related to the sex, duration of pregnancy and zygosity; males and binovular twins tend to be heavier.

There have been numerous studies of the subsequent physical and mental development of low birth weight babies. We showed in Sheffield[13,14,15] that the birth weight was strongly correlated with subsequent weight and height; the smaller the baby was at birth, the smaller he was likely to be in later years before puberty, and the larger he was at birth, the bigger he was likely to be in subsequent build. As a rough guide, a child's weight at any age in the first 10 years was likely to differ from the mean by the difference between his birth weight and the mean birth weight. We found that in older children all the various measurements taken, the sitting height, pelvic girth, chest and calf circumference, standing height and weight, were related to the size at birth. This has been confirmed by many subsequent workers. Unfortunately when we did this work we did not distinguish "small for dates" babies from those prematurely born with a birth weight corresponding to the duration of gestation; there is evidence that the former tend to be smaller.[24,25] Others[7] have shown that low birth weight babies tend to have a lower mean level of intelligence in later years than babies of average birth weight. Singer[25] showed that larger babies have a better rate of growth and better performance in the first year. Crisp[8] made the peculiar observation that adults with anorexia nervosa were more likely to have been large babies than small ones.

It was found that girls weighing over 9 lb at birth (4083 g) and boys weighing over 9 lb 6 oz. (4253 g) had a lower mean intelligence in later years than did babies of average birth weight.[2]

Owing to the tendency of large children to mature early and small ones to mature late, one would have thought that after maturation the adolescent's size would be unrelated to his birth weight. Blegen,[6] however, found that premature babies tended to lag behind in weight and height up to and including puberty. Alm,[1] who compared the physical development of 999 prematurely born boys with that of 1,002 controls, found that the former were statistically significantly smaller in weight and height than the controls at the age of 20. Douglas and Mogford,[9] though conceding that premature babies on the average do not reduce their initial weight handicap in the first 4 years, felt that the best guide to the expected height of a child was the height of his parents.

Subsequent Physical Growth

A child's physical development is so intimately related to his health and nutrition that in any appraisal of these an assessment of his physical development is an essential part of the examination. Perhaps the most important single method of confirming the adequacy of a baby's food is his gain in weight. Frequent weighings are as a rule undesirable and unnecessary because they are liable to worry the mother. She becomes anxious when as a result of a cold, the eruption of a tooth or other simple complaint the weight progress is temporarily slowed. The more intelligent the mother the less necessary are frequent weighings. The less intelligent she is the more important it is to keep a careful watch on the child's progress by means of physical measurements. However intelligent she is, it is always wise to weigh a baby at intervals—say, once a week in the first 2 months, and thereafter at less frequent intervals—probably monthly—in order that in the case of an illness one has previous weights as a base-line from which one can observe the child's progress.

When a mother complains that her child is unwell, is posseting excessively or vomiting, has persistent diarrhœa or severe chronic food refusal, the child's physical development has to be assessed by the doctor in order that he can decide how much importance to attach to her story. When a mother or other person asks for an expert opinion about a child because of his appearance, or because he is unusually small for his age, the doctor must know how to assess his physical development. The child's measurements are then used to reinforce the doctor's clinical observations. When a child is unwell and under treatment or when he is convalescent from an illness, an essential part of his supervision consists of a careful regular examination of his progress in weight gain and other measurements. In the Welfare Clinic and School Medical Service a screening device is constantly needed to enable the nurse or doctor to pick out those children who are in need of expert medical examination.

After infancy, regular weighings are desirable for another purpose— the prevention of obesity. From 1 to 3 or 4 a child should be weighed once every 3 months or so, and thereafter about twice a year. This enables the mother and doctor to detect excessive weight gain, which if unchecked would lead to obesity. It is far easier to prevent obesity than to treat it. It is easy at this stage to reduce sweet eating, and to reduce the intake of carbohydrate and fat.

Much the most important single measurement is that of the weight. Other measurements commonly taken are the height, head and chest circumference, pelvic and calf girth and sitting height. The figures so obtained are compared with average figures obtained from the study of large numbers of children. Much more valuable than isolated readings are serial records showing the rate of increase in growth.

The average weight gain in the first 3 months is 7 oz. per week (196 g), and 5·3 oz. (148 g) in the second 3 months. During the second year the average child gains weight at the speed of about 1½ oz. (42 g) per week. It is wrong to suggest that a child's birth weight should be doubled at 6 months and trebled by a year. That is only true for a child of average birth weight.

I am indebted to Professor J. Tanner for Table III, showing the weights and heights of British children in their first 10 years.

The doctor who is responsible for supervising a child's health should record his weight and height on a centile chart, such as that of Tanner and Whitehouse.[27] It is of particular importance to note any deviation of the line representing the child's growth from the nearby centiles; excessive weight gain should be checked; the cause of a falling off of the child's weight and height should be investigated. The relationship of excessive weight gain in infancy to subsequent weight has been discussed elsewhere.[10]

When a child has an illness or period of starvation, and health is restored, he shows the phenomenon of "catch up growth". The growth rate may be two or three times the usual rate, until he has caught up to the point which he would have reached but for the illness or malnutrition. If the cause of the retardation lasts too long, the child may never catch up. Eid[11] studied the growth of 122 infants who had failed to thrive in the first year, and compared them with controls and siblings measuring the height, weight, head and chest circumference, triceps, subcutaneous fold and skeletal age; the growth of the 122 infants with "failure to thrive" in the first year was significantly less than that of the controls at 1 to 11 years. The longer the illness lasted, the greater was the eventual retardation.

The Prediction of Adult Height

Table III shows the percentage of the expected final adult height reached by the child at different ages. As a rough guide, it may be stated that the height of the adult is twice that of the child at 2 years$\pm$ 2 cm.

In Table IV I have calculated the height which an adult of 5 feet (152·4 cm), 5 feet 6 inches (167·6 cm), and 6 feet (182·9 cm), would probably have reached at various ages in childhood. I find such a table useful in an out-patient clinic, when a parent is worried about the small size of her child. It is useful to be able to reassure her by telling her what the child's eventual height will probably be. It often corresponds exactly with her own height or that of her husband.

Excessive height is usually familial in origin. It is also a feature of gigantism, Marfan's syndrome and Klinefelter's syndrome. Almost all fat children are tall for their age in the early years, on account of adrenocortical overactivity; but the epiphyses fuse prematurely, so that growth ceases early and the eventual height is less than usual. If a fat child is not tall for his age, one suspect's Cushing's disease, the Prader-Willi syndrome, Frohlich's syndrome, Turner's syndrome, or the Laurance Moon Biedl syndrome. There is a secular increase in height; for instance, Glasgow children are on the average 10 cm taller than they were 60 years ago.

Smallness of stature is commonly familial in origin; but a low birth weight baby, especially if he were small for dates, is likely to be smaller than children of average birth weight. Malnutrition and malabsorption retard the growth in height. Children with cretinism are small because of delayed skeletal maturation. The feature of hypopituitarism is a short stature with the growth rate diminishing each year, and a height age considerably less than both chronological and skeletal age. Body proportions are normal. In dwarfism due to emotional deprivation there is retarded linear growth. For the usual causes of defective growth in height or weight see my book "Common Symptoms of Disease in Children".*

For excessive weight gain—see obesity page 265.

The Interpretation of Measurements of Physical Growth

All the methods described above may indicate, some more clearly than others, that a child's measurements are unusual, but none of them tell *why* they are unusual. That depends on the history, clinical examination and clinical judgment, which involves a thorough knowledge of the normal and of the normal variations which may occur and of the various factors, other than disease which affect growth. In all cases the following difficulties and fallacies have to be borne in mind:

Errors in the Measurements. Scales are frequently out of order. It is never wise to compare the weight on one set of scales with the weight on another. In the case of a baby it is always important, in comparing his present weight with a previous one, to know that the conditions of weighing were identical in the two cases. He should be weighed naked in each case. If on one occasion he is weighed before a feed and on another he is weighed after one, a considerable error is introduced. An isolated reading is disturbed by the passage of urine or fæces immediately before weighing.

It is easy to make mistakes in such simple measurements as the head circumference. In older children recumbent length is more accurate than standing height, because it eliminates postural factors.

Fallacies Inherent in Single Measurements. Single measurements are unlikely to give an accurate idea of a child's physical condition. Isolated measurements may be taken at the beginning or end of a period of defective growth. They may reveal unusual features of his physique but they show nothing of his rate of growth. Much more important than single measurements is the growth chart, which shows the child's growth in weight, height and other measurements.

The Average is not the Normal. Any doctor may be able to say what the average weight and height is for a child of given age and sex, but no one can say what the normal is, for it is impossible to define the normal. A child may be pounds below the average in weight and inches below the average in height and yet be perfectly normal. There are great individual variations in body build, but it is impossible to place a dividing line between the normal and the abnormal. All children are individuals, and they have widely differing rhythms of growth. Some have unexplained slow and rapid periods of growth. Some are slow starters; they grow slowly for a few years and then

---

* *Common Symptoms of Disease in Children.* (1971). Blackwell. Oxford.

TABLE III
Percentiles

Height of Boys Age in Years	10 In.	10 Cm	50 In.	50 Cm	90 In.	90 Cm	% of Adult Height
0	20·2	51·4	21·3	54·0	22·3	56·6	30·9
1	28·7	72·8	30·0	76·3	31·4	79·7	43·7
2	32·6	82·7	34·2	86·9	35·9	91·1	49·8
3	35·1	89·3	37·1	94·2	39·0	99·1	53·9
4	37·8	96·1	40·0	101·6	42·1	107·1	58·2
5	40·2	102·2	42·6	108·3	45·0	114·4	62·0
6	42·5	108·0	45·1	114·6	47·7	121·2	65·6
7	44·7	113·5	47·4	120·5	50·2	127·5	69·0
8	46·8	118·8	49·7	126·2	52·6	133·5	72·2
9	48·8	124·0	51·8	131·6	54·8	139·3	75·4
10	50·7	128·8	53·9	136·8	57·0	144·8	78·3

Percentiles

Height of Girls Age in Years	10 In.	10 Cm	50 In.	50 Cm	90 In.	90 Cm	% of Adult Height
0	19·8	50·4	20·9	53·0	21·9	55·6	32·7
1	27·9	70·8	29·2	74·2	30·6	77·7	45·7
2	32·0	81·3	33·7	85·6	35·4	89·8	52·8
3	34·7	88·1	36·6	93·0	38·5	97·9	57·3
4	37·4	94·9	39·5	100·4	41·7	105·9	61·9
5	39·8	101·1	42·4	107·2	44·6	113·2	66·1
6	42·0	106·8	44·5	113·4	47·2	120·0	69·9
7	44·2	112·4	47·0	119·3	49·7	126·3	73·6
8	46·3	117·6	49·2	125·0	52·1	132·4	77·1
9	48·4	122·9	51·4	130·6	54·4	138·3	80·5
10	50·5	128·3	53·7	136·4	56·9	144·5	83·8

Percentiles

Weight of Boys Age in Years	10 Pounds	10 Kg	50 Pounds	50 Kg	90 Pounds	90 Kg
0	6·17	2·8	7·72	3·5	9·04	4·1
0·25	11·05	5·01	13·07	5·93	15·41	6·99
0·5	14·99	6·8	17·42	7·9	20·28	9·2
0·75	17·59	7·98	20·28	9·2	23·43	10·63
1·0	19·40	8·8	22·49	10·2	25·79	11·7
2	24·25	11·0	28·0	12·7	32·19	14·6
3	28·00	12·7	32·41	14·7	37·26	16·9
4	31·52	14·3	36·60	16·6	42·11	19·1
5	34·61	15·7	40·72	18·5	47·4	21·5
6	38·14	17·3	45·20	20·5	52·91	24·0
7	41·89	19·0	49·82	22·6	59·29	26·9
8	46·03	20·9	55·11	25·0	66·13	30·0
9	50·48	22·9	60·62	27·5	73·63	33·4
10	55·56	25·2	66·80	30·3	82·23	37·3

Percentiles

Weight of Girls Age in Years	10		50		90	
	Pounds	Kg	Pounds	Kg	Pounds	Kg
0	6·28	2·85	7·50	3·4	8·71	3·95
0·25	10·6	4·81	12·26	5·56	14·13	6·41
0·5	14·2	6·44	15·21	6·9	18·72	8·49
0·75	16·71	7·58	19·22	8·72	22·09	10·02
1·0	18·52	8·4	21·38	9·7	24·69	11·2
2	22·93	10·4	26·89	12·2	31·09	14·1
3	27·11	12·3	31·52	14·3	36·15	16·4
4	31·09	14·1	35·93	16·3	41·44	18·8
5	35·05	15·9	40·34	18·3	47·17	21·4
6	38·8	17·6	44·97	20·4	53·79	24·4
7	42·33	19·2	49·82	22·6	61·07	27·7
8	46·29	21·0	55·34	25·1	68·78	31·2
9	50·7	23·0	61·07	27·7	78·04	35·4
10	55·34	25·1	68·56	31·1	90·39	41·0

Tanner, J. M., Whitehouse, R. H., Takaishi, M. (1966). "Standard from Birth to Maturity for Height, Weight, Height Velocity and Weight Velocity." *Arch. Dis. Childh.*, **41**, 613.

TABLE IV

Height in Childhood in Relation to Expected Adult Height

Expected Adult Height	5′	150 cm	5′ 6″	165 cm	6′	180 cm
Height of Boys Age in Years	In.	Cm	In.	Cm	In.	Cm
1	25·8	65·5	28·3	72·0	30·9	78·6
2	29·4	74·7	32·1	81·7	35·3	89·6
3	31·8	80·8	35·1	89·2	38·1	97·0
4	34·4	87·3	37·8	96·1	41·2	104·7
5	36·6	93·0	40·3	102·3	43·9	111·6
6	38·7	98·4	42·7	108·4	46·6	118·4
7	40·7	103·5	44·8	113·9	48·9	124·2
8	42·6	108·2	46·9	119·0	51·1	129·9
9	44·6	113·2	49·0	124·4	53·4	135·7
10	46·2	117·4	50·8	129·1	55·5	140·9
Height of Girls Age in Years	In.	Cm	In.	Cm	In.	Cm
1	27·0	68·5	28·3	72·0	32·4	82·2
2	31·1	79·2	34·3	87·1	37·4	95·0
3	33·9	86·0	37·2	94·5	40·6	103·1
4	36·5	92·8	40·2	102·1	43·9	111·4
5	39·0	99·1	43·0	109·1	46·9	119·0
6	41·3	104·8	45·4	115·3	49·6	125·9
7	43·5	110·4	47·8	121·5	52·2	132·6
8	45·6	115·7	50·1	127·3	54·6	138·8
9	47·6	120·9	52·4	133·0	57·1	145·1
10	49·5	125·7	54·4	138·3	59·4	150·9

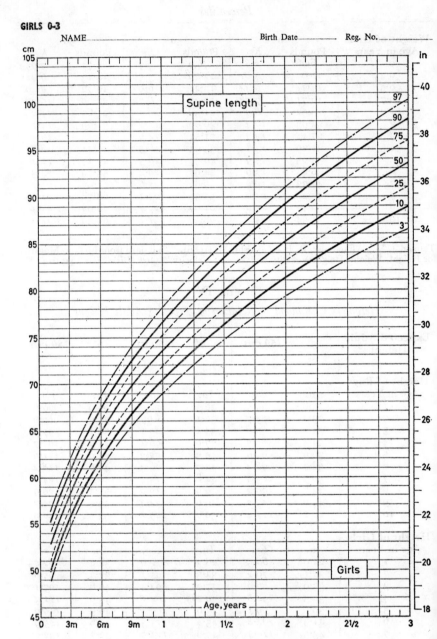

GIRLS 0-3

NAME.. Birth Date.............. Reg. No...................

Supine length

Girls

Age, years

FIG. 2. *Girls 0–3 years—Supine Length.*
(*Figs. 2–13 are reproduced by courtesy of Professor J. M. Tanner.*)

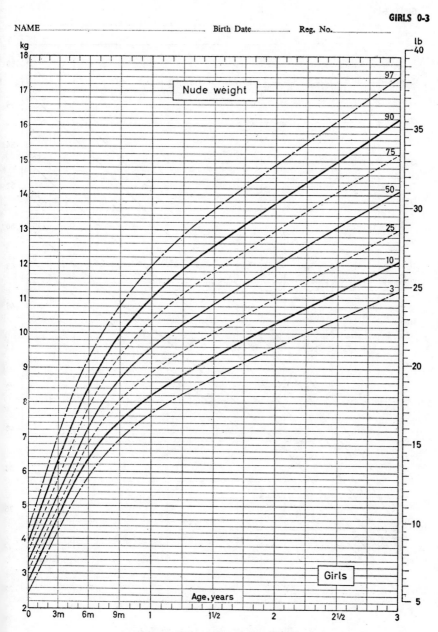

NAME.., Birth Date.............., Reg. No.................

kg

lb

Nude weight

97

90

75

50

25

10

3

Girls

Age, years

FIG. 3. *Girls 0–3 Years: Nude Weight.*

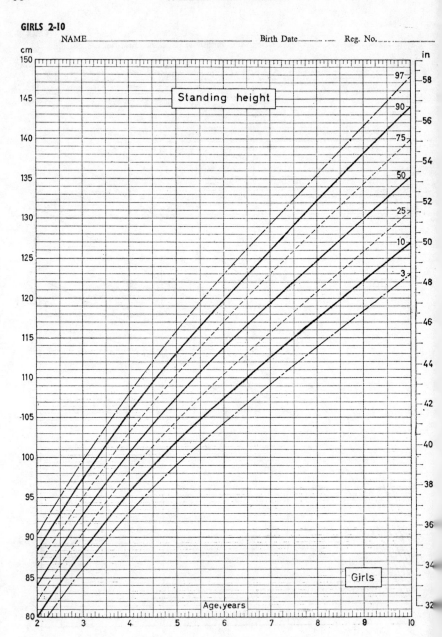

FIG. 4. *Girls 2–10 Years: Standing Height.*

NAME.. Birth Date................... Reg. No..................................

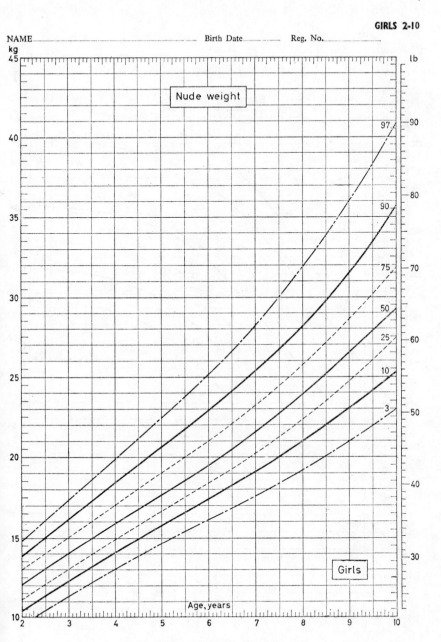

FIG. 5. *Girls 2–10 Years: Nude Weight.*

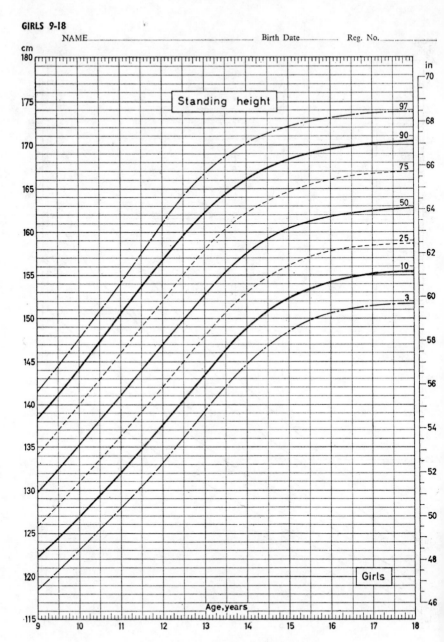

FIG. 6. *Girls 9–18 Years: Standing Height.*

NAME.. Birth Date.............. Reg. No.......................

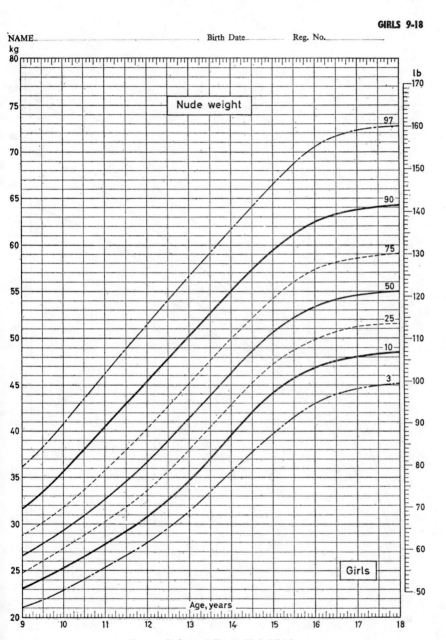

FIG. 7. *Girls 9–18 Years: Nude Weight.*

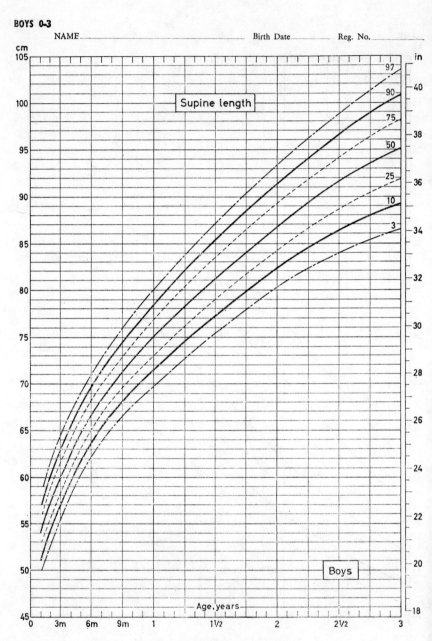

FIG. 8. *Boys 0–3 Years: Supine Length.*

BOYS 0-3

NAME.. Birth Date................. Reg. No.....................

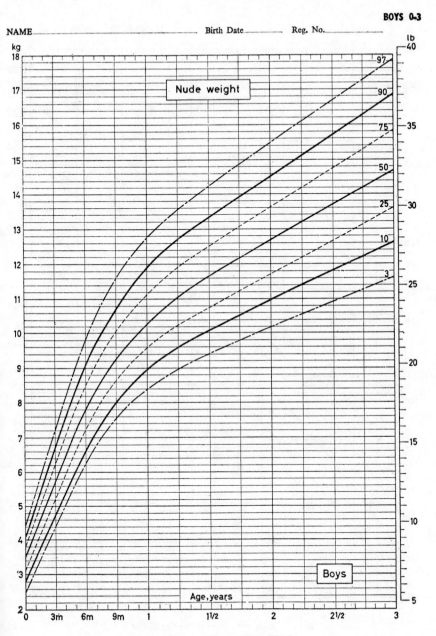

FIG. 9. *Boys 0–3 Years: Nude Weight.*

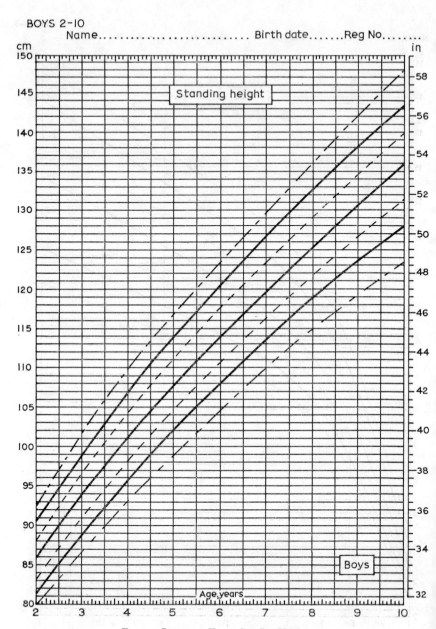

BOYS 2-10

Name............................... Birth date.......Reg No........

Fig. 10. *Boys 2–10 Years: Standing Height.*

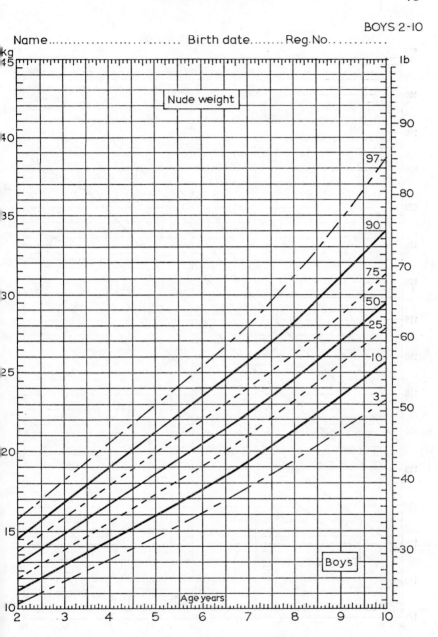

Name........................ Birth date........ Reg.No............

Fig. 11. *Boys 2–10 Years: Nude Weight.*

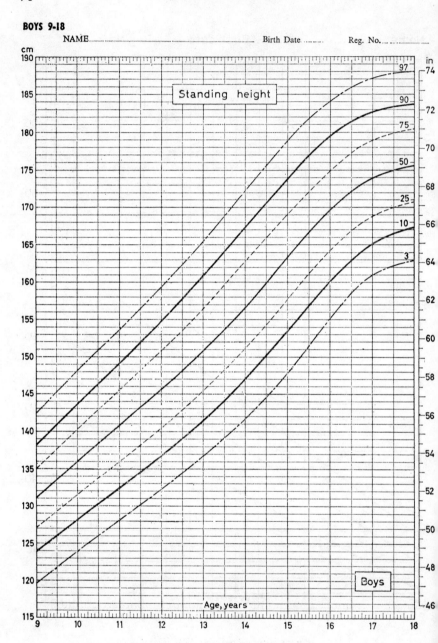

FIG. 12. *Boys 9–18 Years: Standing Height.*

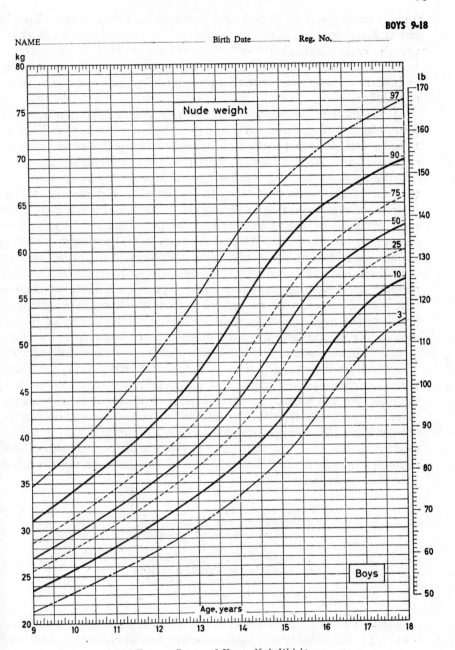

FIG. 13. *Boys 9–18 Years: Nude Weight.*

have a rapid spurt of growth and catch up to their fellows. This is particularly apt to happen at puberty. In general the large child matures early and the small child matures late, so that the small child, by having a longer period of growth, eventually attains the same build as his fellows who were much larger than he was in the earlier years of childhood.

It is logical to assume that the greater a child's deviation from his fellows in any of the measurements of body build the less likely he is to be normal. The fact that a child's weight is below that of 80 per cent. of his fellows of the same age does not prove that he is abnormal.

It cannot be assumed that maximum growth is necessarily the optimum. In the case of the premature baby, for instance, it is dangerous to try to secure a rapid and large weight gain. This may be achieved for a time, but it is apt to be followed by a slowing of the weight gain, and later on by loss of weight. There have been several papers concerning the additional height achieved by giving vitamins in quantities greater than those normally recommended, but no one has proved that the children are healthier on that account. There is nothing to suggest that a child who is 5 or 10 per cent. above the average weight and height at any age is in any way better than a child who is 5 or 10 per cent. below the average, provided that the latter is free from infection or other known illness. Neither is there evidence that a child of 2 or 3 years who is increasing rapidly in weight and height is any healthier than the otherwise well child who is increasing in size at rather less than the average speed. In general, when a doctor is faced with an otherwise well child, who on account of constitutional reasons is smaller than the average, he should direct his efforts not at trying to alter his physique but at trying to persuade his parents and others to accept him as a normal child. One is reminded of the words of John Kendrick Bangs:

> "I met a little Elfman once,
>   Down where the lilies blow.
>   I asked him why he was so small,
>   And why he did not grow.
>   He slightly frowned and with his eyes
>   He looked me through and through.
>   'I'm quite as big for me,' he said,
>   'As you are big for you.' "

Figures used for comparison must be valid ones. It is wrong to use figures obtained in one country as a basis of comparison for children in another. American children for instance, tend to be larger than British ones. In the same way it is unwise to use charts based on figures obtained many years ago. The physique of children varies from decade to decade.

Miscellaneous Factors. Various factors other than disease have an important bearing on the child's physical development, and these must always be borne in mind in the assessment of an individual child. These factors can be summarized as follows:

(*a*) GENETIC FACTORS. It is commonly said that the child's growth potential is decided at the time of the fertilization of the ovum. Environmental factors subsequently may retard growth, but they have little effect in accelerating it. In some families the babies are small at birth, and in others they are large. In some families the children grow comparatively slowly for the first few years, and rapidly later. It should be noted that not infrequently smallness of build in child and parent is due to the effect of malnutrition acting on both.

When a child is unusually small in size, it is essential to note the height of the mother and father. The small stature is commonly nothing more than a familial feature.

(*b*) NUTRITION. Malnutrition has a considerable effect on growth, affecting the weight more than the height. Malnutrition may be due to poverty, ignorance, food fads, food refusal, excessive posseting or rumination as well as to actual disease. There is a voluminous literature on the effect of nutrition on growth, and this is not the place in which to discuss it.

(*c*) THE SIZE OF THE CHILD AT BIRTH. See p. 57.

Conclusion

It will be seen that there is at present no short cut to the assessment of the health of a child. An accurate assessment can only be made by taking a careful history, conducting a careful examination, studying the child's physique and then taking all the various factors which may have affected his growth into account.

Serial weight and height records provide the most useful information about a child's growth. In doubtful cases the figures obtained should be compared with those of others in terms of their percentage distribution. If due allowance is then made for all the various factors other than disease known to effect growth, then the measurements obtained give an invaluable pointer to the child's general state of health.

In the assessment of an individual child whose measurements are unusual, his size at birth and the build of his parents are the chief non-disease, factors, to be considered. *Of far greater importance than his weight and height are his well-being, abundant energy, happiness, freedom from infection and freedom from lassitude.* If he has these he is unlikely to have serious organic disease.

References

1. ALM, I. (1953). "The Long-Term Prognosis for Prematurely Born Children." *Acta Paediat. Uppsala*, Suppl. 94.
2. BABSON, S. G., HENDERSON, N., CLARK, W. M. (1969). "Preschool Intelligence of Oversized Newborns." *Pediatrics*, **44**, 536.
3. BABSON, S. G., BEHRMAN, R. E., LESSEL, R. (1970). "Fetal Growth Liveborn Birth Weights for Gestational Age for White Midle Class Infants." *Pediatrics*, **45**, 937.
4. BAYLEY, N. (1962). "The Accurate Prediction of Growth and Adult Height." *Modern Problems of Pædiatrics*, **7**, 234.
5. BERGNER, L., SUSSER, M. W. (1970). "Low Birth Weight and Prenatal Nutrition; an Interpretative Review." *Pediatrics*, **46**, 946.
6. BLEGEN, S. D. (1953). "The Premature Child." *Acta Paediat. Uppsala*, **42**, Suppl. 88.
7. CHURCHILL, J. A., NEFF, J. W., CALDWELL, D. F. (1966). "Birth Weight and Intelligence." *Obstet. and Gynec.*, **28**, 425.
8. CRISP, A. H. (1965). "Some Clinical and Therapeutic Aspects of Anorexia Nervosa." *J. Psychosomatic Research*, **9**, 67.
9. DOUGLAS, J. W. B., MOGFORD, C. (1953). "The Results of a National Enquiry into the Growth of Premature Children from Birth to 4 Years." *Arch. Dis. Childhood*, **28**, 436.
10. EID, E. E. (1970). "Follow-up Studies of Physical Growth of Children who had Excessive Weight Gain in the First Six Months of Life." *Brit. Med. J.*, **2**, 74.
11. EID, E. E. (1970). "Studies on the Subsequent Growth of Children who had Retardation or Acceleration of Growth in Early Life." Ph.D. Thesis, University of Sheffield.
12. GOLLIN, H. A., ELLIS, A. H., EVANS, E. F. (1958). "The Problem of the Oversized Fetus." *Am. J. Obst. and Gynec.*, **75**, 751.
13. ILLINGWORTH, R. S., HARVEY, C. C., GIN S. Y. (1949). "Relation of Birth Weight to Physical Development in Childhood." *Lancet*, **2**, 598.
14. ILLINGWORTH, R. S., HARVEY, C. C., JOWETT, G. H., (1950). "The Relation of Birth Weight to Physical Growth." *Arch. Dis. Childhood*, **25**, 380.
15. ILLINGWORTH, R. S. (1950). "Birth Weight and Subsequent Weight." *Brit. Med. J.*, **1**, 1.
16. JARVINEN, P. A., PANKAMAA, P., KINNUREN, O. (1957). "The Full-Term Underdeveloped Liveborn Infant." *Études Neonatales*, **6**, 3.
17. Ministry of Health Reports on Public Health and Medical Subjects No. 99 (1959). "Standard of Normal Weight in Infancy." London. H.M.S.O.
18. NISWANDER, K. R., SINGER, J., WESTPHAL, M., WEISS, W. (1969). "Weight Gain During Pregnancy and Prepregnancy Weight." *Obst. Gynec.*, **33**, 482.
19. OUNSTED, M. (1969). "Accelerated Foetal Growth." *Develop. Med. Child Neurol.*, **11**, 693.
20. PRADER, A., TANNER, J. M., VON HARNACK, G. A. (1963). "Catch Up Growth Following Illness or Starvation." *J. Pediat.*, **62**, 646.
21. RANTAKILLIO, P. (1969). "Groups at Risk in Low Birth Weight Infants and Perinatal Mortality." *Acta Paediat. Scand.*, Suppl. 193.
22. SCOTT RUSSELL, C., TAYLOR, R., LAW, C. E. (1968). "Smoking in Pregnancy, Maternal Blood Pressure, Pregnancy Outcome, Baby Weight and Growth and Other Related Factors." *Brit. J. Prev. Soc. Med.*, **22**, 119.
23. SELVIN, S., JANERICH, D. T. (1971). "Four Factors Influencing Birth Weight." *Brit. J. Prev. Soc. Med.*, **25**, 12.
24. SINCLAIR, J. C., COLDIRON, J. S. (1969). "Low Birth Weight and Postnatal Physical Development." *Develop. Med. Child. Neurol.*, **11**, 314.
25. SINGER, J. E., WESTPHAL, M., NISWANDER, K. (1968). "Relation of Weight Gain During Pregnancy to Birth Weight and Infant Growth and Development in the First Year of Life. *Obstet. and Gynec.*, **31**, 417.

26. TANNER, J. M., ISRAELSOHN, W. J. (1963). "Parent Child Correlations from Body Measurements of Children Between the Ages of One Month and Seven Years." *Annals of Human Genetics*, **26**, 245.

27. TANNER, J. M., WHITEHOUSE, R. H., TAKAISHI, M. (1966). "Standard from Birth to Maturity for Height, Weight, Height Velocity and Weight Velocity." *Arch. Dis. Childh.*, **41**, 613.

28. WARKANY, J., MONROE, B. B., SUTHERLAND, B. J. (1961). "Intrauterine Growth Retardation." *Am. J. Dis. Child*, **102**, 249.

CHAPTER 5

THE HEAD

The Size of the Skull

The routine examination of any baby, in a well-baby clinic, hospital, or at home, must include the measurement of the maximum circumference of the skull. The reason is that the size of the skull depends in large part on the growth of the cranial contents. If there is hydrocephalus, a subdural hæmatoma, hydranencephaly, or megalencephaly (a large brain of poor quality), the head is likely to be too large; if the brain does not grow adequately, as in mental deficiency, the skull is usually small (microcephaly). Rarely there is premature closure of the

TABLE V

Head Circumference*

Percentiles

Girls	10		50		90	
Age in Years	In.	Cm	In.	Cm	In.	Cm
0·25	15·0	38·1	15·6	39·7	16·1	40·9
0·50	16·2	41·2	16·9	42·9	17·4	44·2
0·75	17·0	43·2	17·6	44·6	18·1	46·2
I	17·5	44·4	18·0	45·7	18·6	47·2
2	18·1	46·2	18·9	48·0	19·4	49·3
3	18·5	47·1	19·4	49·2	19·9	50·5
4	18·9	48·0	19·6	49·9	20·2	51·4
5	19·1	48·6	19·8	50·4	20·4	51·9
6	19·3	49·1	20·0	50·8	20·6	52·2
7	19·5	49·5	20·1	51·1	20·7	52·5
8	19·6	49·8	20·2	51·3	20·8	52·8
Boys	10		50		90	
Age in Years	In.	Cm	In.	Cm	In.	Cm
Birth	13·1	33·5	13·8	35	14·1	36
0·25	15·5	39·3	16·0	40·6	16·6	42·1
0·50	16·5	42·0	17·2	43·8	17·7	45·0
0·75	17·1	43·6	18·0	45·7	18·6	47·2
I	17·5	44·5	18·4	46·8	19·1	48·5
2	18·5	47·1	19·3	49·1	20·0	50·9
3	19·0	48·2	19·8	50·2	20·5	52·0
4	19·3	48·9	20·0	50·8	20·7	52·5
5	19·4	49·4	20·2	51·3	20·9	53·0
6	19·6	49·9	20·4	51·8	21·0	53·4
7	19·8	50·3	20·5	52·1	21·1	53·8
8	19·9	50·6	20·6	52·4	21·3	54·2

* Through the courtesy of Professor J. M. Tanner.

cranial sutures (craniostenosis), which will not permit the skull to enlarge, so that the skull remains small. As some of the above conditions, notably the subdural hæmatoma, hydrocephalus and craniostenosis are amenable to treatment, early diagnosis is important.

The head of a prematurely born child is larger, relative to the rest of the body, than that of a full term child. I have seen the diagnosis of hydrocephalus wrongly made in premature babies because of ignorance of this fact.

It was shown in Africa that the relationship between the head size and the circumference of the chest was useful for assessing children with severe malnutrition. Normally the circumference of the head is greater than that of the chest until the age of 6 months, and smaller thereafter. Dean[4] found that in malnutrition the measurement least affected was the head circumference, and that the head is nearly always larger than usual in relation to the size of the infant as a whole. I have frequently seen hydrocephalus suspected because of the relatively large head in a severely malnourished baby.

Table V shows the percentile distribution of figures for the maximum head circumference at various ages.

The head circumference of premature babies was determined by Mary Crosse.[3] They correspond closely to those given by Lubchenco.[7] Her figures were as follows:

Weeks of Gestation	Head Circumference	
	Ins.	Cm
28	10	25
32	11·5	29
36	12·8	32
40	14	35

Usher and McLean[9] provided useful figures for the mean head circumference in relation to birth weight. (Page 82.)

In the interpretation of any measurement, the normal variations must be fully understood and the difficulties in assessment must be recognized. The first point to remember is that an unusually large or small head may be nothing more than a familial feature, the child merely taking after his mother or father.

The second point to remember is the obvious fact that a large baby is likely to have a larger head than a small baby, and vice versa. In other words it is always essential to relate the child's head size to his weight. This can be done in one of two ways; his head size can be plotted on the head circumference chart and his weight on the weight chart. The two should more or less correspond in relation to the appropriate centile position. Even then the familial factor applies. It should be noted that a child who is small in weight, but whose head circumference corresponds exactly to the fiftieth percentile, may well have hydrocephalus; and a heavy child, whose head circumference corresponds to the fiftieth percentile, may well be a microcephalic idiot. A rapid increase in head circumference may correspond simply to a rapid increase in the weight and physical growth of the child as a whole.

TABLE VI

Relation of Head Circumference to Weight

(Usher and McLean[9])

Weight at Birth (grams)	Mean head Circumference (cm)
1000	24·5
1200	26·2
1400	27·7
1600	29·0
1800	30·1
2000	31·0
2200	31·8
2400	32·5
2600	33·1
2800	33·6
3000	34·1
3200	34·5
3400	34·9
3600	35·2
3800	35·5
4000	35·8

The child's head measurement can be related to his size in another way.[5] In a study of 1,000 babies seen at the Jessop Hospital, Sheffield, we related the head circumference to the weight at four age periods—birth, 6 weeks, 6 months and 10 months. We found that one could calculate the average head circumference for unusually small or large babies by subtracting or adding the following to or from the head circumference for each pound above or below the average weight:

	Boys		Girls	
	In.	*Cm*	In.	*Cm*
Birth	$\frac{1}{3}$	*0·8*	$\frac{1}{4}$	*0·6*
6 weeks	$\frac{1}{4}$	*0·6*	$\frac{1}{4}$	*0·6*
6 months	$\frac{1}{8}$	*0·3*	$\frac{1}{8}$	*0·3*
10 months	$\frac{1}{10}$	*0·3*	$\frac{1}{10}$	*0·3*

When in doubt about a head size, the child should be reexamined after a short interval so that serial measurements can be made. When these are plotted on a chart, it is immediately obvious whether the head is enlarging at an unusually slow or fast rate or whether the increase in size merely corresponds to the growth of the baby as a whole.

Palpation of the sutures for undue separation or for the thickened rim of craniostenosis, and palpation of the fontanelle for undue separation and bulging, are essential parts of the physical examination if hydrocephalus or other abnormality is suspected. It should be remembered that the effect of moulding in birth usually disappears in 2 or 3 days.

The diagnosis of microcephaly does not depend merely on the relation of the head size to the size of the baby. It depends on the shape of the head. The microcephalic head tapers off towards the vertex, and the forehead is often sloping.

It must be remembered that if a child's mental deficiency develops after a period of normal growth, the head size may be relatively normal, for the brain reaches half the adult size by the age of 9 months and three-quarters by the age of 2 years. The earlier in the first year the mental deficiency develops, the more obvious will be the microcephaly.

It is reasonable to expect that there will be some correlation between head circumference in relation to weight and subsequent intelligence, bearing in mind the fact that if the brain does not develop normally, the head circumference is likely to be small. In one study[8] it was found that the I.Q. at four years of age varied directly with head circumference and body length. In a study of 9379 children, no one-year-old with a head circumference of less than 43 cm or girl with a head circumference of less than 42 cm had a four-year-old I.Q. score of 120 or more.

The causes of variations in the size of head can be summarized as follows:

Large head—big baby
familial feature
hydrocephalus
megalencephaly
hydranencephaly

Small head—small baby
familial feature
mental subnormality
craniostenosis

As in all measurements involving the use of a tape measure, one must ensure that the tape measure is accurate, and is of the nonelastic variety. I have seen the measurement of a head by two tape measure differ by a whole inch, because one tape had stretched.

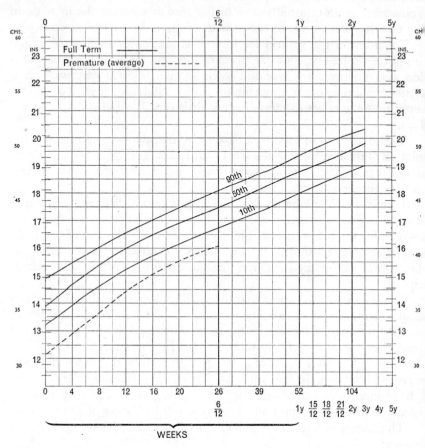

FIG. 14. Head circumference chart as used at The Children's Hospital, Sheffield.

The Shape of the Head

A common source of worry to the mother and doctors is a flattening of the skull of the baby on one side and a corresponding bulge on the other. This is perfectly normal and is simply due to the baby always lying on one side. Babies often prefer one side, and it is pointless to attempt to make them lie on the other side. The peculiarity disappears shortly after the first birthday.

When other peculiarities of shape are noted, the first step is to see both parents. Often the peculiarity in the shape of the skull is familial

It is not due to moulding at birth, because the effect of moulding disappears a few days after birth.

Sometimes the peculiarity of shape is such that one thinks of craniostenosis, or premature closure of the cranial sutures. This condition is rare, but early diagnosis is important for successful operative treatment. Expert radiology confirms the clinical diagnosis.

Asymmetry of the face may be due to the condition known as hemiatrophy or hemihypertrophy.

The Fontanelle

The anterior fontanelle is small at birth, and enlarges considerably during the first 2 or more months. After this period it decreases until it is closed on palpation. Early closure of the anterior fontanelle (e.g. by 4 or 5 months) may be an entirely normal variation in healthy babies.

Unusually late closure, in the absence of bulging, rarely indicates disease; I have seen normal children at the age of three or four with an open fontanelle. Nevertheless, delayed closure occurs in hydrocephalus, rickets, hypothyroidism and cleidocranial dysotosis.

The age of closure may be associated with certain diseases. Premature closure occurs in microcephaly and craniostenosis. The posterior fontanelle is usually closed to palpation after the second month.

There may be a third fontanelle situated between the anterior and posterior fontanelles.[2] A third fontanelle was found in 6·3 per cent. of 1020 newborn infants. Ten were mongols, one had the rubella syndrome and one had congenital dislocation of the hip, but the rest were normal. It is not a true fontanelle, but a bony defect related to the parietal bones.

The Setting Sun Sign

A child with hydrocephalus may show the so called "setting sun sign"—a rim of sclerotic seen above the pupil without retraction of the eyelid by the examiner.

It is important to note that this is commonly seen in normal infants. One must not diagnose hydrocephalus because of this sign when other signs are absent—a bulging fontanelle, unduly separated sutures, an excessive head circumference in relation to his weight, or a too rapidly increasing head size.

The Caput Succedaneum

This is an exudation of serous fluid in the soft tissues of the presenting part during delivery. It disappears by the second or third day. There may be some residual blood pigment for a few days but no permanent mark is left even if the caput is over the face.

Cephalhæmatoma

Cephalhæmatomata occur in up to 1 per cent. of deliveries. They are rare in premature babies. They consist of an extravasation of blood between the bone and periosteum. The swellings are therefore limited by the sutures. They may be unilateral or bilateral. They are usually found in the region of the parietal bones, but may be elsewhere. During the first few days the cephalhæmatoma is often obscured by an overlying caput. This disappears after a day or two, revealing the underlying cephalhæmatoma. It may increase in size in the first few days as a result of further hæmorrhages. By the second or third week a rim of bone may be felt round the periphery of the cephalhæmatoma due to new bone formation at the site of the detachment of the periosteum. The hæmatoma is cystic and an erroneous diagnosis of a depressed fracture is readily made.

Small swellings subside by the third or fourth week, but large ones may be visible for 3 months or more. When extensive ossification occurs the swelling may be visible for many months or even years. They are thought to be due to the tearing of veins as a result of the to-and-fro movement of the scalp with the uterine contractions. They are more likely to occur if the pelvis is roomy than if it is a constricted one. Though they may occur in forceps deliveries, they are sometimes found after Cæsarean section and they bear little relationship to difficult labour. They are very occasionally associated with hæmorrhagic disease of the new born or other blood diseases, or with an underlying fracture.

The treatment is entirely conservative, except in the rare case in which bleeding persists after birth, necessitating transfusion. Even if there is an underlying fracture, nothing is done about it. They should on no account be aspirated. They disappear if left alone and do no harm to the baby. Suppuration is a rare occurence if they are not tampered with. If they are in the mid-line in the occipital region they have to be distinguished from occipital encephaloceles. The rim of calcium which can be seen in the X-ray in most cephalhæmatomata after 2 or 3 weeks helps to establish the diagnosis.

Craniotabes

This condition was reviewed by Bille.[1] He found that one in three infants who had no rickets at all, had craniotabes at some time in the first year. He ascribed it to pressure of the skull against the pelvic bones of the mother, on the grounds that it is rare after breech or Cæsarian deliveries, and the craniotabes is found on the right in right vertex presentations and on the left in left presentations. It is three times

commoner in first-born children than in subsequent ones, presumably because of the lower position of the head *in utero* in the last few
weeks of pregnancy. Though admitting that craniotabes is common in
rickets, Bille regarded it as a normal condition in the great majority of
infants.

References

1. BILLE, B. S. V. (1955). "Non Rachitic Craniotabes." *Acta Paediat. Uppsala*, **44**, 185.
2. CHEMKE, J., ROBINSON, A. (1969). "The Third Fontanelle." *J. Pediat.*, **75**, 617.
3. CROSSE, V. M. (1957), *The Premature Baby*. Edinburgh and London. Churchill. Livingstone.
4. DEAN, R. F. A. (1965). "Effect of Malnutrition, Especially of a Slight Degree, on the Growth of Young Children." *Courrier*, **15**, 73.
5. ILLINGWORTH, R. S., LUTZ, W. (1965). "Head Circumference of Infants Related to Body Weight." *Arch. Dis. Childh.*, **40**, 672.
6. ILLINGWORTH, R. S., EID, E. E. (1971). "The Head Circumference in Infants and Other Measurements to which it may be Related. *Acta Paediat. Scand.*, **60**, 333.
7. LUBCHENCO, L. O., HANSMAN, C., BOYD, E. (1966). "Intrauterine Growth in Length and Head Circumference as Estimated from Live Births at Gestational Ages from 26 to 40 Weeks." *Pediatrics*, **37**, 403.
8. NELSON, K. B., DEUTSCHBERGER, J. (1970) "Head Size at One Year as a Predictor of Four Year I.Q." *Develop. Med. Child Neurol.*, **12**, 487.
9. USHER, R., McLEAN, F. (1969). "Intrauterine Growth of Live Born Caucasian Infants at Sea Level. Standards obtained from Measurements in 7 Dimensions of Infants Born Between 25 and 44 Weeks of Gestation." *J. Pediat.*, **74**, 901.

4

CHAPTER 6

THE MOUNT

The Teeth

Normal Dentition

There are considerable variations in the age at which teeth erupt. On the one hand, the child may be born with a tooth or teeth; on the other hand, the first tooth may not appear until the child is 13 or 14 months old. In neither case is there a need to suppose that there is any disease. As a milestone of development teething is useless. It is true that dentition is sometimes late in mentally retarded children, but more often the time of dentition is normal. The eruption of a deciduous tooth may be delayed by an eruption cyst, which presents a bluish swelling on the gum. It is useful to know the average age at which teeth appear, as long as one remembers that individual variations are considerable. Table VII shows the average age of eruption of the first teeth.

TABLE VII

Average Age of Eruption of First or Deciduous Teeth*

	Months		Months
Lower central incisor .	6	Upper first molar . .	14
Lower lateral incisor . .	7	Lower cuspid . .	16
Upper central incisor .	7½	Upper cuspid .	18
Upper lateral incisor .	9	Lower second molar .	20
Lower first molar . .	12	Upper second molar .	24

* Finn, S. B. (1963). *Clinical Pedodontics*. Philadelphia. Saunders.

It is said that deciduous teeth are shed earlier in the upper social classes than the lower ones, and in boys earlier than in girls.

Teeth in the New-born

Julius Cæsar, Hannibal, King Louis XIV, Mazarin, Mirabeau, Napoleon and Richelieu were said to be born with teeth. According to Shakespeare, King Richard III was born with teeth "such that he could gnaw a crust at two hours old." In Poland, India and China a new-born baby with a tooth was viewed with fear and superstition, and in parts of Africa such a child was killed. Approximately 1 in 2,000 children are born with a tooth.

The subject of teeth in the new-born has been reviewed by Gardiner, at Sheffield.[4] He followed children for 10 years in order to observe the effects of the teeth on subsequent alignment. Nearly all new-born teeth are normal deciduous teeth. They are loose at first, because the root is not well formed, but they become firmly fixed if left. They may cause ulceration under the tongue. Because they bend in the gum when the baby sucks, they are unlikely to hurt the mother's nipple. Owing to deficiency of the enamel, they often appear to be yellow in colour and they wear down more easily than other teeth. In 85 per cent. of 359 examples observed by Bodenhoff and Gorlin,[3] the neonatal teeth were lower central incisors; in 14·5 per cent. there was a family history of the same condition. Certain congenital anomalies may be associated.

The teeth should be left if possible. Removal may be followed by hæmorrhage owing to physiological hypoprothrombinæmia. Their removal may lead to malformation of subsequent teeth, but does not usually do so.

The cause of this condition is unknown. In 10 of 24 examples observed by Gardiner, there was a family history of the same thing.

The Symptoms of Dentition

The symptoms of teething have occupied the attention of writers for generations. Guthrie[8] wrote an interesting review of the subject. Hippocrates* in the twenty-fifth aphorism of his third book said that: "Teething children suffer from itching of the gums, fever, convulsions, diarrhœa, especially when they cut their eye teeth, and when they are very corpulent and costive." Jean Scultet (1675)* treated the pain of teething by application of the actual cautery to the occiput. Popular remedies of the Middle Ages included necklaces made of the roots of henbane, peony, the wild gourd and other vegetables; blistering and leeches behind the lower jaw; rubbing of the gums with hare's brain and the hanging of the tooth of a dog or wolf round the neck. Ambroise Paré introduced gum lancing in the sixteenth century as an improvement on the practice of nurses "who with the nails and scratchings tear and rend the children's gums in order to liberate their teeth." Hurlock* nearly 200 years later alluded to the mischief caused by "meaner people who with their thimbles and monstrous wedding rings hack and bruise the gums in attempting to bring the teeth out." Clendon* in 1862 wrote: "Trace the nerve to its source in the Pons Varolii and floor of the fourth ventricle, where it is in close proximity to the glossopharyngeal, pneumogastric and spinal accessory and spinal

* Quoted by Guthrie.[8]

nerves, and at once the whole train of evils—difficult breathing, immoderate diarrhœa, convulsions, squinting, effusion on the brain are easily accounted for." Arbuthnot* in 1732 wrote that "above one-tenth part of all children die in teething by symptoms proceeding from the irritation of the tender nervous parts of the jaws, occasioning inflammation, fevers, convulsions, looseness with green stools, not the worst symptoms, and in some gangrenes." Charles West in 1842 quoted the Registrar-General's reports that teething was the registered cause of death in 4·8 per cent. of all children who died in London under 1 year old, and in 7·3 per cent. of those who died between the age of 1 and 3 years. Guthrie wrote that the Registrar-General's report of 1839 showed 5,016 deaths in England and Wales attributed to teething. Guthrie concluded that there was no proof that any of the constitutional symptoms were due to dentition.

It has been said that teething produces nothing but teeth. This is not quite true, for it may cause the baby to be a little irritable, to salivate excessively, and oddly enough, to refuse temporarily to sit on the pottie (as Gesell pointed out). Nevertheless, a great deal of the crying and sleep disturbance ascribed by mothers to teething is due simply to bad habit formation. It is convenient, however, to be able to blame teething for a child's bad behaviour. When the gums are painful, hard items of food may be refused by the baby, and sometimes he may refuse almost everything.

It is still said by many that teething causes bronchitis, diarrhœa, a rash, convulsions and fever. I searched through the whole of the world literature for evidence of this and found none. It would indeed be surprising if the eruption of a tooth should cause a virus infection of the respiratory or alimentary tract. It is easy to understand how the idea has arisen. Children are teething from about 6 months to 6 years, and parents have naturally ascribed any untoward event in the child to teething. *No general condition should ever be ascribed to teething.* Many serious mistakes have been made as a result of putting convulsions and other symptoms down to "teething."

Arvi Tasanen, of Oulu, North Finland,[15] wrote an excellent thesis on the subject, after fully utilizing unrivalled opportunities of day to day study of 126 normal infants. When they were teething there was no increase of infections, diarrhœa, fever, convulsions, rash or bronchitis, nor of ear-rubbing. There was some restlessness by day and some increase of salivation, with an increase of thumb sucking and gum rubbing.

Teething should be regarded as a natural though sometimes painful process, and no specific treatment is required. Teething powders are

* Quoted by Guthrie.[8]

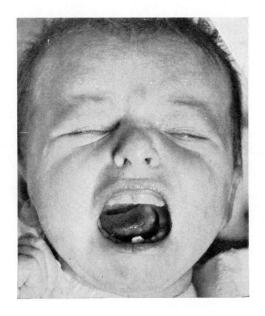

Fig. 15. Lower central incisor tooth in new-born baby.

To face p. 90

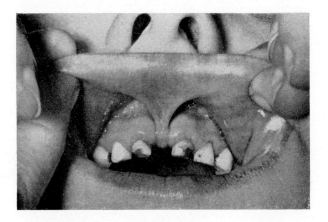

Fig. 16   Alveolar frenum.

useless. Lancing of the gums is always wrong. It is dangerous and may cause infections of the mouth. The diet should be suitably modified if the baby shows reluctance to eat hard foods. If the baby cries because of pain he should be picked up even though there is some risk of habit formation.

The Prevention of Dental Caries

For at least 3,000 years man believed that caries was due to gnawing by worms. This was believed in ancient Egypt and Mesopotamia, right through Roman times and in the Middle Ages. Jaques Houllier (1498–1562)[11] first cast doubt on the existence of dental worms, but Gottfried Schulz, who lived at the same period, declared that the gastric juice of a pig would expel worms, some even as large as an earthworm, from a decayed tooth.

Caries is caused by bacteria acting on fermentable carbohydrates in contact with the surface of the tooth. This liberates organic acids which dissolve the inorganic portions of the teeth. Refined carbohydrates are more harmful than starch. Sweets given between meals, and especially toffee, which is in contact with the teeth for prolonged periods, are harmful. Lollypops, biscuits and acid drinks are particularly bad for the teeth. There was a sharp drop in the incidence of caries during the war years, when sugar was rationed, followed by a rise subsequently.

There are other factors which govern the child's susceptibility to caries. These include genetic and developmental factors.

The role of fluorine in the prevention of caries is now firmly established.[9,14,16] Fluoridation of water supplies reduces the incidence of caries by 50 to 65 per cent. Topical application of stannous fluoride at intervals of about 3 years gives a 40 per cent. reduction in dental caries. Dietary fluoride supplements in the form of sodium fluoride provide some protection if the water is not fluoridated.[14] Fluorine is now incorporated in certain toothpastes. The value of fluoridation has been endorsed by the World Health Organization, the U.S. Public Health Service, the American Medical Association, the American Dental Association, the American Academy of Pediatrics, and the American Society of Dentistry for Children.[16]

Other essential methods of preventing caries are as follows:

(1) Avoidance of sweets between meals, because of the fermentation of the sugar and acid formation, and the avoidance of excessive amounts of refined carbohydrates at any time. Pacifiers sweetened with honey, rosehip syrup or glycerine are particularly harmful to the teeth. In a study of 2,468 Australian children,[6] it was found that there was a statistically significant excess of tooth decay over a two year period in

children attending schools which sell sweets in the canteen, as compared with those attending schools which did not sell sweets.

Fruit syrups are harmful because of their viscosity with high sugar content, low pH, and the chelating action of citric acid.

(2) Removal of fermentable carbohydrates from the mouth before conversion into acid. The care of the teeth should begin when the first tooth comes through. It is brushed morning and night. By the age of three the child learns to brush his teeth without help, but under supervision.

(3) Elimination of areas where food stagnation occurs, and of developmental defects on the surface of the enamel.

(4) The prevention of overcrowding.

Orthodontics

A child should be taken to a dentist shortly after his second birthday. This enables dental caries to be treated promptly so that the deciduous teeth can be preserved, for the premature loss of deciduous teeth is a major cause of malocclusion; and if malocclusion is found, or teeth are becoming overcrowded, steps can be taken to remedy the defect. One frequently sees older children and adults with unsightly malocclusion and with seriously overcrowded teeth, defects which could readily have been prevented.

Alveolar Frenum

The midline membranous labial frenum, which normally extends from the upper lip to the labial surface of the upper gum, may continue on between the upper central incisors to the lingual side of the upper gum, and may lead to spacing between the central incisors (*Fig. 16*). As the alveolar ridge grows downward in later childhood, the attachment of the frenum normally migrates from the alveolar margin so that the spacing of the incisors is corrected. Occasionally plastic surgical treatment is required, but this must be very rare. The condition nearly always cures itself. Treatment is rarely necessary before the age of 11 years.

Tongue Tie (Ankyloglossia)

The frenum linguæ arises from a thickening of the geniohyoglossus muscles meeting in the midline of the tongue to form a vertical fold. Tongue tie ranges from only a mucous membrane band to a fibrosed frenulum and genioglossus muscle, or even fusion of the tongue to the floor of the mouth.[10] The tongue is always short at birth, but as the infant grows the tongue becomes longer and thinner towards the tip until eventually the frenum is placed well behind the tip. Many mothers ascribe their child's feeding difficulties, lateness in speaking or indistinctness of speech to tongue tie. This diagnosis is almost invariably wrong. In my experience true tongue tie, sufficient to produce symptoms, is rare, but I certainly do not deny its existence.

Some think that if the child is unable to protrude the tongue or to touch the palate with the tongue, he may have difficulty in pronouncing the letters N, L, T, D and Th, especially if the palatal arch is high. It has been said that intelligent emotionally stable healthy people can overcome such a slight physical handicap without operation or speech therapy. Dyslalia is common and it is easy to ascribe indistinctness of speech to tongue tie when it is due to no such thing. I have certainly never seen any feeding difficulty in the first year as a result of tongue tie, and I doubt whether it is ever necessary to carry out an operation on it till the age of 2 or 3. The operation should certainly not be performed if the tongue can touch the palate. A guide to the severity of the tongue tie is a marked midline depression at the tip and the child's inability to lick his upper lip.

There are still doctors who cut the frenum in the new-born period. This is always wrong. There is apt to be hæmorrhage from the profunda linguæ vein, and infection may complicate the operation. The operation in the new-born period is always due to ignorance of the normal appearance of the tongue of the new-born. If it has to be done at all the operation should be done by a pædiatric or plastic surgeon when the child is 2 or 3 years old.

Cullum[5] wrote an interesting historical account of the condition.

White Tongue

One often sees a uniformly white furred tongue in a baby in the first few weeks of his life. There is no sign of stomatitis. It is quite unlike the appearance of a monilia infection, in which the white areas are discrete. It is of no significance and disappears as the baby grows older.

Black Tongue

Some infants have a black coating on the tongue. It is a harmless condition requiring no treatment. It is due to an overgrowth of the tongue papillæ.

Geographical Tongue

This is characterized by small, round grey areas on the dorsum of the tongue. The advancing margin is somewhat elevated, and the desquamating centre presents a reddened surface. On coalescing, the areas resemble a map.

On the basis of a study of 1,246 cases, it was concluded that geographical tongue is related to seborrhœic dermatitis and spasmodic bronchitis; 17·1 per cent. of 775 cases had seborrhœic dermatitis as well.[12]

Tonsils and Adenoids

The tonsils are often quite large by the age of 3 or 4, but there is practically never any need to remove them in a child as young as that. They tend to become smaller after the age of 6 or 7.

Adenoids may cause trouble, even in an infant. They may lead to postnasal obstruction, excessive snoring, a persistent nasal discharge, a nasal speech, with substitution of B for M, a troublesome cough on lying down, and recurrent otitis media. If they cause these symptoms, they should be removed.

Uvulectomy

According to Apffel[1] uvulectomy is performed amongst the Berbers of North Morocco on infants of both sexes by the caretaker or sexton of the neighbouring mosque, or by the barber. The operation is performed by a wooden spatula or reed or falciform bistoury. The operation is intended to facilitate breast feeding and to improve speech and health.

Mouth Breathing

In a study of mouth-breathers, it was found that over 6 per cent. of children with an habitually open mouth breathe only through the mouth. Thirteen per cent. breathe through nose and mouth. Eighty-one per cent., though the mouth is constantly open, breathe entirely through the nose.

Habit formation is clearly a factor.

Halitosis

This is an unusual but occasional complaint in normal children. Halitosis of recent onset in a well child should arouse the suspicion of a foreign body in the nose. In an ill child it may be due to tonsillitis, Vincent's infection or diphtheria. Chronic halitosis may be associated with bronchiectasis or a pulmonary abscess or it may be due to atrophic rhinitis. The halitosis resulting from the eating of onions and garlic is well known.

It is fair to say that it is commonly impossible to determine the cause of minor degrees of halitosis. .

Slobbering and Drooling

Mentally normal children mostly control their saliva by the age of about fifteen months. Drooling continues long after that in children with mental subnormality or cerebral palsy. In some normal children, however, drooling continues long after the age of fifteen months, without any apparent reason. Sometimes, but not always, it is associated with mouth breathing.

Drooling is occasionally a symptom of familial dysautonomia, stomatitis, and iodide or mercury poisoning.

The Lips

In the first few weeks of life one often sees so-called "sucking pads" or "sucking blisters" on the lips. They are well demarcated areas of cornified epithelium separating off from the underlying mucosa. As they are shed, new ones are formed. They are normal.

The Gums

Inclusion cysts ("epithelial pearls") and sometimes larger mucous cysts may be found on or near the margin of the gum in young babies. They shed themselves spontaneously in a few weeks, and require no treatment.

Of 209 one to five day old full term infants,[4] 80 per cent. had cysts of the alveolar or palatal mucosa or both; in 65 per cent. they were located on the median palatine raphé, in 36·5 per cent. on the maxillary alveolar mucosa, and in 9·9 per cent. on the mandibular alveolar mucosa. It was suggested that the median palatal cysts may arise from epithelium entrapped during development. They all disappeared spontaneously in a few months.

One sometimes sees a fringe of membranous material with a serrated edge extending along the gum margin in a new-born baby. It disappears if left alone.

The Palate

Inclusion cysts (Epstein's pearls), mostly pinhead size, commonly form close to the median raphé of the palate in new-born babies. They last a few weeks, and are of no importance.

Snoring

Snoring may be due to vibrations of the thin edge of the velum of the soft palate and the posterior faucial pillars.[13] Birch[2] wrote that while snoring is often attributed to vibrations of the soft palate, pharyngoscopy has shown that the main fault lies in the cage of the posterior pillars of the fauces, which vibrate noisily. The noise is aggravated by mouth-breathing and supine sleeping.

References

1. APFFEL, C. A. (1965). "Uvulectomy." *J. Am. Med. Ass.*, **193**, 164.
2. BIRCH, C. A. (1969). "Snoring." *Practitioner*, **203**, 383.
3. BODENHOFF, J., GORLIN, R. J. (1963). "Natal and Neonatal Teeth." *Pediatrics*, **32**, 1087.
4. CATALDO E., BERKMAN, M. D. (1968). "Cysts of the Oral Mucosa in Newborns." *Am. J. Dis. Child.*, **116**, 44.
5. CULLUM, I. M. (1959). "An Old Wives' Tale." *Brit. med. J.*, **2**, 497.
6. FANNING, E. A., GOTJAMANOS, T., VOWLES N. (1969). "Dental Caries in Children Related to Availablity of Sweets at School Canteens." *M. J. Australia*, **1**, 1131.
7. GARDINER, J. (1961). "Teeth in the Newborn." *Proc. roy. Soc. Med.*, **54**, 504.
8. GUTHRIE, L., (1908). Teething. *Brit. med. J.* **2**, 468.
9. H.M.S.O., London, 1962. "The Conduct of the Fluoridation Studies in the United Kingdom and the Results Achieved after Five Years." M.O.H. Scottish Office, Min. of Housing and Local Government.
10. HORTON, C. E., CRAWFORD, H. H., ADAMSON, J. E., ASHBELL, T. S. (1969). "Tongue Tie." *Cleft palate*, **6**, 8.
11. *Lancet* (1955), Annotation. "The Mystery of Dental Caries." **1**, 1009.
12. RAHAMIMOFF, P., MUHSAM, H. V. (1957). "Some Observations on 1,246 Cases of Geographical Tongue." *Am. J. Dis. Child.*, **93**, 519.
13. ROBIN, I. G. (1968). "Snoring." *Proc. Roy. Soc. Med.*, **61**, 575.
14. SCHLESINGER, E. R. (1963). "Dental Caries and the Pediatrician." *Am. J. Dis. Child.*, **105**, 1.
15. TASANEN, A. (1968). "General and Local Effects of the Eruption of Deciduous Teeth." *Ann. Paediat. Fenniae.*, **14**, Suppl. 29.
16. WEECH, A. A. (1964). "Fluoridation." *Am. J. Dis. Child.*, **108**, 571.

CHAPTER 7

THE SKIN AND UMBILICUS

Perianal Soreness

Sooner or later the majority of babies develop some perianal soreness or ammonia dermatitis, however careful the management. Perianal soreness is particularly common in the new-born period, especially in artificially-fed babies. When the baby is older, and therefore more tolerant of a wet or soiled napkin than he is in the earlier weeks, he may lie or sit with a soiled napkin for a long period, especially in the night, before it is removed. In the new-born period the best treatment is exposure of the buttocks to the air, the baby being kept in the prone position. This, however, can only be done in a warmed room. An alternative treatment is the liberal use of a baby cream or zinc and castor oil ointment. With this treatment the skin usually rapidly clears.

Ammonia Dermatitis

This is a dermatitis affecting the napkin area, and therefore largely avoiding the creases in the groin and the perianal region. The prepuce is often severly involved. At first there is a simple erythema, but subsequently the skin becomes thickened and rough, resembling the skin of the scrotum, and it often desquamates and cracks. Vesicles may form, and they may become secondarily infected and even form ulcers. There may be a great deal of swelling and local heat. Sometimes with secondary infection oozing of serum occurs and scabs form. In the circumcied baby there may be ulceration at the urinary meatus, which causes severe pain on micturition especially if the urethral orifice is unusually high on the end of the glans. Meatal ulceration only rarely occurs in uncircumcised babies, because the prepuce usually fully projects the glans. The ulceration is followed by scabbing and scarring, and sometimes by narrowing of the urethral orifice.

Ammonia dermatitis is due to urea-splitting organisms, including the *Bacillus ammoniagenes*, which is a normal inhabitant of the fæces. The organisms cause the liberation of ammonia from the urine, and the napkins smell strongly of ammonia. The condition should be distinguished from simple erythema due to contact with alkalies or soap residue in the napkins.

The treatment of the condition should begin with a discussion with the mother about the washing of the napkins and the frequency with which they are changed. It is wise to ask her in the first place how many napkins she possesses. Some mothers from particularly poor social conditions only own a dozen napkins in all because of their high cost. Even two dozen would not really be enough, because of the frequency with which babies pass urine or stools and the time taken to dry the napkins after they have been washed. Some mothers do not always wash them out when they have only been wetted. They merely hang them up to dry and reapply them to the baby. It is important also to advise the mother about the thorough rinsing of the napkins after they have been washed, for no alkali soap material must be left in them. The babies' buttocks should be sponged after they have been wet with urine, then thoroughly dried and powdered. It is particularly important to remove all traces of a stool from the buttocks. Simple exposure to the air, leaving the baby lying on a napkin, is often effective without other measures. Baby cream or zinc and castor oil ointment applied to the affected part will, with these steps, rapidly cure the mild cases. In the severe forms a lotion containing 4 per cent. tannic acid with 0·1 per cent. proflavine, applied several times a day, is useful. Waterproof pants are undesirable because they retain moisture and aggravate the condition. A plastic napkin holder avoids this difficulty. In the severest forms, with acute inflammation and oozing, simple saline dressings are desirable until the inflammation has subsided. The tannic acid lotion may then be applied. In all cases the mother must be instructed to change the napkin as soon as she reasonably can after it has been wet.

Boracic crystals should never be used, either in solution or worse still, sprinkled into the napkin, bacause of the serious risk of boric poisoning. This is a highly dangerous condition, manifested by diarrhœa and vomiting, generalized erythema with desquamation, especially of the palms and soles, meningism, hæmorrhages, convulsions, circulatory collapse and death. The mortality in one series of 113 cases was 55 per cent. Boracic ointment should never be used, especially when the skin is macerated or excoriated. On the other hand, the small amount of boric acid (5 per cent.) in dusting powders does not do any harm, though it might be unwise to use it if there were severe excoriation.

A meatal ulcer should in addition be treated by the application of Tulle Gras. If there is severe pain on micturition a local anæsthetic ointment (e.g. Nupercaine 1 per cent.) may be applied to the ulcerated area. An older child may be persuaded to pass urine in his bath if pain is severe. As meatal ulcers are merely a part of the ammonia dermatitis this must be treated as already described.

Thrush Dermatitis

When ammonia dermatitis proves resistant to treatment, a monilia infection should be suspected. Flat superficial vesicles may be found on the buttocks, thighs or genitalia. These are often followed by desquamation. Flexural intertrigo or seborrhœic dermatitis predisposes to the infection. Scrapings of the skin lesions should be cleared of debris by partly heating with 10 per cent. potassium hydroxide, and examining under the microscope without staining, when the yeastlike cells and branching mycelia may easily be seen. Scrapings may also be cultured on Sabouraud's medium. Treatment consists of the application of nystatin ointment.

It has been found that when babies are nursed in the prone position, there is less tendency to ammonia dermatitis.

Psoriasiform Dermatitis

This begins as an erythema, but spreads to other parts of the body, including the face. The lesions are discrete, with a clear margin, which distinguishes it from seborrhœic dermatitis. It may be a response of a seborrhœic individual to infection by monilia. It responds to a corticosteroid ointment such as Betnovate, with equal parts of Lassar's paste. It is a self-limiting condition, disappearing in one to three months without treatment.

Seborrhœic Dermatitis or Eczema

This can be distinguished from ammonia dermatitis by the fact that seborrhœic dermatitis involves the creases, while ammonia dermatitis spares them. The seborrhœic rash is a smoother more shiny rash than ammonia dermatitis. It commonly involves other parts of the body.

Intertrigo

For intertrigo 1 per cent. brilliant green, applied three or four times a day, is an effective treatment, though it is a nuisance for the mother on account of the colour.

Scurfy Scalp

Some scurfiness of the scalp occurs in most babies in the first few weeks of life. In the mildest forms no treatment is necessary. In the rather more severe forms the scalp should no longer be washed in soap and water; the scalp should be washed daily in a lotion of 1 per cent. cetrimide. If more severe, it is treated by the application of ung. salicyl et sulph. N.F. on two nights.

Nævi

Small capillary dilatations or nævi on the inner corner of the upper eyelid, on the forehead above the nose and on the back of the neck are so common that they should be considered to be normal. I there is one on the forehead, there is almost always one on the back o the neck. They always disappear in a few months, and no treatment i required.

In a study of 2171 Scandinavian children aged 6 to 17 years,[16] næv were found on the back of the neck of 42·6 per cent. of the boys anc 35·1 per cent. of the girls; telangiectases were found in the inter scapular region of 39·9 per cent. of the girls and 32·3 per cent. of the boys

Strawberry nævi are crimson raised nævi on any part of the body They are hardly ever, if ever, present at birth. A few days after birtl strawberry nævi begin as a pinhead mark and grow—for a period of uj to 5 to 6 months. Growth then stops, and they become grey in the centre and gradually heal from the centre outwards. Over half disap pear without trace within 5 years, and the remainder disappear within about 10 years. No treatment is required and, in fact, treatmen should be avoided, for it is liable to leave a scar (or even a keloid) Very rarely a hæmangioma, especially one at a mucocutaneou junction, begins to grow excessively. Such a nævus should be excisec promptly.

Spider nævi are found in normal children and are of no significance.[1,] They were found in 47·5 per cent. of 1,138 healthy school children a Bristol. They are more common in older children than in younge ones. Some spider nævi disappear spontaneously, and treatment i not advised.

Mongolian Pigmentation

This consists of greyish-blue pigmentation mainly over the sacrum but also sometimes on the thighs and legs, and sometimes in the bucca mucosa, shoulder and hand. It is exceedingly common in dark-skinnec people, and it is said to be common in Eskimos. It occurs infrequentl) in white children, and is then apt to be confused with bruising. It wa originally described in Japan, and viewed with superstition, the mal not being allowed to see it. These pigmented areas have been termec "Tâches Bleuâtres" by French workers. They disappear in 2 or 3 year and are of no significance.[11]

Other Skin Lesions in the New-born Period

Most new-born babies show white or yellow punctate pinheac lesions on the nose ("Milia"). They are due to the retention of secretior in the sebaceous glands and should not be confused with pustules. The)

may occur elsewhere on the face, and the distinction from pustules is not always easy. A red areola round them should suggest an infection.

Peeling of the skin, especially of the hands and feet, is normal in the new-born period. It sometimes occasions some in mothers.

It is normal for hair to fall out after 2 or 3 weeks. Baldness over the occipital region should not cause alarm. It will be temporary only. Some normal babies are born with an unusually large amount of hair.

Petechiæ may be seen on the face in a new-born baby as a result of delivery. They should not cause alarm. Splinter hæmorrhages were found in 10·3 per cent. of patients without subacute bacterial endocarditis admitted to a general medical ward. Most of these were adults, but some were children.[13]

Hypertrichosis

Forbes[6] wrote a comprehensive review of the subject of hypertrichosis. One is occasionally concerned by the excessive hair on a child's body. It may be purely a racial matter. It is commonly caused by drugs—phenytoin, ethosuccimide and corticosteroids. It is commonly seen in children who are malnourished for any reason, as from severe debilitating diseases. It occurs in cretins and in virilizing conditions, such as adrenocortical hyperplasia.

The Effect of Tight Mittens

Mann[14] described cases of finger-tip necrosis as a result of tight mittens.

Cyanosis

Cyanosis may be due to conditions other than serious organic diseases. There have been several papers on cyanosis in babies due to methæmoglobinæmia resulting from nitrites from well water, and from the marking ink used in laundries to mark napkins and other clothes. It only occurs if the laundry mark is applied after washing, instead of before. It is rapidly cured by an intravenous injection of 1·5 mg methylene blue per kilogram as a 0·1 per cent. solution. Cyanosis may result from eating spinach which has been fertilized by nitrates.

There is sometimes local cyanosis of the face for a few days after birth. The cyanosis of the head and neck may be quite marked, especially where there has been delay in delivery of the shoulders after the birth of the head. The cyanosis disappears spontaneously after a few days.

A new-born baby may have marked cyanosis of the arms below the elbow, and the legs below the knees, the hands and feet being particularly blue. It is of no importance and disappears in a few days.

Harlequin Colour Change

Neligan and Strang[15] described episodes lasting up to 20 minutes in which an exact half of a new-born baby became paler than the other half. The distribution of colour appeared to be related to gravity, for the picture became reversed by turning the baby on to the opposite side during an attack. The attack was brought to an end by turning the baby on to his back. There was no evidence that it was associated with any particular disease, and it appeared to have no particular clinical or pathological significance.

The Umbilicus

The umbilical cord usually separates by the fifth to the ninth day. It tends to separate early if it is kept dry and there is no daily bathing. It sometimes separates later than the ninth day in spite of being kept dry and free from infection. Moistness after separation should be dealt with by cleansing with spirit, and in some cases by the application of tetracycline in kaolin powder. Small granulations should be touched with a silver nitrate pencil. Bright red polypi with a mucoid secretion may represent the end of the omphalomesenteric duct. A bright red polyp with a sinus is likely to be a persistent vitelline duct (with a Meckel's diverticulum at the other end.) Another type may be connected with a patent urachus. Hence unless an umbilical polyp is clearly no more than granulation tissue, a pædiatric surgeon should be asked for advice.

The umbilicus should be covered up at birth and kept covered until the cord has separated.

Umbilical hernias are so common that they can be considered normal, especially in premature babies. The vast majority cure themselves, if left alone.

Halpern[8] studied 147 premature infants with an umbilical hernia. He found that strapping delayed healing, whether the hernia was large or small. Large hernias healed three times more quickly when left alone than when strapped. Healing normally occurred between 7 and 12 months, but in some it did not occur till 3 years of age.

A controlled study of 201 Australian children showed that strapping was useless.[2]

On the other hand Hawarth[10] thought that large hernias disappeared more quickly if strapped. My advice is that umbilical hernias should be left to cure themselves without strapping. This accords with the opinion of Denis Brown.[5]

Strangulation of umbilical hernias is exceedingly rare.[4] In a series of 514 infants with umbilical hernia, strangulation occurred in one case only.

Inguinal Hernias should be operated on without delay, especially when found in the first year, because of the serious risk of strangulation.

Absence of one umbilical artery. It should be a routine practice to count the umbilical vessels of every newborn infant, because a single umbilical artery is associated with a considerable risk of other congenital anomalies.[2] The incidence of a single umbilical artery is about one per cent. of live births[7]; the incidence is said to be many times higher in low birth weight babies and could be related to fœtal malnutrition[12] Froehlich and Fujikura[7] found a single artery in 1·22 per cent. of white babies and 0·44 per cent. of negro infants; there were associated abnormalities in 23·0 per cent. of the white babies and 42·1 per cent of the negro infants—giving an overall incidence of abnormalities of 28·6 per cent. In another series 33 per cent. of the babies with a single artery had renal anomalies.[9]

Epicanthic Folds

Epicanthic folds are common in normal children and lead many to make the mistake of diagnosing mongolism. According to Solomons[17] they are found in a third of all new-born infants. They commonly disappear as the child grows older, and are unusual in normal children after the age of ten. The epicanthic fold in normal infants is placed across the canthus in such a way that portions of the upper and lower eyelids are covered, the concavity of the semi-lunar fold itself looking outwards. In mongols there is an oblique fold of loose skin just above the inner angle of the eye, impinging on the eye-lashes.

Congenital Dermal Sinus

A glance down the midline of the back is part of the routine examination of any infant. A congenital dermal sinus may be found in the midline of the scalp or anywhere else in the midline. The most common site is the upper end of the natal cleft. Those above the natal cleft are apt to be important, because they may communicate with the subarachnoid space and lead to meningitis. Any such sinus should be operated upon. Those in the natal cleft are only important if they remain deep, because then they may become infected. If they remain deep after the age of two, they should be excised, because of the difficulty of keeping them clean, and therefore the risk of infection.

Sweating Around the Head

Some infants and small children sweat profusely around the head when asleep. It is of no significance and is not associated with any particular disease.

References

1. ALDERSON, M. R. (1963). "Spider Nævi: Their Incidence in Healthy School Children." *Arch. Dis. Childh.*, **38**, 286.
2. ANGEL-LORD, G. (1971). "Infantile Umbilical Hernia." *Med J. Australia*, **1**, 83
3. BEAN, W. B. (1960). "Notes on the Natural History of Vascular Spiders in Healthy Persons." *Arch. Int. Med.*, **106**, 35.
4. BRANDON, S., WHITEHOUSE, D. (1960). "Two Unusual Complications of Umbilical Hernia in Childhood." *Brit. med. J.*, **2**, 1935.
5. BROWNE, D. (1952). "Abdominal Hernia in Childhood." *Brit. med. J.*, **2**, 1144.
6. FORBES, A. (1965). "Hypertrichosis." *New. Engl. J. Med.*, **273**, 602.
7. FROEHLICH, L. A., FUJIKURA, T. (1966). "Significance of a Single Umbilical Artery." *Am. J. Obstet. and Gyn.*, **94**, 274.
8. HALPERN, L. J. (1962). "Spontaneous Healing of Umbilical Hernia." *J. Amer. med. Ass.*, **182**, 851.
9. HARRIS, R. J., VAN LEEUWEN, G. (1968). "Single Umbilical Artery. *J. Pediat.*, **42**, 98.
10. HAWORTH, J. (1956). "Adhesive Strapping for Umbilical Hernia in Infants." *Brit. med. J.*, **2**, 1286.
11. HAYWARD, R. (1964). "Mongolian Blue Spots." *Brit Med. J.*, **2**, 679.
12. JEAN C., DUPRÉ, A., CARRIER C. (1969). "Single Umbilical Artery. Study of 112 Cases." *Can. Med. Ass. J.*, **100**, 1088.
13. KILPATRICK, Z. M., GREENBERG, P. A., SANFORD, J. P. (1965). "Splinter Hemorrhages: Their Clinical Significance." *Arch. Int. Med.*, **115**, 730.
14. MANN, T. P. (1961). "Finger-tip Necrosis in the Newly Born: a Hazard of Wearing Mittens." *Brit. Med. J.*, **2**, 1755.
15. NELIGAN, G. A., STRANG, L. B. (1952). "Harlequin Colour Change." *Lancet*, **2**, 1005.
16. ØSTER J., NIENSEN, A. (1970). "Nuchal Nævi and Interscapular Telangiectases." *Acta Paediat, Scand.*, **59**, 416.
17. SOLOMONS, G., ZELLWEGER, H., JAHNKE, P. G., OPITZ, E. (1965). "Four Common Signs in Mongolism." *Am. J. Dis. Child.*, **110**, 46.

CHAPTER 8

THE BREASTS AND GENITALS

Changes in the New-born

It is common for the breasts of babies of both sexes to be enlarged in the newborn period. This does not usually occur in premature babies. The exact frequency cannot be stated, because minor degrees are often overlooked. It is certainly not an inflammatory condition, as the term "neonatal mastitis" would imply. It is probably related to the secretion of œstrogenic substances from the ovary, and prolactin from the anterior pituitary gland. The breasts secrete a fluid closely resembling colostrum, commonly called "witches' milk." The swelling may persist for several weeks. No treatment is ever required, because it is a normal condition, and no attempt should be made to massage the breast.

Enlargement of the external genitalia is equally common in the new-born period. In the female the labia and clitoris are often so prominent that it may even be suggested that the baby is a pseudo-hermaphrodite. The enlargement subsides by a month or so of age. Smith[26] described the occurrence of small tags or excrescences about the inner surfaces of the labia, which are sometimes so prominent that the question of their surgical removal arises. They always disappear if left alone. The vulva becomes moist and congested and there is a thin glairy discharge from the vagina, becoming thicker and milky white after 2 or 3 days, disappearing by the fourth to the fourteenth day. At about the seventh day there may be some blood in the vaginal discharge of a full-term baby. This arises from the endometrium. The vaginal discharge is due to the hypertrophy of the vaginal epithelium in the new-born period and the subsequent desquamation of the squamous cells. It is also associated with the invasion of the vagina by organisms. The genital changes are due to œstrogenic substances received from the mother via the placenta. No treatment is indicated, because the changes are normal.

Circumcision

Historical. An excellent review of the subject of circumcision was written by Gairdner.[6] An interesting section on the historical aspects of the operation was written by Gordon.[8] According to Gairdner the operation is practised over a wide area of the world by about one-sixth of its population. It is probably the oldest surgical operation known to man, dating some 6,000 years back to antiquity. According to Herodotus, the Egyptians were the first to circumcise. The operation was performed by priests or barbers.[7] The fact that the operation was practised by the ancient Egyptians was shown by wall carvings in the Temple of Karnak, near Luxor. According to Voltaire, circumcision among Jews arose from an earlier Egyptian religious custom, and later it became a blood covenant. It was a form of tribal marking, enabling the nomadic Jews to produce a secret sign of the fact of belonging to one tribe.[13] The Arabs practised it before the time of Mohammed. There is no reference to the operation in the Koran. It is said that Pythagoras had to submit to circumcision before he was allowed the privilege of studying in the Egyptian temples. Moses made his wife circumcise him with a stone implement. According to the Bible, God ordered Abraham to circumcise all male infants at the age of 8 days. Abraham performed the operation on himself when he was 99 years old. Bergmann holds that circumcision was originally a method of marking slaves, which was a development from an earlier practice or amputating the organ. Saul instructed David to bring 100 foreskins as evidence of killing that number of Philistines, in order that he should prove that he was worthy to be his son-in-law. He brought 200. According to Schlossman[23] the 12th century rabbinical scholar Marmonides declared that the purpose of the operation amongst Jews was to weaken the penis and so limit intercourse. In various African tribes and in New Guinea circumcision is part of an initiation ceremony at puberty. After puberty, it is part of the ritual of mutilation, by which the young male, and less often the young female, is called upon to give proof of courage, by which they are admitted to the privileges of the tribe or estate of manhood or womanhood.

Bolande[1] compared the operations of circumcision and tonsillectomy with the knocking out of teeth as a manhood initiation rite, female pubertal rite, or a propitiatory sacrifice to the dead. He discussed other rites, such as infibulation, castration and uvulectomy. Morrison[20] discussed the origin of the practice in the Australian aborigines and the extension of the operation by incision under the entire shaft of the penis. Jomo Kenyatta stated that it is taboo for a Kikuyu woman to have sexual relations with someone who has not been circumcised. The uncircumcised cannot build a house of his own. In feasts there are certain "joints" of which he cannot partake. Circumcision is the only qualification which gives a man the recognition of manhood and the full right of citizenship.

Morgan[18] wrote that "perhaps not least of the reasons why American mothers seem to endorse the operation with such enthusiasm is the fact that it is the one way an intensely matriarchal society can permanently influence the physical characteristics of its males." Elsewhere[19] he wrote that "the American public has come to view circumcision as the other essentials of life—namely superhighways, refrigerators and T.V. sets. As well deprive these citizens of their birthright as suggest that they retain their prepuce. It has become imperative to lop it off to keep up with the Joneses, for in the affluent society, status and a foreskin are incompatible". Leitch, writing about the widespread practice of routine circumcision in Australia, wrote that "the undressed penis stands as a social symbol, and the foreskin is still a schoolboy curiosity, viewed with wonder and awe".

Normal Development. Gairdner, after a study of the embryological development of the prepuce, showed that the prepuce is still in the course of development at birth, and so is usually incompletely separated from the glans penis. Prior to birth, there is no separation of the prepuce from the glans. The term "preputial adhesions" is therefore a misnomer. Gairdner studied 100 new-born babies and 200 boys of varying ages up to 5 years, and found that only 4 per cent. of the new-borns had a fully retractable prepuce. In 54 per cent. the glans could be uncovered enough to reveal the external meatus, and in the remaining 42 per cent. even the tip of the glans could not be uncovered. The prepuce is non-retractable in 4 out of 5 normal males of 6 months, and in half of normal males of 1 year. By 2 years about 20 per cent., and by about 3 years about 10 per cent., of boys still have a non-retractable prepuce.

Schoenfeld, Freud and others have suggested[23, 24] that circumcision is a factor in the causation of antisemitism, in that circumcision becomes equated in the subconscious mind with castration.

It is a common practice to perform circumcision on young babies without an anæsthetic. This is a cruel practice.

More than a third of circumcisions are performed in the first month of life at a time when faults or diseases of the prepuce itself are practically non-existent.

There is no need for the mother to retract the foreskin in the first year or two. Gentle efforts may be made by the time the boy is 2 or 3, and if by the age of 3 or 4 it is still not retractable, then a blunt instrument may be passed through the orfice in the prepuce and round the glans to separate the strands of tissue remaining between the two structures. It is only in a very small number of children that this manœuvre fails, and circumcision may then have to be considered in order that smegma can be removed and the glans can be kept clean. A surgeon can always retract a child's foreskin. If he does this in a very young boy, he applies Vaseline so that micturition is not painful in the next day or two.

Incidence. In a National Sample of 2,428 children 24 per cent. had

had the operation by the age of 4 years.[17] It is likely that 100,000 operations for circumcision are carried out in the United Kingdom every year. In the United States the corresponding figure is 2,000,000. It is interesting that the operation has the same sort of social incidence as that of tonsillectomy, affecting as it does the upper classes more than the lower ones; 84 per cent. of 73 students at Cambridge, coming from the best-known public schools, had been circumcised, compared with only 50 per cent. of 174 coming from grammar or secondary schools.

Complications. Most practising pædiatricians have seen unfortunate consequences from the operation of circumcision, and seen or personally heard of death directly resulting from it. The Registrar-General's returns show that every year there are about 16 deaths from the operation. Browne[2] described some of the operations which he has had to do in order to correct mistakes made by others. The mistakes included: (i) Removal of too much skin. Browne said that he had known a case in which skin grafting was necessary to relieve pain on erection due to this cause. (ii) Removal of too little mucosa, causing obstruction to the flow of urine. (iii) Untidy tags of skin. (iv) Eight cases of fistula of the urethra. (v) Amputation of part of the glans. (vi) Amputation through the body of the organ. (vii) Sewing the skin edge to the glans, with consequent burying of the corona. (viii) Circumcision in a case of hypospadias. This removes the reservoir of skin on which the surgeon depends for making a new urethra.

I have twice seen partial amputation of the glans during the operation, several cases of severe hæmorrhage and prolonged sepsis, and various strange cosmetic results. Freud[5] and others have shown that meatal ulcer is almost confined to circumcised male infants and is only occasionally seen in the uncircumcised child when the prepuce is unusually lax and the glans is consequently exposed.

Gangrene of the penis has occurred as a result of over-enthusiastic bandaging of the organ by the parents. In the Thousand Family Survey[27] at Newcastle, 22 per cent. of the children circumcised developed complications from the operation, including infections, and hæmorrhage severe enough to necessitate transfusion.

Enthusiastic efforts to stretch the foreskin by forcibly opening sinus forceps inserted into the preputial orifice are painful and completely unjustified. Efforts forcibly to withdraw the foreskin cause bleeding, and are unjustified and unnecessary, considering the fact that it is not usual for separation of the prepuce from the glans to have been completed by the time the baby is born. Every casualty department is well used to seeing babies with paraphimosis, which results from the mother's efforts to retract the foreskin on someone's wrong advice.

Indications. The operation should certainly not be done because of enuresis. There is not the slightest reason to believe that the operation will help. It should not be done because the foreskin is a long one. There is no justification for this. It should never be done on account of masturbation. It will make no difference. It should not be done because the foreskin is involved in ammonia dermatitis (unless it has resulted in scar formation. Even then circumcision should not be performed until the dermatitis has been cured). This dermatitis has nothing to do with the uncircumcised state of the child. The operation should never be done because the mother or the father or the general practitioner has asked that it should be done. The child is the only one who matters in this regard. It is he who should be considered and no one else. If it is in his interests that the operation should be performed, it should be done. If there is no particular reason from his point of view for doing the operation, it is quite unjustified to do it. The child has to suffer the pain and discomfort of the operation and the unpleasantness of the anæsthetic. If the technique is faulty and there are any of the unfortunate results described by Denis Browne, which have been seen by most other pædiatricians, then it is the child who is the sufferer and no one else.

I cannot agree with Benjamin Spock, who wrote: "I think that circumcision is a good idea, especially if most of the boys in the neighbourhood are circumcised: then a boy feels regular."

It is commonly stated that cancer of the penis is confined to uncircumcised men, and that cancer of the cervix is more common in wives of those who have not been circumcised. Investigation has shown that the statements are incorrect.[4,9,10,12,16] Preston,[22] and Cook and Burkitt[3] showed that there is a marked geographical pattern of carcinoma of the penis in non-circumcision areas; the high risk in some areas is lost when the tribes move to low frequency areas—unlike carcinoma of the œsophagus, in which migrant groups carry the high risk with them. They wrote that there is no association in Africa between carcinoma of the penis and carcinoma of the cervix; in parts of Africa carcinoma of the penis is virtually unknown, while carcinoma of the cervix is exceedingly common. The world's highest incidence of penile carcinoma is in the circumcised men of Java. The wives of the circumcised Ethiopians have an unusually high incidence of carcinoma of the cervix. Some ethnic groups who never practice circumcision have the lowest incidence of carcinoma of the cervix. The American National Cancer Institution found that smegma has no carcinogenetic action. Even if it had, if the penis is kept clean by daily washing, the smegma would not have an irritant action.

Other reasons which I have seen adduced for circumcision include the prevention of venereal disease and the reduction of sexual desire.

It used to be performed to make men better warriors, to make men more chaste husbands, to increase their libido, to reduce masturbation, to give them longevity and increased physical vigour.

Some consider that the operation has to be done because the prepuce causes obstruction to the flow of urine. In the last 30,000 babies born in the Jessop Hospital at Sheffield, we have not seen one such case. Ballooning of the prepuce on micturition is normal and is certainly not an indication for circumcision. It is simply due to part of the foreskin lying in front of the meatus at the time of micturition.

After the first 5 or 6 months it may be found that a neglected chronic ammonia dermatitis has, as a result of secondary infection caused such severe scarring in the prepuce that retraction when he is older will be impossible. Circumcision is then indicated. Rarely a baby develops a balanitis (apart from that due to ammonia derma titis) and pus formation may occur behind the prepuce. Circumcision is then necessary to drain the infected parts. Recurrent paraphimosis may be another indication, but this is usually due to unwise and deter mined efforts on the part of the mother to retract the foreskin before separation of the prepuce from the glans is complete. Occasionally the orifice in the prepuce is so small that it is obvious that retraction will never be possible. Circumcision should be performed in such a case.

Finally, the Editor of the *Lancet* has given me permission to reproduce a letter from the late Sir James Spence[28] to a family doctor. "Your patient C.D. aetat 7 months, has the prepuce with which he was born. You ask me, with a note of persuasion in your question, if it should be excised. Am I to make this decision on scientific grounds, or am I to acquiesce to a ritual which took its origin at the behest of that arch-sanitarian Moses?

"If you can show good reason why a ritual designed to ease the penalties of concupiscence amidst the sand and flies of the Syrian deserts should be continued in this England of clean bed linen and lesser opportunity, I shall listen to your argument; but if you base your argument on anatomical faults, then I must refute it. The anatomists have never studied the form and evolution of the preputial orifice. They do not understand that nature does not intend it to be stretched and retracted in the Temple of the Welfare Centres or ritually removed in the precincts of the operating theatre. Retract the prepuce and you see a pinpoint opening, but draw it forward and you see a channel wide enough for all the purposes for which the infant needs the organ at that early age. What looks like a pinpoint at 7 months will become a wide channel of communication at seventeen.

"Nature is a possessive mistress, and whatever mistakes she makes about the structure of the less essential organs such as the brain and tomach, in which she is not much interested, you can be sure she nows best about the genital organs."

Paraphimosis

When a mother herself forcibly retracts a child's foreskin because f unwise advice given to her, she may find that she cannot restore it o its original place, so that œdema occurs (paraphimosis).

A doctor can usually reduce it immediately. The penis is grasped 1 the hand, and the fingers and thumb of the other hand squeeze and longate the glans in order to compress it under the constriction ring. he other hand eases the skin of the shaft over the glans. If this fails, ne ampoule of hyaluronidase (1,500 I.U.) is dissolved in 4 ml of 1 per ent. plain Xylocaine. It is injected into four sites round the clock into he œdematous ring, and the penis is then wrapped in gauze wrung out f iced water. In 10 minutes the swelling will have gone.[21]

Manipulation of the Penis—Erection

When a baby learns to grasp objects it is natural that he should rasp the penis and pull at it. No attempt should be made to stop it. It 1ay be seen in very young babies, and it is certainly common by a year r two. Usually there is no discoverable cause. It certainly should not ause any alarm.

Erection of the penis is commonly seen in babies. It is short 1sting, and is not connected with any stimulation of the glans. It has o significance.

Undescended Testes

It has been said that the commonest cause of undescended testes is old hands. Cold hands cause contraction of the cremaster muscles and he testes are then retracted.

Most surveys of the incidence of undescended testes are meaning-ess, because of observer errors. It is easy to conclude that testes re undescended when another more experienced doctor can readily ush them down into the scrotum. It is commonly stated that testes re undescended in 3 to 10 per cent. at birth, and in 0·1 to 0·2 per cent. n leaving school.

In a study of 4,500 Copenhagen boys[29], the testes were found to be ndescended in 1·8 per cent. of full term babies at birth, but in 17·2 er cent. of those prematurely born. At the age of 3 years the figure for 1ll term babies was 0·8 per cent., and that for premature babies 2·3 er cent. Three-quarters of those babies with undescended testes at irth had normally placed testes at one year. Scorer[25] studied 3,612 oys, and found that testes were undescended in 2·7 per cent. of full term babies and 21 per cent. of those prematurely born. By 9 months 89 per cent. had descended.

The prognosis for unilateral maldescent of the testis is not good It is useful to note that the scrotum is commonly undeveloped on th same side.

Complete undescent (usually associated with a malformed scrotum may be a manifestation of Klinefelter's syndrome, testicular agenesis pituitary dwarfism, and male intersex.

It is now a widespread practice to operate on undescended teste between the age of three to four. Hormone treatment is useless and potentially harmful.

There is no satisfactory evidence that maldescent predisposes to malignant change.

Labial Adhesions

The opposing epithelial surfaces of the labia minora may stic together without any union of deeper tissue. It is harmless, but th mother's anxiety is allayed if 0·1 per cent. dienoestrol cream is applied the labia separate in 10 to 14 days. Alternatively the adhesions ma be separated by a probe and the labia then smeared with "Vaseline" so that they do not reunite.

Precocious Puberty

Precocious puberty may occur in the pre-school child. In boys i is likely to be due to a tumour involving the hypothalamus, adrenal, o testes. In girls, the condition is usually a physiological variant and no due to disease. I have discussed the causes of delayed and early pubert elsewhere.[11]

A child with this condition should always be seen by an expert.

References

1. BOLANDE, R. P. (1969). "Ritualistic Surgery—Circumcision and Tonsillectomy." New Engl. J. Med., 280, 591.
2. BROWNE, D. (1950). "Fate of the Foreskin." Brit. med. J., 1, 181.
3. Cook, P. J., Burkitt, D. P. (1971). "Cancer in Africa." Brit. Med. Bull., 27, 14
4. FOLEY, J. M. (1961). "The Male Prepuce." J. Amer. med. Ass., 175, 118:
5. FREUD, P. (1947). "The Ulcerated Urethral Meatus in Male Children." J. Pediat., 31, 131.
6. GAIRDNER, D. (1949). "The Fate of the Foreskin." Brit. Med. J., 2, 1433.
7. GHALIOOUNGUI, P. (1963). Magic and Medical Science in Ancient Egypt. Londor Hodder and Stoughton.
8. GORDON, B. L. (1945). The Romance of Medicine. Philadelphia. Davis.
9. GREENBLATT, J., MORGAN, W. K. C. (1966). "Circumcision of the Newborn. Am. J. Dis. Ch., 111, 448.
10. HUTT, M. S. R., BURKITT, D. (1965). "Geographical Distribution of Cancer i East Africa: A New Clinicopathological Approach." Brit. Med. J., 2, 720.

ILLINGWORTH, R. S. (1971). *Common Symptoms of Disease in Children*. Blackwells. Oxford.

JONES, E. G., BRESLOW, L., MACDONALD, I. (1958). "A Study of Epidemiologic Factors in Cancer of the Uterine Cervix." *Am. J. Obst. and Gynec.*, **76,** 1.

KENNEDY, D. A. (1953). "Circumcision." *Lancet*, **2,** 734.

KENYATTA, JOMO (1956). *Facing Mount Kenya*. London. Secker & Warburg.

LEITCH, I. O. W. (1970). "Circumcision. A Continuing Enigma." *Australian Paed. J.*, **6,** 59.

LILIENFELD, A. M. (1965). "Circumcision." *J.A.M.A.*, **193,** 223.

MCCARTHY, D., DOUGLAS, J. W. B., MOGFORD, C. (1952). "Circumcision in a National Sample of 4-year-old Children." *Brit. med. J.*, **2,** 755.

MORGAN, W. K. C. (1965). "The Rape of the Phallus." *J.A.M.A.*, **193,** 223.

MORGAN, W. K. C. (1967). "Penile Plunder." *Australian Med. J.*, **1,** 1102.

MORRISON, J. (1967). "The Origins of the Practices of Circumcision and Subincision Among the Australian Aborigines." *Australian Med. J.*, **1,** 1125.

PENDER, B. W. T. (1958). "Paraphimosis." *Practitioner*, **180,** 628.

PRESTON, E. N. (1970). "Whither the Foreskin." *J.A.M.A.*, **213,** 1853.

SCHLOSSMAN, H. H. (1966). "Circumcision as Defence." *The Psychoanalytic Quarterly*, **35,** 340.

SCHOENFELD, C. G. (1966). "Psychoanalysis and Antisemitism." *Psychoanalytic Review*, **53,** 24.

SCORER, C. G. (1964). "The Descent of the Testes." *Arch. Dis. Childh.*, **38,** 605.

SMITH, C. (1951). *Physiology of the Newborn*. Springfield. Thomas.

SPENCE, J. WALTON, W. S., MILLER, F. J., COURT, S. D. (1954). *A Thousand Families in Newcatle-upon-Tyne*. London. Oxford Univ. Press.

SPENCE, J. C. (1950). In *Lancet* (1964), **2,** 902.

VILLUMSEN, A. L., ZACHAU-CHRISTIANSEN, B. (1966). "Spontaneous Alteration in Position of the Testes." *Arch. Dis. Childh.*, **41,** 198.

CHAPTER 9

PREVENTION OF THE COMMON
INFECTIOUS DISEASES

The Role of Quarantine

The term quarantine implies the restriction of movements of contac of a case of infectious disease for a period equal to the longest incuba tion period of that disease. This must be distinguished from su veillance, which implies the practice of observing contacts during tl incubation period without imposing restrictions on their movement It is now widely recognized that quarantine has proved an ineffectiv weapon in the prevention of infectious disease.

The wide difference of practice in countries abroad is shown by World Health Organization report.[23] For instance, in the case of rul ella, quarantine for 16 days was advised in France, while in Iowa an Pennsylvania quarantine is not advised at all. In the latter Stat mumps, chickenpox, and rubella are no longer notified or subject t quarantine.

It is a matter of opinion whether quarantining of contacts advisable in the case of poliomyelitis. The difficulty is the fact tha the relative importance of the different modes of spread of infection ar not known. Contacts of a case of poliomyelitis in the home are likely t harbour the organism in the nasopharynx and to excrete it in the stool and excretion in the stools may continue for some weeks—long afte the quarantine period has expired, so that isolation hardly seen rational.

In New York, quarantine for poliomyelitis is not practised.[23] O the other hand, knowing the frequency with which contacts harbou the organism in the nasopharnyx, there is something to be said for th quarantining of child contacts of a case in the home, and adult contac of such a case if they come into contact with other children. This wou! accord with the recommendations of the Ministry of Health that child contact should be isolated for 21 days. In other diseases, with th possible exception of smallpox, there is no case for the use of quarar tine. It is certain that in no other disease should contacts who hav themselves suffered from the disease be quarantined.

It is now widely recognized that quarantine achieves little, and tha in the past it led to a great deal of unnecessary absence from school. I seems much more sensible to tell parents when their child has been i

ntact with a case of infectious disease, to keep him under special
rveillance at the time when the disease is liable to develop (e.g. in the
se of mumps, any time after the twelfth day until about the twentieth
y after exposure). It is not necessary to take the temperature if the
ild is well. Unless he is unwell, he should be allowed normal activity,
ough friends should be warned that the child may be about to develop
 infectious disease.

An important point against quarantine is the fact that however
reful the precautions most children will acquire whooping cough and
easles unless immunized. By the age of 14 about 90 per cent. of school
ildren have had measles, 70 per cent. have had chickenpox and
hooping cough, and 50 per cent. have had rubella and mumps. In
y case there is much to be said for acquiring the infectious diseases
uring childhood. Mumps, for instance, rarely causes orchitis before
uberty, but it frequently does later. Rubella is well known to cause
rious anomalies in the fœtus if a woman acquires the infection in the
rst 3 months of pregnancy. Chickenpox, measles, rubella and other
fectious diseases are often more severe in adults than they are in
ildren.

The classical study of quarantine was that of R. E. Smith at Rugby.[18]
ver a 16 year period, 203 boys who had been exposed to infectious
isease were allowed back to school, and only one developed the
pected disease. There were no secondary cases. If strict quarantine
ad been imposed, 4,224 days would have been lost. If only the
sceptible boys had been quarantined, 2,123 days would have been
st.

Another fallacy in the practice of isolating children from a nursery
 other school lies in the fact that such children are likely to mix
ith the others at and around the home at play. In poor social
rcumstances with overcrowding, strict isolation is almost impossible
 achieve.

When a child acquires one of the acute infectious diseases, one has
 decide what policy to adopt with regard to isolating him from his
blings. Each case has to be decided on its merits. It should be
orne in mind that the most infectious period is probably the day or
vo before the rash develops in the case of the exanthemata, or before
e parotid swelling develops in the case of mumps, or before the signs
 poliomyelitis develop in the case of that disease; in other words,
 is likely to be too late to achieve anything by isolation. Isolation is apt
 lead to quite a lot of unpleasantness except in the case of older
ildren, because it is difficult to prevent younger ones going to the
edroom of a sibling. One should not normally try to prevent contact
etween an infectious child and his siblings.

The Duration of Infectivity

Table VIII shows the incubation period of the common infectic diseases, with the duration of infectivity. In the case of chickenpox, used to be held that a child was infectious until all scabs have separate

TABLE VIII

Incubation Period and Duration of Infectivity of Common Infectious Diseases

Disease	Incubation Period (Days)	Period of Infectivity
Chickenpox	15–18	1 day before rash to 6 days after start of ra
Diphtheria Scarlet fever	2–5	Till swabs negative.
Enteric group	7–21 (especially 14)	2 days before symptoms, till stools and uri negative.
Measles	10–15	5–6 days before rash till 5 days after tempe ture becomes normal.
Mumps	12–26 (especially 18)	2 days before swelling, till swelling has su sided.
Poliomyelitis	4–30 (especially 7–14)	3 days before symptoms start to 2 weeks af onset if temperature is normal.
Rubella	10–21 (especially 18)	1 day before rash till 2 days after start of ra
Whooping cough	7–10	2 days before start, 5 weeks after start.

A joint memorandum of the Ministry of Health and the Ministry Education considered that a child should be regarded as infectious f 14 days after the appearance of the rash, but one feels that there is need for such excessive caution. Elsewhere it is commonly thought th infectivity is absent 6 days after the appearance of the rash.

In the case of rubella, girls who have not had the infection should immunized against it; at least they should not be protected from co tact with it. The same applies to mumps in the case of boys.

The duration of infectivity of poliomyelitis may be longer than th mentioned in Table VIII, because the virus may be excreted in t stools for some weeks. It is felt that the chief periods of infectivity a the day or two before onset of symptoms and the 7 to 10 days after.

Infectivity within the Home

The infectivity of the common exanthemata varies considerabl The Newcastle Survey[19] found that 87 per cent. of those exposed hooping cough in the home acquired the infection. The corresponding gure for measles (in the first year of life) was 71 per cent., and for hickenpox 64 per cent. Measles is rare in the first 6 months. About 5 per cent. of contacts of chickenpox in the home will acquire the nfection, as compared with a figure of 20 per cent. of those exposed to numps.

Secondary cases of poliomyelitis in the home are common. When he first case is paralytic, three-quarters of contact cases are paralytic; when the first is nonparalytic, most contact cases are nonparalytic.

Pertussis, Diphtheria, Tetanus

Children should be protected against pertussis, diphtheria and etanus; immunization is usually given in the form of the triple vaccine ("DPT"). There are varied opinions as to the age at which the vaccine hould be given. A suggested scheme is outlined on p. 122. It is now known hat antibody formation is more effective if the first and second doses re separated by six to eight weeks, instead of the four weeks previously dvocated, and the second and third doses by a still longer interval. The factors against earlier immunization are interference with antibody ormation by passive antibodies from the mother, less effective antibody ormation by the child if the vaccine is given before about three months f age, and the fact that severe reaction to the pertussis component is ess common when the baby is older. The difficulty is the fact that almost ll deaths from pertussis occur in the first year, and the younger the hild, the higher is the mortality; children can acquire whooping cough within a week or two of birth.

If a dose of the triple vaccine is missed, the gap does not matter if it s not much greater than a year; the remaining doses are given in the usual way without starting again.

If a child has a febrile reaction with an injection of the triple vaccine, it is wise to give one-tenth of the dose next time, and to give spirin and an antihistamine drug (e.g. mepyramine maleate) half an our before the injection. Febrile convulsions are a rare complication of immunization, occurring in about 0·1 per cent. of children. If his occurs, I would not risk giving another injection of the vaccine.

Encephalitis is a rare complication of any immunization procedure. There was no case in 50,000 immunizations in the Medical Research Council trial of the whooping cough vaccine.

It is unwise to immunize the child when he has a cold. Mothers refer to wait until the child has recovered. The immunization may dd to the irritability caused by the cold. Any complication of the cold vould be ascribed to the immunization.

There is no agreement as to immunization of a child who is spastic mentally defective or who has fits. Some say that there is no increase risk of complications in such children if immunization is carried out i the usual way. It is probably wiser, however, to postpone immunizatio for a year and then to immunize for diphtheria and tetanus only starting with a tenth of the usual dose, and then two months late giving the remainder of the normal first dose, before proceeding with th remaining injections. The first dose should be preceded by aspirin an phenobarbitone. This is a counsel of caution, probably excessive. I hav given the triple vaccine to numerous children falling into the abov categories without untoward effect.

All children should be immunized against tetanus; they have fre quent falls and the danger of tetanus is ever present. Tetanus anti toxin is now no longer given for prophylaxis; it is no substitute fo proper wound toilet and antibiotic cover; antitoxin is not effective an there is always a risk of a serious reaction to it, even though one ha given a test dose. Furthermore, if tetanus antitoxin has been given, second dose subsequently would carry a much greater risk of anaphy laxis, and and in any case it would be ineffective because it is rapidl excreted.

If an injured child has been immunized with tetanus toxoid he i given a booster dose of toxoid only if he has not had a booster dos within the last three years, and the immunization was completed mor than three years ago; for children may have an adverse reaction t tetanus toxoid if there is already a high level of circulating anti toxin.[5,10,17,20]

Unless there is an injury there is no need to give booster doses c toxoid more frequently than every 10 years.[17] Reactions to toxoi include angioneurotic œdema, asthma, urticaria and the Arthu phenomenon. If an unimmunized child is injured, there must as alway be proper wound toilet and if necessary antibiotic cover; an active immunization should simultaneously be commenced an completed.

If a child has not been immunized against tetanus, the triple vaccin should not be given as a booster, for interference may lead to an unsatis factory response to the tetanus component, unless the mixture has bee preceded four weeks or more previously by tetanus toxoid.

Smallpox
Until recently, it has been the practice to vaccinate for smallpo during the first year. Owing to the publication of figures indicating th possibility that encephalitis was slightly more frequent in thos

vaccinated in the first year than in the second year, it is now advised that vaccination should be postponed until the second year.

It was shown in England that the risk of complication of vaccination in the first year was 1 in 18,000, as compared with an incidence of 1 in 40,000, if it was carried out in the second year. The corresponding figures in the United States were 1 in 7,000 and 1 in 23,000.[11,12]

There is a disagreement as to whether there should be universal vaccination in countries such a Britain, the United States and Scandinavia, where smallpox is rare, because of the fear that the small risk of complications of vaccination outweighs the risk of smallpox.[11,12,16] In the United States the last documented case of smallpox occurred in 1949, but since that date there have been 111 deaths from vaccination. In 1968 there were 572 confirmed complications of the vaccine, with 9 deaths. The mortality and morbidity resulting from vaccination is highest in infancy. The Department of Health and Social Security now no longer recommend universal vaccination in infancy in the U.K.

In order to decide whether vaccination in infancy should be universal, one would need to know the extent to which vaccination in infancy protects against encephalitis resulting from vaccination in later years, by comparing the incidence of encephalitis at various ages in previously vaccinated or unvaccinated persons.

Complications of vaccination include encephalitis, erythema multiforme, periarteritis, vaccinia gangrenosa, allergic and erythematous rashes, accidental secondary vaccination (especially of the eyelid), chronic progressive vaccinia, hyperthermia, thrombocytopenic purpura, myocarditis, periostitis.[1,6]

Vaccination is contraindicated in pregnancy, or for patients receiving corticosteroid or other immunosuppressants, or patients with hypogammaglobulinæmia. It is absolutely contraindicated for children with infantile eczema. Vaccination should not be performed if there has been immunization with any live virus in the previous three weeks. There have been reports of fœtal death as a result of vaccination during pregnancy; but in one study 65 placentas were examined after maternal vaccination[22] and no evidence of abnormality was found; there has been no increased incidence of stillbirths or abortions. Nevertheless, there is a risk and it should be avoided.

Vaccination should never be carried out on a baby with eczema, or who has had eczema in the past, even though there is now no sign of it. It would be unwise to vaccinate a child with any other significant rash at the time, such as a severe nappy rash. Vaccination should on no account be carried out on a sibling if there is a child in the house with eczema; the latter would be in grave danger of generalized vaccinia.

5

There is no doubt that children living in areas where smallpox is endemic should be vaccinated in infancy. In many countries it is the practice to vaccinate such babies in the newborn period.

Vaccination is performed either by a single linear scratch $\frac{1}{8}$ to $\frac{1}{4}$ inch long, or by multi-puncture. Revaccination is performed at 5 years, 10 to 12 years, and two or three further times in adult life. A "take" consists of a vesicle one week after the vaccination. The so called "immediate" or "immune reaction" 48 hours after a second or subsequent vaccination is purely an allergic response to virus protein, dead or alive, and has nothing to do with immunity.

Poliomyelitis

All children should be immunized against poliomyelitis. The live oral vaccine is now the only vaccine used. It is given in 3 doses each of 3 drops at 3 months, 5 months and 11 months, along with the DPT vaccine, with a booster at 5 years and 15 to 19 years. The vaccine must not be given within 3 weeks of smallpox vaccination, or when the child has diarrhœa or other illnesses. Tonsillectomy should not be performed at the time.

Measles

Passive immunization is achieved best by gamma globulin. The dose depends on whether complete prevention is desired or merely an attenuated attack. If complete prevention is achieved, no active immunity is developed by the child. If the child has an attenuated attack he develops full immunity to the disease. Normally, therefore, it is desirable to give a child a modified attack. The dose recommended is as follows:

	Dose in Milligrams		
	Modification Desired	Prevention Desired	Prevention Essential
Age 6 to 23 months .	150–225	450	675
„ 24 „ 59 „ .	225–300	675	900

These doses must be given within 72 hours of the appearance of the rash in the primary infecting case. The danger of hepatitis as a result of gamma globulin is almost *nil*.

Active immunization against measles is now widely carried out. In an African study of 2,000 children immunized, 7 developed measles, and there were no deaths. Of 2,000 controls, 464 developed measles, and 25 died.

Dudgeon wrote in 1969[3] that in the previous four years 35 million doses of measles vaccine had been given in the United States and elsewhere. It confers approximately 98 per cent. immunity.

In countries where there is malnutrition, measles may carry a high mortality, and wherever possible, immunization should be carried out. In other countries high risk children should be immunized; those include children suffering from any chronic debilitating disease, and children in institutions. Otherwise the main indication is the prevention of post-measles encephalitis. This occurs in one in about 250 to 500 cases of measles; the incidence of encephalitis resulting from the measles vaccine is about 1 in 1 million. An even rarer complication is subacute sclerosing pan-encephalitis due to a slow virus.

Measles vaccine is contraindicated for children receiving cortico-steroids or other immunosuppressants, or those suffering from lymph-adenoma, leukæmia or hypogammaglobulinæmia. It should be avoided in pregnancy.[14]

Live attenuated measles vaccine is given in a single dose of 0.5 ml at 13 months. It should not be given at the same time as poliomyelitis vaccine. The killed measles vaccine is now no longer used. After the measles vaccine, 5 to 10 per cent. have elevated temperature and some malaise. There may be a slight rash. A febrile convulsion occurs in approximately 2 per 1000, as compared with a figure of about 7 per 1000 in unvaccinated children developing measles.

Rubella

In Britain rubella vaccine is given to girls aged 10 to 14 years—preferably only if they have no circulating antibodies to rubella.[4] It is inadequate to rely on a history of rubella.[13] In one study of 275 women aged 15 to 56, 92 per cent. of those giving a history of rubella had a significant antibody level, but 50 per cent. of those not giving a history of it had antibodies; but the important finding was the fact that 7 of 38 (18 per cent.) with no antibodies reported that they had had rubella. In the United States the vaccine is given to girls and boys between 1 and 12 years of age.[8] Boys are included in the programme in order to reduce the pool of infection. We do not know how long active immunity will persist, so that the danger of immunizing early is the possibility that immunity will be lost by women in early adult life. The vaccine is reconstituted with 0.5 ml of diluent and must be given subcutaneously within an hour of mixing.

Side effects are few.[9,15] There is occasionally an elevation of temperature, rash, mild respiratory symptoms, lymph node enlargement, arthritis, or paræsthesiæ 10 to 28 days after vaccination. Kilroy *et al.*[7] described 32 cases of pain and paræsthesiæ in the wrists, hands and knee following an immunization campaign. They ascribed it to a transient polyneuropathy.

Contraindications to rubella immunization are corticosteroid or other immunosuppressant treatment, leukæmia, lymphadenoma, hypogammaglobulinæmia or pregnancy.

An Immunization Scheme.

There is no universally agreed immunization scheme. The following accords with[2] recommendations of the Department of Health and Social Security.

3 months	Diphtheria, pertussis, tetanus(DPT), poliomyelitis.			
5 months	„	„	„	„
11 months	„	„	„	„
13 months	Measles			
5 years	Diphtheria, tetanus, poliomyelitis.			
10–13 years	B.C.G. (if tuberculin negative)			
15–19 years	Poliomyelitis, tetanus.			

Allow three to four weeks between any two live vaccines, or between DPT and a live vaccine other than poliomyelitis.

Infective Hepatitis

Gamma globulin gives some protection. The dose recommended is 0·04 ml. per kg. intramuscularly within 7 days of exposure. It reduces the severity of the attack, but may not prevent one.

Tuberculosis

Though the usual measures for the prevention of tuberculosis are essential, there is much to be said for the protection of young children against tuberculosis by the use of the B.C.G. vaccine. It should certainly be given to the infant or child of any person who has had tuberculosis in the past, even though it is stated to be inactive. It should certainly be given if the child is known to be going to come into contact with any such person, whether a relative or not.

In Britain all school children have a tuberculin test at the age of 10 to 12 years, and negative reactors are given B.C.G. vaccination.

It is recommended that B.C.G. vaccination should be separated from other immunization procedures.

Cholera, Typhoid and Paratyphoid

This vaccine is administered to children about to live in certain countries abroad, or those about to travel there.

It is now recognized that immunization against paratyphoid A and B is unsatisfactory. For a child about to travel abroad on holiday 0·1 ml of typhoid vaccine is given intradermally, with a second dose four to six weeks later. It is wise to avoid giving a booster dose sooner than three years later, because more frequent doses increase the risk of reactions.[21]

Rheumatic Fever

When a child is found by throat swab to have a streptococcal tonsillitis, he should be given penicillin for 10 days, partly to prevent rheumatic fever.

When a child has had rheumatic fever, he should be given penicillin (200,000 units twice a day) continuously until well into adolescence. It is known that this greatly reduces the relapse rate.

Colds and Sore Throats

We know of no way of preventing colds. Vaccines so far have not proved effective. Vitamins and ultra-violet light are of no value.

Not more than half of all sore throats with tonsillitis are streptococcal in origin. If they are streptococcal, frequently recurrent attacks can often be prevented by giving continuous pencillin prophylaxis by mouth (200,000 units twice a day). This should certainly be given to a child who has had acute nephritis, until the urinary findings have returned to normal, and to a child who has had rheumatic fever.

Immunization Record Cards

Mothers of children who have been immunized should be given an immunization record card, and told to have it filled in when immunization is carried out. Mothers should also be instructed to show the card to the doctor if the child is injured, so that tetanus antitoxin will not be given in error instead of the much safer tetanus toxoid.

References

1. DICK, G. (1969). "Immunisation of Children Against Virus Disease." *Brit. J. Hosp. Med.*, **2**, 463
2. *Drug and Therapeutics Bulletin* (1969). "The New Immunisation Schedule." **7**, 85.
3. DUDGEON, J. A. (1969). "Measles Vaccine." *Brit. Med. Bull.*, **25**, 153.
4. DUDGEON, J. A. (1969). "Rubella Vaccine." *Brit. Med. Bull.*, **25**, 159.
5. EDSALL, G., ELLIOTT, M. W., PEEBLES, T. C., LEVISE, L., ELDRED M. D. (1967). "Excessive Use of Tetanus Toxoid Boosters." *J. Am. Med. Ass.*, **202**, 17.
6. HALLETT, P. (1969). "Complications of Smallpox Vaccination." *M. J. Australia*, **1**, 898.
7. KILROY, A. W., SCHAFFNER, W., FLEET, W. F., LEFKOWITZ, L. B., KARZON, D. T., FENICHEL, G. M. (1970). "Two Syndromes Following Rubella Immunisation." *J. Am. Med. Ass.*, **214**, 2287.
8. KRUGMAN, S. (1971). "Present Status of Measles and Rubella Immunization in the United States; A Medical Progress Report." *J. Pediat.*, **78**, 1.

9. LAMBERT, H. P. (1971). "Rubella Immunisation." *Practitioner.*, **206,** 467.
10. *Lancet.* (1967). "Tetanus Toxoid." Leading Article. **2, 662.**
11. LANE, J. M., RUBEN, F. L., NEFF, J. M., MILLER, J. D. (1969). "Complications of Smallpox Vaccination 1968." *New Engl. J. Med.*, **281,** 1201.
12. LANE, J. M., MILLER. J. D. (1969). "Routine Child Vaccination against Smallpox Reconsidered." *New Engl. J. Med.*, **281,** 1220.
13. LERMAN, S. J., LERMAN L. M., NANKERVIS, G. A., GOLD, E. (1971). "Accuracy of Rubella History." *Ann. Int. Med.*, **74,** 97.
14. *Measles Vaccine Committee.* (*M.R.C.*) (1971). "Vaccination against Measles." *Practitioner*, **206,** 458.
15. MEYER, H. M., PARKMAN, P. D. (1971). "Rubella Vaccine." *J. Am. Med. Ass.*, **215,** 613.
16. NEFF, J. M., LANE, J. M., PERT, J. H., MOORE, R., MILLAR, J. D., HENDERSON, S. A. (1967). "Complications of Smallpox Vaccination." *New. Engl. J. Med.*, **276,** 125.
17. PEEBLES, T. C., LEVINE, L., ELDRED, M. C., EDSALL G., (1969). "Tetanus Toxoid Emergency Boosters." *N. Engl. J. Med.*, **280,** 575.
18. SMITH, R. E. (1963). "Quarantine." *Brit. med. J.*, **2,** 374.
19. SPENCE, J., WALTON, W. S., MILLER, F. J. W., COURT, S. D. M. (1954). *A Thousand Families in Newcastle-upon-Tyne.* London. Oxford Univ. Press.
20. STEIGMAN, A. J. (1968). "Abuse of Tetanus Toxoid." *J. Pediat.*, **72,** 753.
21. WALKER, J. H. (1971). "Typhoid and Paratyphoid Immunisation." *Practitioner*, **206,** 478.
22. WENTWORTH, P. (1966). "Studies on Placentæ and Infants from Women Vaccinated for Smallpox during Pregnancy." *J. Clin. Path.*, **19,** 328.
23. World Health Organization (1959). "Communicable Diseases in School." *A Survey of Recent Legislation*, **10,** 193.

CHAPTER 10

MISCELLANEOUS PHYSICAL CONDITIONS

Snuffles

A nasal discharge, other than that associated with coryza, or following a spell of crying, is common in young babies. The problem has been well reviewed by Apley, Laurence and MacMath.[2] They studied 99 babies with snuffles in the new-born period, and observed them until the discharge cleared up. In most of them it began between the age of 2 and 12 weeks. The discharge was usually serous, but in some it was purulent or serosanguineous. None were due to syphilis. In most of them there was no evidence of infection. In only a few was there any evidence of allergy, and there was no seasonal variation. Cultures of nasal swabs failed to grow pathogenic organisms. They suggest that some babies have a larger than usual amount of mucus in the nose, without any apparent reason, and that this is responsible for the "snuffles." The condition was not responsible for any other symptoms of note. It may be concluded that in the young baby snuffles, in the absence of coryza, is of little significance.

Depressed Bridge of Nose

Depression of the bridge of the nose is a feature of many normal children, and may be familial. It should not arouse the suspicion of congenital syphilis. It is a common feature of achondroplasia.

Impatency of the Nasolachrymal Duct

Incomplete patency of the nasolachrymal duct in young babies is so common that it can hardly be regarded as an abnormality. Most babies do not produce tears till about the age of 3 weeks, though there is considerable variation in this. When tears are produced and the duct is not patent, epiphora occurs and the eye may become infected (dacryocystis or conjunctivitis). For some months after birth epiphora is apt to occur when the child has a cold, presumably as a result of swelling of the nasal mucosa and consequent obstruction of the ostium of the duct.

There is a difference of opinion about the treatment of this condition. Many ophthalmologists advise that the duct should be probed as soon as the condition is diagnosed before secondary changes in the mucosa occur from chronic or repeated infection. It should be noted that ophthalmologists are apt to see the severe cases only, the mild cases of epiphora never reaching them. Others strongly advise conservative treatment. Kendig and Guerry[23a] advised that no probing should be carried out for 6 months, any infection which occurs being controlled by massage upwards over the duct and the use of penicillin ointment three times a day (1,000 units per gram of ointment). Many ophthalmologists advise that the child should be observed for a full year before operative treatment is carried out. The vast majority treated in this way clear spontaneously.

I prefer to leave these cases for at least 6 months in the hope that they will cure themselves, as the great majority do. I have not yet had to refer a baby to the ophthalmologist for probing of the duct. Probing necessitates the use of a general anæsthetic. I have seen one death from post-anæsthetic pneumonia after an operation for this condition. In my opinion the condition would have cured itself if only the child had been left alone.

Absence of Tears

Some normal babies do not produce tears for some months after birth. It was found that 13 per cent. of 1,250 full term infants produced tears within 5 days of birth.[30] It must be borne in mind that in the rare condition termed familial dysautonomia (Riley's syndrome) there is an absence of tears, in association with excessive salivation and drooling, severe pulmonary infection and various other manifestations.

Puffiness of the Eyelids

Puffiness of the eyelids may be merely the result of crying. It is sometimes noted when a baby wakes up after a sleep. It may be a sensitivity reaction to aspirin, or be due to rubbing of the eyes when they itch with hay fever, or angioneurotic œdema, nephritis or even infections near the eyes.

Blue Sclerotics

Sclerotics in babies for the first few months are often notably blue. This should not lead one to diagnose osteopetrosis, or osteogenesis imperfecta.

Retinal Hæmorrhages in New-born Babies

These are said to occur in about 20 per cent. of normal new-born babies. They are not related to other hæmorrhages in the new-born period.

Brushfield's Spots

Brushfield's spots, the depigmented areas in the iris, are by no means specific for mongolism. They were found in 18 per cent. of 95 clear eyed normal children and in 1·8 per cent. of normal dark eyed children.[35]

Squint

Infants in the first few weeks of life commonly show slight degrees of strabismus, but it disappears by the age of 5 or 6 months. If strabismus is noted after the age of 6 months, the baby should be examined and treated by an ophthalmologist. It is a common mistake to postpone treatment till later, thereby delaying the resolution of the squint, and so causing blindness in the squinting eye.

A fixed squint should be referred to the ophthalmologist long before six months; it is always pathological and one important cause is a retinoblastoma.

Epicanthic folds give an impression of a convergent squint. When one eye is covered, and the cover is removed, there should be no movement of the eye. Eye movements in all directions are normal.

Setting Sun Sign

By the term "setting sun sign" one refers to the sign commonly found in infants with hydrocephalus. The white sclerotic is seen above the pupil without the eyelid having been retracted.

One commonly sees the sclerotic above the pupil in normal infants.

Transitory Fever of the New-born ("Dehydration Fever")

By transitory fever of the new-born is meant a sudden rise of temperature, especially on the third or fourth day, with an equally rapid subsidence of the temperature within 12–13 hours or less, in a baby who is otherwise well and free from infection. The fever hardly ever lasts beyond the fifth day. The maximum temperature is usually 100°–102° (37·8°–38·9°C). The child may be apparently unaffected or be a little sleepy and lethargic. The fever corresponds with the lowest point of the weight curve, after the loss of weight characteristic of the new-born period. It is probably related to dehydration.

It will probably never be recognized unless routine temperatures are taken. Treatment consists of giving boiled water.

Temperature Variations after the New-born Period

Pædiatricians are sometimes faced with the problem of the child who appears to be perfectly well but has been found to have a slightly raised axillary or sublingual temperature (99°–99·8°F) (37·2°–37·7°C). When a careful history has been taken and a thorough examination has been performed, the finding has to be checked by personal observation.

One then has to do various special investigations, including the tuber
culin reaction, x-ray of the chest, blood sedimentation rate, red and
white cell count, culture of the urine, culture of the stools for patho
genic organisms, and agglutinations for brucellosis and other infections
All investigations are usually completely negative, and one is safe in
telling the mother to stop taking his temperature. The boy is then seen
at intervals to check progress and to weigh him.

The cause of this abnormality is not known. It seems that for som
children the "normal" temperature is a little above the usual figure o
98·4°F (37°C). Van der Bogert and Moravec[6] discussed the temperatur
variations in normal children. They conducted a series of experiment
to show the effect of excitement and exertion in causing a rise of tem
perature. They concluded that oral readings slightly above 99°F and
rectal readings over 100°F need not in the absence of other findings b
considered to be evidence of disease.

The various fallacies in temperature recording were fully set ou
in Talbot's monograph.[36] He showed the differences in temperature in
different parts of the body (e.g. trunk, face, extremities), the relation
of the skin temperature to the environment, the rise of temperatur
after exertion and other factors. Talbot stated that the rectal tem
perature varies with the depth to which the thermometer is inserted
It should be inserted 5 cm in infants. He mentioned the well-know
effect of hot and cold drinks on the oral temperature.

Heart Murmurs in the New-born Period

Routine examination of new-born babies sometimes reveals
precordial murmur, which naturally suggests the possibility of con
genital heart disease. In the majority the murmur is heard all over th
precordium, but it is usually loudest at the apex or in the third lef
space close to the sternum.

In about 85 per cent. of cases the murmers disappear—in abou
half by the third or fourth day. In some babies no murmur is heard o
the first day, but a murmur is heard in the following week or two
Richards et al.[32] found that murmurs heard at birth carry a 1 in 1
chance of being due to congenital heart disease. The chance was in
creased to 1 in 3 if it was heard again at 6 months. When a murmur i
first heard at 6 months and it persists till 12 months, the chance of it
being organic is 1 in 7. When a murmur is first heard at 12 months, th
chance of it being organic is 1 in 50.

Burnard[9] found that murmurs in the new-born are often related t
anoxia, and that they probably represent an increased flow through th
ductus arteriosus. When the temperature of the baby was reduced, th
murmur disappeared.

Venous Hum

A common source of confusion in ausculating a heart is a continuous nasal hum, passing right through systole into diastole, and therefore simulating the murmur of a patent ductus arteriosus. It is heard best in the erect position, and it decreases or disappears when the child lies down. It can be heard on both sides, and the point of maximum intensity is usually the supraclavicular region. It is accentuated on inspiration, and on turning the head to the opposite side, especially if the chin is raised. It is obliterated by compression of the jugular vein. It is distinguished from the murmur of a patent ductus arteriosus by the change in intensity on rotating the head, and by its diastolic accentuation. It is heard to some extent in 50 per cent. of children under the age of 9, and is of no significance.

Intracranial Bruits

Hughes and Todd[21] heard an intracranial bruit in 15 per cent. of children under 5 years of age suffering from common clinical conditions. The murmur was best heard in the temporal region, and in some it could only be heard when the child stopped breathing.

The importance of this observation lies in the fact that when an intracranial vascular anomaly is suspected, the finding of a bruit does not prove the presence of such an anomaly.

Respirations in the New-born Period

The average respiration rate in the first 2 weeks is about 45 per minute, but there are great individual variations. The rate under ordinary resting conditions may be as low as 20 per minute. I noted a respiration rate of over 150 per minute in a normal 3-month baby who was feeling pleased at the time.

Irregularity and periodicity of the respirations is common. If there is marked irregularity in the new-born period the baby should be given oxygen. This usually increases the breathing volume and restores regular respiratory rhythm.

A young baby in the first two or three months frequently grunts in breathing when asleep. Mothers are often worried by this and think that the baby has "catarrh" or some obstruction at the back of the throat. The noise is not that of a snore. It is possibly due to vibrations produced by the soft palate in respiration.

Hiccough is almost universal in young babies after a feed.

Sneezing is frequent in young babies and should not suggest that the child has acquired an upper respiratory tract infection.

The Blood Pressure

The mean blood pressure at birth was found to be 69. At 6 month it was 93.[19] The blood pressure was lower in premature babies and in full-term babies who were anoxic or who had been delivered by Cæsarean section.

The Pulse Rate

The average pulse rate on the first day is 123 to 126.[34] At the age of 2 months it is 130. At 6 or 12 months it is 113–127 per minute.

An uncommon condition in normal babies is sinus tachycardia resulting in a pulse rate of up to 200 per minute.[23] The baby is entirely well and there are no signs of heart failure. It may persist for years. No treatment is required.

Postmaturity

The importance of postmaturity lies in the heavy fœtal risk with which it is associated. Clifford[10] in his full review of the subject found that after 300 days of gestation in a primipara, the fœtal death rate is 1 in 10. In this section the problem is discussed only in so far as it affects the living baby. Clifford described three stages in the development of the features characteristic of the postmature child. In the first stage there is a loss of vernix, and the skin is dry and parchment like. The child looks old and worried, long and thin, with skin too big for the body, as if he has recently lost weight. The skin late peels. In the second stage there is a large quantity of meconium in the amniotic fluid, so that the skin is covered by meconium. In the third stage the nails are bright yellow, as a result of changes in the colour of the meconium.

The birth weight is not necessarily a large one. In one series 25·5 per cent. were under 7 lb. at birth, and 40 per cent. weighed between 7 and 8 lb.

Travel Sickness

Travel sickness is common in children. It occurs particularly on car and train journeys, and it causes considerable inconvenience to the parents. Sea-sickness is also common in small children. According to Bakwin it has been estimated that under severe condition only 20 per cent. of unacclimatized children will remain entirely free from sea-sickness. Sea-sickness is said to occur in dogs, cats, horses, monkeys and birds. Brooks* said that fish transported from the Galapagos Islands to the New York acquarium were sea-sick! The usual age at which travel sickness begins is the second o

* Quoted by Bakwin.[3]

hird year, but it may begin in the earliest infancy. The child becomes
)ale, quiet, looks unwell and then vomits. The excitement which is so
.ommon before a journey predisposes to it and may even cause vomiting
)efore the journey begins.

Glaser and McCance[16] have shown that hyoscine is the best drug
)r short periods: it can be given in the form of "Kwells" or "Ellan-
,ee." Antihistamines had some value, cyclizine ("Marzine") proving
omewhat better than an inert control substitute.

In my experience hyoscine, given in the form of "Kwells," is effec-
ive when given half an hour before a journey. A child of 7 takes
.alf a tablet, and a child of 3 to 7 a quarter of a tablet. Each tablet
ontains 0·0046 gr. of hyoscine hydrobromide. The Kwell should be
aken half an hour before the journey starts. The makers recommend
hat a quarter to a half of a tablet should be repeated every 6 hours, but
he child under 7 should not take more than $1\frac{1}{2}$ tablets in the 24 hours,
.nd the child over 7 should not take more than 3 tablets in that period.

On a boat, the child should lie down until the drug has taken effect,
.nd should then, if possible, get up and about.[16,17]

It is probable that a stuffy atmosphere and reading in the car
)redispose to sickness, and so they should be avoided. It has been
aid that the child should be encouraged to look forward rather than
hrough the side window.

When vomiting is threatening, the child's attention should be
mmediately distracted and if possible the car should be stopped so
hat he can have a walk before continuing the journey. Every effort
hould be made to avoid suggesting sickness by anything one says. When
ickness occurs there should be a minimum of fuss about it, for vomiting
eadily becomes an attention-seeking device. The less that is said
.bout it either before a journey or after an attack of vomiting the less
ikely he is to have trouble again.

Travel sickness is due to a disturbance of the vestibular system.
'sychological factors such as excitement play a part, so that condi-
ioning occurs (e.g. to the sight of the sea or to smells).

It is important not to suggest nausea by talking about the matter.

Edema of an Arm

Œdema of an arm often occurs in young babies in the first month
.f their life. The mother is dismayed when she picks her baby from
.is cot in the morning and finds that one arm is swollen, cold and
)erhaps blue. It is not due to the baby lying on the arm, for it may
)e found when he is lying on his back and when one knows that he has
)een on his back all night. It is more likely to occur in cold weather
han the hot. In a series of 25 cases[14] the attacks occurred in the winter

in 24. It occurs in the arm which has been uncovered by bedclothe
and not in the arm which has been under the blankets. It seems to b
due partly to posture and partly to cold, but the part played by eacl
is not clear. The œdema usually subsides in a few hours but occasion
ally it may last for a day or two. It may recur night after night. N
treatment is necessary.

Physiological Jaundice

It is not possible to give the exact frequency of physiologica
jaundice, neither would it help to make a precise statement on th
matter. At least 50 per cent. of all babies show it. It is detectable i
doubtful cases if the skin is pressed with a glass slide. Jaundice usuall
appears on the second to the third day and reaches a maximum by th
third or fourth day. Physiological jaundice usually disappears by th
end of the first week, but it may last longer. If it lasts beyond th
second week, serious doubts about the accuracy of the diagnosis shoul
be entertained. The colour of the urine and stools is unchanged
a feature which immediately eliminates neonatal hepatitis or othe
obstructive lesion. The liver and spleen are not enlarged. The jaun
dice is due to a combination or slight hæmolysis with immaturity o
the liver. There is an excess of bilirubin in the blood of every infant a
birth, and this reaches a peak on the second to the fourth day.

It should be remembered that prolonged physiological jaundice i
sometimes the first sign of hypothyroidism.

The Urine of the New-born Baby

It is commonly stated that the urine of new-born babies frequentl
contains albumin. Doxiadis[12] showed that this is not the case. Whe
urates are removed before the urine is heated it is found that there i
either no albumin at all or that there is a mere trace.

Haworth and McCredie[18] tested the urine of 50 normal mal
babies for reducing substances by paper chromatography, and foun
that 24 excreted either lactose, galactose, or xylose, or a combinatio
of these, at some time during the first 7 days.

About 1 in 10 babies do not pass any urine for the first 24 hours.

Red urine may be due to the child taking blackcurrant juice, or t
beeturia following the eating of beetroot. The red colour is due to th
pigment betanin; the colour changes to yellow on adding alkali an
returns to red on acidification.

Bleeding from the Bowel in Normal Children

Blood in the stool of a new-born baby is usually due either t
swallowed blood from the mother, or to hæmorrhagic disease of th

new-born. The same applies to vomited blood (hæmatemesis). The vomitus or stool is filtered, and a few drips of N/5 NaOH are added to the pink filtrate. If the colour remains pink, it is due to the baby's blood, because the baby's hæmoglobin is more resistant to alkali, but if the colour changes to yellow, it is the mother's blood.

Blood in the stool of a baby or older child may be due to the insertion of a thermometer into the rectum. This is a thoroughly undesirable procedure, and many cases of perforation of the rectum have been reported.[15]

In the case of older infants and young children, the commonest cause of blood in the stool is constipation, with or without an anal fissure. The stools are hard and the child feels pain on passing them.

A rare cause of melæna in a well child is milk allergy.

Melæna otherwise is associated with disease—such as dysentery, ulcerative colitis, intussusception, Meckel's diverticulum, and other rare conditions. It may be due to administration of aspirin. Purple or red stools may be due to rose hip syrup.

A Large Abdomen

After a child has begun to walk and until the age of about 3 the abdomen often seems to be unduly large, and this often worries the mother. As long as a simple physical examination reveals no abnormality, the large size of the abdomen should be ignored. It is normal.

Cold Injury

Mann and Elliott[25] drew attention to the condition termed "cold injury" in babies. The syndrome is manifested by the onset of lethargy, swelling of the extremities with œdema or sclerema, a deceptive facial erythema, and often by hæmatemesis and pulmonary hæmorrhages. The skin temperature is found to be very low (e.g. 88°F). A series of 70 cases were described by a Birmingham team.[7] The children lose their appetite and pass little urine. There is a marked depletion of glycogen reserves and the blood sugar may drop to such a low level that convulsions occur.

The obvious cause of the condition is exposure to cold. It has been described in association with thyroid deficiency. It is frequently associated with infections and may sometimes be a response to an infection.

The treatment consists of very slow re-warming in a room with a temperature of 65° to 70°, fully clothed. Rapid re-warming is apt to cause convulsions and hyperthermia. The child is given a glucose drink to counteract the hypoglycæmia.

The mortality is probably about 26 per cent.

Bow-legs and Knock-knee

The normal bowing of the legs of the toddler nearly always rights itself without treatment. No treatment is ever needed if there is no more than half an inch separating the knees when the child is standing with the malleoli touching, and if there is no abnormal weight bearing, as shown by abnormal shoe wear. If there is doubt about the bow legs, the child should be seen again in three months, and if necessary an ortho-pædic opinion should be sought. Rickets should be considered in severe cases, as should the rare condition known as Blount's disease, a condition involving the proximal tibial metaphysis and epiphysis, with severe bowing. Rickets can be confirmed by x-ray and biochemical investiga-tions, and Blount's disease by x-ray.

The great majority of children with knock-knee cure themselves by six. It is normal for a toddler to have a gap of two to three inches between the malleoli when the knees are in contract. No orthopædic surgery is ever performed on these children below the age of eight, and it would be exceedingly rare unless there is abnormal weight bearing, as shown by abnormal shoe wear, and unless there is obvious organic disease.

Farrier and Lloyd Roberts[13] wrote that "On the evidence provided, there seems no justification for treating knock-knee in young children unless it can be shown that the outcome in treated patients followed for a comparable period of time is superior to that to be expected in un-treated patients". Not having found such evidence, they declared that attempts at surgical correction are contraindicated.

Knock-knee beginning at the age of seven or eight is a different condition. It is progressive and orthopædic surgery may be required at the age of eleven or twelve years.[33]

Flat Foot

A flat foot is normal in infancy and in the toddler, because the arch is filled with a fatty pad. This obscures the contour of the medial aspect of the longitudinal arch, and suggests that the foot is flat.[37] The fatty pad disappears when walking is learnt.

When a child first stands, the feet are spread apart and everted. By the end of the second year, the heel should show maximum wear on the outside of the midline. If there is pain in the foot, and the inner side of the heel shows wear, while the arch is poor when the child is on tip toes, then and then only should the heel be wedged by 3/16 of an inch.

Lloyd Roberts[24] wrote that if the foot is painless, capable of full movement and supported by muscles of normal power, the condition is normal and no treatment is required.

Asymmetrical Thigh Creases

Asymmetry of the thigh creases, though commonly found when there is dislocation of the hip, is not a reliable sign of that condition, for it is found in many normal babies. Palmen[29] found asymmetry of the thigh creases in 32·8 per cent. of 500 new-born babies; in 27·6 per cent. there were no folds at all; in 39·6 per cent. the folds were symmetrical.

Toeing In

When a young child turns his toes in when walking, the question of corrective measures arises. Nothing is done if it is found that there is a full range of ankle movements. The condition corrects itself.

Toe Walking

Toe walking occurs in some normal children, especially around the age of one or two. It may be a habit. The child can stand on his heel without difficulty, and ankle movements are full.

The organic causes of toe walking are the spastic form of cerebral palsy, congenital shortening of the tendo Achilles, muscular dystrophy, infantile autism and dystonia musculorm deformans.

Curly Toes

If toes are merely curly without overlapping, they are normal and require no treatment; but if toes overlap and in addition begin to cause soreness when shoes are worn, surgical treatment may be required. Strapping is useless.[33]

The Prevention of other Foot Deformities

An important step towards the prevention of foot deformities in later life is the provision of properly fitting shoes. Shoes should only be obtained from a good firm which measures the foot. It is essential to ensure that the feet are measured at frequent intervals, so that the shoes being worn are not allowed to become too tight. Owing to radiation hazards, x-ray apparatus should not be used in shops. Children's feet should be measured when they are standing, because the foot lengthens in that position.

Round-toe shoes tend to displace the terminal phalanx of the great toe towards the midline.

Single Palmar crease

It is wrong to suppose that the single transverse palmar crease denotes mongolism or other form of mental deficiency. It can occur in normal children. Davies[11] found that it was twice as common in boys as in girls. He found a single crease in 3·7 per cent. of 6299 newborn infants; 13·9 per cent. were small for dates; 8·6 per cent. weighed less than 2500 g; 3·3 per cent. had congenital anomalies.

Incurving Little Finger

Though usual in mongols, an incurving little finger is more often a feature of normal children.

Clicking Hip

Part of the routine examination of any baby or toddler includes testing for congenital dislocation of the hip, using the method described by Barlow[4] or others.

When testing the new-born baby, a click during the manœuvre may be felt and heard. Barlow wrote that a click may be due to (1) a flattened or oval sectioned ligamentum teres rotating under the femoral neck. (2) Tendons moving over each other in the region of the great trochanter. (3) An unduly lax hip. In the first two, the femoral head and the pelvis move together. If one holds the pelvis with a thumb over the symphysis and the fingers over the sacrum, and attempts to move the femoral head backwards and forwards on the side of the pelvis, in a normal hip it is found that the two move together; as the femur goes backwards so the pelvis rotates with it, and a click occurring during this manœuvre is of no importance. When the joint is lax, the manœuvre shows that the femoral head is moving backwards and forwards, but that the pelvis is not moving. Treatment for a lax hip is needed.

After 4 or 5 weeks, the main sign of dislocation of the hip is limited abduction with the hip flexed to 90°. The degree of abduction in normal babies depends on muscle tone; when the baby is somewhat hypertonic, abduction at the hip is less than usual, and dislocation may be suspected. An X-ray should be taken where there is doubt.

Hula Hoop Syndrome

Newman[27] and Zaidi[37] have described this syndrome, which consists of pain in the side of the neck and upper part of the abdomen, aggravated by movement. Pain in the chest may resemble pleurisy. There may be spasm and tenderness of the sternomastoid and trapezius, neck rigidity and spasm and guarding of the abdominal muscles.

Similar pains may follow over-indulgence in the "twist" and similar dances.

Stitch

According to Adolph Abrahams,[1] stitch is due to strain on peritoneal ligaments attached to the diaphragm. The pain usually disappears when the child lies down. It is more common on the right than the left. It is especially liable to occur when exercise is taken after a large meal.

Pigeon Chest

Some degree of forward angulation of the sternum may be regarded as normal and does not merit the term pigeon chest. The cause is uncertain. It is suggested that it is due to inadequate segmentation of the sternum in fœtal life, with resultant obliteration of the sternal sutures and forward angulation.[26] Others have suggested that the deformity is due to a congenital abnormality of the diaphragm.

Howard,[20] after studying 50 patients, distinguished primary and secondary pigeon chest. He thought that the primary type was genetic and related to funnel chest, which may affect other members of the family and may be due to the sternum being abnormally long in the anteroposterior or transverse diameter, giving certain diaphragmatic fibres sufficient mechanical advantages to produce sternal protrusion or depression. He thought that the secondary type was due to respiratory obstruction as in asthma, or to increased bulk of the thoracic contents, as in congenital heart disease or diaphragmatic hernia.

Funnel Chest (Pectus Excavatum)

The funnel chest consists of a longitudinal indentation in the lower part of the sternum. The cause is unknown. It may be due in some to shortness of the central tendon of the diaphragm. It has been ascribed in others to rickets or to respiratory obstruction. In severe cases the heart may be displaced, and the lung volume is decreased. It may cause embarrassment.

There is disagreement as to whether any children with pectus excavatum should be operated on.[22,28,31] Some advocate that surgery should be performed on the more severe cases at the age of eight to twelve, before the rib cage becomes relatively inelastic, partly for cosmetic reasons, and partly because it has been suggested that the deformity may reduce cardiovascular efficiency. Others[5] found that the incidence and nature of complaints arising from the deformity bear no correlation with the degree of funnel chest nor with the results of cardiopulmonary investigation, and have concluded that there is no definite indication for surgical intervention.

Harrison's Sulcus

Harrison's sulcus consists of depression of the sixth and seventh costal cartilage at the site of the attachment of the anterior part of the diaphragm. It was thought by Brodkin[8] to be due to abnormal contractions of the diaphragm during infancy, due to respiratory obstruction, when the chest wall is soft and yielding. It used to be ascribed to rickets.

References

1. ABRAHAMS, A. (1959). "Stitch in the Side." *Practitioner*, **182**, 771.
2. APLEY, J., LAURANCE, B., MACMATH, F. (1954). "Snuffles." *Lancet*, **2**, 1048.
3. BAKWIN, H. (1949). "Motion Sickness in Children." *J. Pediat.*, **35**, 390.
4. BARLOW, T. G. (1966). "Early Diagnosis and Treatment of Congenital Dislocation of the Hip in the Newborn." *Proc. Roy. Soc. Med.*, **59**, 1103.
5. BAY, V., FARTHMANN, E., NAEGELE, U. (1970). "Unoperated Funnel Chest in Middle and Advanced Age; Evaluation of Indications for Operation." *J. Pediat. Surgery*, **5**, 606.
6. BOGERT, F., MORAVEC, C. L. (1937). "Body Temperature Variations in Apparently Healthy Children." *J. Pediat.*, **10**, 466.
7. BOWER, B. D., JONES, L. F., WEEKS, M. M. (1960). "Cold Injury in the Newborn. A Study of 70 Cases." *Brit. med. J.*, **1**, 303.
8. BRODKIN, H. A. (1956). "Etiology and Mechanism of Harrison's Groove." *J. Amer. med. Ass.*, **161**, 1555.
9. BURNARD, E. D. (1959). "The Cardiac Murmur in Relation to Symptoms in the New-born." *Brit. med. J.*, **1**, 134.
10. CLIFFORD, S. H. (1954). "Postmaturity with Placental Dysfunction." *J. Pediat.*, **44**, 1.
11. DAVIES, P. A. (1966). "Sex and the Single Palmar Crease in Newborn Singletons." *Develop. Med. Child Neurol.*, **8**, 729.
12. DOXIADIS, S. A., GOLDFINCH, M. K., COLE, N. (1952). "Proteinuria in the Newborn." *Lancet*, **2**, 1242.
13. FARRIER, C. D., LLOYD ROBERTS, G. C. (1969). "The Natural History of Idiopathic Knock Knee in Children." *Practitioner*, **203**, 789.
14. FELDMAN, G. V., FORRESTER, R. M. (1955). "Swollen Arms in Infancy." *Brit. med. J.*, **2**, 722.
15. FONKALSRUD, E. W., CLATWORTHY, H. W. (1965). "Accidental Perforation of the Colon and Rectum in Newborn Infants." *New England J. Med.*, **272**, 1099.
16. GLASER, E. M., MCCANCE, R. A. (1959). "Effect of Drugs on Motion Sickness Produced by Short Exposures to Artificial Waves." *Lancet*, **1**, 853.
17. GLASER, E. M. (1959). "Prevention and Treatment of Motion Sickness." *Proc. roy. Soc. Med.*, **52**, 965.
18. HAWORTH, J. C., MCCREDIE, D. (1956). "Chromatographic Separation of Reducing Sugars in the Urine of New-born Babies." *Arch. Dis. Childhood*, **31**, 189.
19. HOLLAND, W. W., YOUNG, I. M. (1956). "Neonatal Blood Pressure in Relation to Maturity, Mode of Delivery and Condition at Birth." *Brit. med. J.*, **2**, 1331.
20. HOWARD, R. (1958). "Pigeon Chest." *Med. J. Aust.*, **2**, 664.
21. HUGHES, R., TODD, R. M. (1953). "Intracranial Bruits in Infants and Children." *Arch. Dis. Childhood*, **28**, 198.
22. JENSEN, N. K., SCHMIDT, W. R., GARAMELLA, J. J., LYNCH, M. F. (1970). "Pectus Excavatum. The How, When and Why of Surgical Correction." *J. Pediat. Surgery*, **5**, 4.
23. KEITH, J. D., ROWE, R. D., VLAD, P. (1958). "Heart Disease in Infancy and Childhood." *New York*. Macmillan.
23a. KENDIG, E. L., GUERRY, D. (1950). "The Incidence of Congenital Impotency of the Nasolachrymal Duct." *J. Pediat.*, **36**, 212.
24. LLOYD-ROBERTS, G. C. (1964). "Orthopaedic Problems in Childhood." *Practitioner*, **193**, 634.

25. MANN, T. P., ELLIOTT, R. I. K. (1957). "Cold Injury." *Lancet*, **1**, 229.
26. MARTIN, L. W., HELMSWORTH, J. A. (1962). "The Management of Congenital Deformities of the Sternum." *J. Amer. med. Ass.*, **179**, 82.
27. NEWMAN, J. O. (1958). "Hula Hoop Syndromes." *Brit. med. J.*, **2**, 1530.
28. ORZALESI, M. M., COOK, C. D. (1965). "Pulmonary Function in Children with Pectus Excavatum." *J. Pediat.*, **66**, 898.
29. PALMEN, K. (1961). "Preluxation of the Hip Joint." *Acta Pædiat Uppsala*, **50**, Suppl. 129.
30. PENBHARKKUL, S., KARELITZ, S. (1962). "Lachrymation in the Neonatal and Early Infancy Period of Premature and Full Term Infants." *J. Pediat.*, **61**, 859.
31. POLGAR, G., KOOP, C. E. (1963). "Pulmonary Function in Pectus Excavatum." *Pediatrics*, **32**, 209.
32. RICHARDS, M. R., SAMUELS, M. H., MERRITT, K. K., LANGMANN, A. G. (1955). "Frequency and Significance of Cardiac Murmurs in the First Year of Life." *Pediatrics*, **15**, 169.
33. SHARRARD, W. J. W. (1971). "Paediatric Orthopaedics and Fractures." Oxford. Blackwell Scientific Publications.
34. SMITH, C. A. (1959). *The Physiology of the New-born Infant.* Oxford. Blackwell.
35. SOLOMONS, G., ZELLWEGER, H., JAHNKE, P. G., OPITZ, E. (1965). "Four Common Signs in Mongolism." *Am. J. Dis. Childh.*, **110**, 46.
36. TALBOT, F. (1931). "Skin Temperatures in Children." *Am. J. Dis. Childh.*, **42**, 965.
37. ZAIDI, Z. H. (1959). "Hula Hoop Syndrome." *Canad. med. Ass. J.*, **80**, 715.

CHAPTER 11

TWINS

Twins and Superstition

Twins are always viewed with interest and in the past have been viewed with superstition. There was a wide-spread belief that they have a magic power over nature, and especially over rain and weather.[3] They are supposed to have other supernatural powers to predict the sex of an unborn child, to be immune from poisons of serpents and scorpions and to possess the ability to stop water boiling over from a pot.

Some cultures assume that no man can father more than one at a time and that the mother has, therefore, been unfaithful. Elsewhere, one or both twins are killed.

British Columbia Indians are said to fear twins, because it is thought that their wishes are always fulfilled so that they can harm those they dislike. Some Indian tribes think that they are transformed salmon and will not allow them to go near water, lest they are changed back to fish. In many countries they are thought to have the power to make good or bad weather.

In New Guinea it is thought that if a woman consumes two bananas growing from a single head, she would give birth to twins. The Guarani Indians of South America thought that a woman would become the mother of twins if she ate a double grain of millet.

Parents of twins are believed by the Baganda of Central Africa to be so fruitful that they can increase the fruitfulness of the plantain trees, which provide the staple food. They hold a ceremony to transmit the reproductive virtue to the plantains.

In New Guinea, when one dies, the survivor is given a wooden image of his sibling.[12,27] Twins are welcomed and placed in a special dwelling built by twin workmen. They must refrain from certain foods, such as the Iguana lizard. Twins are decorated with white beads.

Famous twins include Castor and Pollux, Jacob and Esau, Romulus and Remus, Viola and Sebastian and Tweedledum and Tweedledee.

Incidence

The incidence of twins in this country is approximately 1 in 87, that of triplets is 1 in 87^2 and that of quadruplets is 1 in $87.^3$

The incidence of twins varies from country to country, and in Western Nigeria 10·1 per cent. of all new-born infants are from multiple pregnancies.[22] In the United States, there is a higher incidence in negroes.[13] The incidence of twinning is particularly low in Japan. These differences are in the incidence of dizygotic twins, that of monozygotic twins remaining constant—3 per 1,000 maternities. Dizygotic twins are more frequent after the second pregnancy, and with advancing maternal age. Mothers of 35 to 40 are three times more likely to have twins than mothers under 20, and after the fifth birth they are five times more likely to have twins.[33] There is a higher incidence of dizygotic twinning in the lower classes. It is thought that the tendency to give birth to dizygotic twins is inherited mainly through the female, probably as a recessive.[26] There is a two or three times greater incidence of twinning in relatives of twins than in the normal population. In the case of monozygotic twins environmental and genetic factors appear to be unimportant. If a mother has a twin, there is a 3 to 10 times greater likelihood of further twin pregnancies than in the normal population, especially if the twins are dizygotic.

Twinning among sheep is more common if mating occurs in October.

Identical and nonidentical Twins

Mongozygotic twins must be of the same sex, with certain rare exceptions.[10,29] They have the same appearance, the same hair whorls, texture, distribution and colour, and the same colour of eyes, the same iris pattern, ear configuration, dental morphology,[22a] and closely similar weight and height. Two thirds of monozygotic twins have a common chorion. Monozygosity is proved by detailed examination of the blood groups (ABO, MNS, Rhesus, Duffy). The final proof is cross transplantation of tissue, but this is a test which is more theoretical than practical. Other features which have been used for diagnosis include dermal patterns, dental morphology, the retinal vascular pattern and the haptoglobin, phosphoglucomutase and transferrin systems. Examination of the placenta is not an acceptable method of distinguishing uniovular from binovular twins.[2]

Triplets are uniovular, binovular or triovular. The Dionne quintriplets were monozygotic.

If twins are of opposite sex, they are nearly always dizygotic; if they are enclosed in a single chorion, they are probably monozygotic whether or not they are monoamnionic or diamnionic. Seventy per cent. of monozygos twin pregnancies have monochorial placentas—and in these vascular anastomoses are common. They may be responsible for future differences in growth and development. If the twins are of the same sex and enclosed in separate chorions, no conclusion can be reached from examination of the placenta and membranes. It is wrong to assume that twins of the same sex with a single placenta are monozygotic.[6,9]

Birth Weight

McKeown and Record[25] found that the mean birth weight of twins was 2395 g (mean duration of gestation 262 days); that of triplets 1818 g (gestation 247 days); that of quadruplets 1395 g (mean duration of gestation 237 days). The largest known total weight of stillborn twins was 35 lb, 8 oz. Leonard[24] described live born twins weighing 8 lb 15 oz and 11 lb 7 oz respectively. Identical twins tend to be smaller than nonidentical ones.[16]

Pregnancy and Labour Difficulties

The perinatal mortality of monozygotic twins is eight times that of singletons and four times that of dizygotic twins. The mean length of gestation of monozygotic twins is less than that of dizygotic twins.

Twin pregnancies are associated with a sixteen times greater incidence of hydramnios than that found in single pregnancies, and with more toxæmia, placenta prævia, antepartum hæmorrhage, prolapse of the cord, abnormal presentation, premature labour and uterine inertia than single pregnancies, and this may be a factor in the relatively poor prognosis of twins.[8] Furthermore, the smaller of twins is more liable to hypoglycæmia in the newborn period, and this may be a factor responsible for the lower mean I.Q. of the smaller of twins. The differences in size of twins is probably related to the size of the placenta. Monochorionic twins are more likely to suffer fœtal growth retardation, discordance of birth weight and congenital malformations than same sex dichorionic and opposite sex twin pairs. The cause may lie in the abnormal process responsible for monochorionic twinning.[15]

In about 47 per cent. of twin pregnancies both are born by vertex delivery; in 37 per cent. one is born by breech, and in 8 per cent. both are breech.

The twin transfusion syndrome has been the subject of several papers. In this condition one twin bleeds into the other, so that one is born plethoric, and therefore liable to thrombosis, while the other is exsanguinated. Jacob and Esau were probably examples of this syndrome. Rausen et al.[30] found the syndrome 19 times in 130 monochorial twin pregnancies. They found that there may be persistent differences in the growth and development of the twins.

Prognosis

There is a higher incidence of mental subnormality and of cerebral palsy in twins.[3a,29] In institutions for mental defectives, there is often a relatively high incidence of twins. In a series of 651 children with cerebral palsy the incidence of twins was 8·4 per cent., and in 729 children with mental subnormality without cerebral palsy the incidence

twins was 3·8 per cent.[20]—the incidence of twins in the normal
population being 1·2 per cent. In other studies the incidence of twins in
cerebral palsy has been given as, 9, 10 and 10·4 per cent.[1,4,17,32]

The smaller of twins tends to have the lower level of intelligence,[21]
and to be relatively worse in verbal tests than in performance.[7] This
only applies to nonidentical twins. This presents severe psychological
problems in the less intelligence twin.

Because of the findings of various authors that the mean I.Q. of
twins was somewhat less than that of singletons, McKeown and his
colleagues[31] studied the mean verbal scores in the "11 plus" examination
of Birmingham multiple births. The mean score was 95·7 for 2164
twins, 91·6 for 33 triplets and 100·1 for 48,913 singletons. The low
score of twins was not explained by the mother's age, the birth order,
birth weight, duration of gestation, the delivery of the second twin or by
monozygosity. They suggested that the difference in the performance
of twins as compared with singletons was due more to postnatal environment than to prenatal factors. They then studied 148 twins whose
co-twins had been stillborn or who had died in the first four weeks; the
mean score was 98·8–compared with a score of 99·5 for singletons when
singletons were standardized for mother's age and the birth rank
distribution of twins. They therefore concluded that the low score of
twins, as indicated by poor verbal reasoning, was of postnatal origin
and was not due to prenatal factors.

Twins tend to be later than singletons in learning to speak. It is
argued by many that this is because twins learn each other's language
and understand each other, so that they do not communicate with
others. I think that it is much more likely that it is a developmental
matter which we do not understand; and that the mother of twins has
less time to read to them and talk to them than the mother of singletons.

Left handedness is more common in univular twins than in binovular
twins, and more common than in singletons.

Psychological Studies

None of the studies of monozygotic twins reared apart have been
entirely satisfactory. For instance, Shields[34] described 44 pairs of
monozygotic twins reared apart. All such studies are open to the
criticism that even if they are reared apart, a similar environment may
be chosen for them because they are twins, so that the effects of heredity
and environment cannot be separated. Erlenmeyer-Kimling and
Jarvik[11] reviewed 52 genetic studies carried out over 50 years in 8
countries, and including 1082 identical and 2052 nonidentical twin
pairs. The mean correlation in the score of nonidentical twins was
0·53; for identical twins reared together it was 0·87; for identical twins

reared apart it was 0·75; while for unrelated persons living together was 0·23. Burt[5] studied 53 pairs of identical twin school children reare apart, and found a correlation coefficient of 0·87.

If identical twins have a neurosis, it is more likely to be of tl anxiety neurosis type,[9] but there is no excess of neurosis or personali disorders in identical twins.[35] There is no difference between identic and nonidentical twins with regard to juvenile delinquency,[23] a fa which suggests that environmental factors are more important tha genetic ones, but in the case of adult crime there is a high concordan in identical twins. Twin studies have shown that there may be genetic predisposition in homosexuality.[18]

There have been numerous studies of the genetics of schizophr nia.[14,35] The identical twin of a patient with schizophrenia is 42 tim more likely to suffer from schizophrenia than the normal populatior the nonidentical twin is only 9 times more likely to have schizophreni. It is commonly thought that there are both genetic and environment factors in schizophrenia.

According to Zazzo,[37] twins tend to be unsociable, introverted an timid, especially when they are uniovular. They marry less often tha singletons.

It has been said[36] that the first born is likely to be more adu oriented, more likely to be the leader, to take responsibility, to t ambitious and aggressive, while the second born is more gay, cheerfu stubborn, lighthearted and gentle.

Burlingham[4] wrote that twinning may produce an overstrong bor between the two children and an accompanying weakness of relatior ship with the parents. They are more likely to be jealous of each oth than singletons, and the rivalry may be so severe that difficulties ari at school, so that they have to be separated. They decide always to wa the same thing so that neither can have an advantage over the othe Burlingham thought that it was unwise to dress them alike, to give the the same presents and to treat them as if they are one individual. The should be given the opportunity to go out alone with either the moth or father. They should be treated as individuals, though the clo relationship of the twins to each other should be preserved within reaso

It is important that one should emphasize the unique traits ar abilities of twins. They should be encouraged to develop apar Failure to manage them in this way may lead to serious emotional di turbances later, in adolescent or adult life, when they have to separat

Not only are twins likely to be jealous of each other, but the siblings are apt to be jealous of them, partly because others pay much attention to them, and partly because they take so much of the parents time.

For a fascinating account of the life of Siamese twins, the reader is ferred to the biography of Chang and Eng written by Hunter.[19]

References

. ALBERMAN, E. D. (1964). "Cerebral Palsy in Twins." *Guy's Hosp. Rep.*, **113**, 285.
. ALLEN, G., HARVALD, B., SHIELDS, J. (1967). "Measures of Twin Concordance." *Acta Genet. Basel*, **17**, 475.
. BABSON, S. G., KANGOS, J., YOUNG, N., BRAMHALL, J. L. (1964). "Growth and Development of Twins of Dissimilar Size at Birth." *Pediatrics*, **33**, 327.
. BERG, J. M., KIRMAN B. H. (1960) "The Mentally Defective Twin." *Brit. med. J.*, **1**, 1911.
. BURLINGHAM, D. (1952). *Twins*. London. Imago.
. BURT, C. (1966). "The Genetic Determination of Differences in Intelligence; A Study of Monozygotic Twins Reared Together and Apart." *Brit. J. Psychol.*, **57**, 137.
. CARTER, C. O. (1969). "Genetics in the Aetiology of Disease." *Lancet*, **1**, 1014.
. CHURCHILL, J. A. (1965). "The Relationship between Intelligence and Birthweight in Twins." *Neurology*, **15**, 341.
. DUNN, P. M. (1965). "Some Perinatal Observations on Twins." *Develop. Med. Child Neurol.*, **7**, 121.
. EDWARDS, J. H. (1968). "Multiple Pregnancy." *Proc. Roy. Soc. Med.*, **61**, 227.
. EDWARDS. J. H., DENT, T., KAHN J. (1966). "Monozygotic Twins of Different Sex." *J. Med. Genet.*, **3**, 117.
. ERLENMEYER-KIMLING, L., JARVIK, L. F. (1963). "Genetics and Intelligence." *Science*, **142**, 1477.
. FRAZER, J. G. (1933). *The Golden Bough*. London. Macmillan.
. GEDDA, L. (1961). *Twins in History and Science*. Springfield. Charles Thomas.
. GOTTESMAN, I. I., SHIELDS, J. (1966). "Schizophrenia in Twins; 16 Years' Consecutive Admissions to a Psychiatric Clinic." *Brit. J. Psychiat.*, **112**, 809.
. GRUENWALD, P. (1970). "Environmental Influences on Twins Apparent at Birth." *Biol. Neonat.*, **15**, 79.
. GUTTMACHER, A. F., KOHN, S. G. (1958). *Obstet. and Gynæc.*, **12**, 528.
. HENDERSON, J. L. (1961). *Cerebral Palsy in Childhood and Adolescence*. Edinburgh. Livingstone.
. HESTON, L. L. (1968). "Homosexuality in Twins." *Arch. Gen. Psychiat.* **18**, 149.
. HUNTER, N. (1964). *Duet for a Lifetime*. London. Michael Joseph.
. ILLINGWORTH, R. S., WOODS, G. E. (1960). "The Incidence of Twins in Cerebral Palsy and Mental Retardation." *Arch. Dis. Childhood*, **35**, 333.
. KAELBER, C. T. PUGH, T. (1969). "Influence of Intrauterine Relationships on the Intelligence of Twins." *N. Engl. J. Med.*, **280**, 1050.
. KNOX, G., MORLEY, D. (1960). "Twinning in Yoruba Women." *J. Obstet. Gynæc. Brit. Emp.*, **67**, 981.
A. KRAUS, B. S. (1957). "The Genetics of Human Dentition." *J. Forensic Sc.* Oct.
. LANGE, J. (1931). *Crime and Destiny*. London. Allen and Unwin.
. LEONARD, M. W. E. (1957). "Large Twins—Report of a Case." *Obstet. and Gynæc.*, **9**, 219.
. McKEOWN, T., RECORD, R. G. (1952). "Observations on Fœtal Growth in Multiple Pregnancy in Man." *J. Endocr.*, **8**, 386.
. NANCE, W. E. (1959). "Twins—An Introduction to Gemellology." *Medicine*, **38**, 403.
. NEWMAN, H. H. (1940). *Multiple Human Birth*. New York. Doubleday Doran.
. PENROSE, L. S. (1966). "Heredity, Environment and Mental Subnormality." *J. Ment. Subnormality*, **12**, 55.
. PENROSE. L. S. (1966) "Identical Twins of Different Sex." *J. Ment. Subnormality*, **12**, 56.

30. RAUSEN, A. R., SEKI, M., STRAUSS, L. (1965). "Twin Transfusion Syndrome" *J. Pediat.*, **66**, 613.
31. RECORD, R. G., McKEOWN, T., EDWARDS, J. H., (1970). "An Investigation the Difference in Measured Intelligence Between Twins and Single Births" *Annals of Human Genetics*, **34**, 11.
32. RUSSELL, E. M. (1961). "Cerebral Palsied Twins." *Arch. Dis. Childhood*, **36**, 32
33. SCHEINFELD, A. (1968). *Twins and Supertwins*. London. Chatto and Windus.
34. SHIELDS, J. (1962). *Monozygotic Twins*. London. Oxford Univ. Press.
35. SLATER, E. C. "Psychotic and Neurotic Illnesses in Twins." Spec. Rep. Se Med. Res. Coun. (Lond.) No. 279.
36. VERY, P. S., HINE, N. P. V. (1969). "The Effect of Birth Order Upon Personali Development of Twins." *J. Genet. Psychol.*, **114**, 93.
37. ZAZZO, R. (1960). *Les Jumeaux, Le Couple et la Personne*. Paris. Presses Unive sitaires de France.

CHAPTER 12

DEVELOPMENTAL TESTING

Introduction

pædiatric practice there are numerous common conditions which
se the question of whether a child's mental development is normal
abnormal. Every normal parent has a natural curiosity and interest
wanting to know whether his child is normal or not. There is all
e more reason for his interest if there has been a previous unfortunate
perience, such as the birth of a mentally or physically defective child,
if there has been some noxious influence in pregnancy, such as a
us infection or rhesus incompatibility. An odd facies or a peculiarity
the shape or size of the skull may raise the question of mental
ficiency. One of the commonest conditions which raises doubts
out a child's normality is retardation in one field of development,
ch as walking, talking or sphincter control. When a child suffers
m epilepsy or physical defects, such as hypothyroidism, it is parti-
larly important to assess his development. When he shows unusually
d and unco-operative behaviour one needs to assess his intelligence
order to decide whether the basic trouble is mental deficiency.
hen a child is examined for the purposes of adoption it is vital to be
le to express an opinion as to the likelihood that he is mentally
rmal, for it is a tragedy if he turns out to be mentally defective.
would be tragic for a baby if an incorrect diagnosis of mental re-
rdation were made on the basis of impression rather than thorough
velopmental assessment, for this might well mean that he is regarded
unsuitable for adoption, with consequent relegation to an institution.
l too often babies are passed for adoption without any developmental
amination at all. A great deal of anxiety and unhappiness is caused
an incorrect diagnosis of mental deficiency—a diagnosis which is
en too lightly made.

For practical purposes one does not want to know whether an
fant will at school age have an intelligence quotient of 100 or 105.
at can be only of academic interest. What one does want to know
whether a child is likely to be of average intelligence or not. It
uld certainly be of very great interest if one could predict the future
telligence more accurately, but it might not be of advantage to the
ild. Routine intelligence testing of any kind is undesirable because
uch more reliance is apt to be placed on the findings than the accuracy

of the tests warrants. They may well cause totally unnecessary anxie in the minds of parents.

The Prediction of Intelligence

There is a difference of opinion as to whether development studies in the first 3 years have any predictive value. It would see reasonable to suppose that if careful detailed observations were ma of the course of development of a sufficiently large number of babi record being made of the age at which various skills were learned, should be possible to establish some relationship between records obtained and their subsequent progress through childhood. Though is impossible to say what is "normal," there is no difficulty in defini the "average," and it should be easy to determine the sequence ai rate of growth in the average child and to note the frequency wi which deviations from the usual growth pattern occur as a result known or unknown factors. Having determined the development pattern of average children, it should be possible to determine wheth an individual child has developed as far as the average one of his ag taking into account all factors which might have affected his develo ment. By making further examinations at intervals in order to ass his rate of development, and by taking into account all possible factc in the child and his environment which might affect the future cou of his development, one ought to be able to make a reasonable pred tion of his future progress provided that one knows the frequency abnormal growth patterns. Arnold Gesell and his staff at the Y Clinic of Child Development made such studies for 40 years or mo and they were convinced that such prediction is in fact possible.

In 1930 Gesell[3] wrote that 10,000 infants had been examin by his staff, most of them at repeated intervals. Many thousands mc were examined subsequently. By following them up into later childho he was able to determine what reliance could be placed on the develc mental examination in the first 3 years for the prediction of futu development. He established norms by selecting children born a homogeneous group of apparently normal parents, chosen wi the aid of a careful socio-economic survey. All children were exclud who had a history of birth injury or other disease. He followed t children up in later years in order to make sure that no abnorn children had been included. The examination of the children was very full one and included every aspect of their behaviour, includi the development of locomotion, manipulation, feeding, play and soc behaviour, the development of speech and of sphincter control. I pointed out that with the aid of "norms" so established one c determine how far an individual child has developed in relation to I

;e. He said "attained growth is an indicator of past growth processes
id a foreteller of growth yet to be achieved." He emphasized the
awfulness" of growth, the constancy of the sequence of development,
iinting out that "where there is lawfulness there is potential predic-
in."* Having completed the developmental examination, he
en considered all the environmental factors and relevant personality
aits which might have affected his development in order that a fair
sessment can be made.

It is obvious to anyone that the great majority of infants do conform
ith their norms at various ages, and that on following them up
ey turn out to be normal children. It is equally obvious that when
fants lag seriously behind in all fields of development they grow
) to be mentally defective, unless there is an associated physical
indicap. When one goes back on the history of mentally defective
iildren, such as mongols, there is always a history of lateness in
:hieving the various skills described by Gesell, while in going back on
e history of normal children there is no such retardation. The only
:ception to this is the tragic mental deterioration which may result
)m encephalitis, meningitis or other cause, in a child who had pre-
ously been normal and had passed the milestones at the usual age.
is obvious to all that the mentally defective child throughout his first
years shows defective interest and concentration in his surroundings.
e is late not only in the more obvious aspects of development, such
locomotion and manipulation, but also in dropping the practice of
outhing objects and in ceasing to slobber. In infancy he shows a
:rsistence of primitive reflexes, such as the reciprocal kick, long after
e normal child has lost them.

It would indeed be surprising if some children did not show unusual
itterns of development. These deviations are responsible for much
the difficulty of developmental diagnosis. Gesell and his co-workers[3]
ive collected together some of these unusual patterns. They should
: studied by all who are interested in the diagnosis and prediction of
iormality." He described some children who were low average in
fancy and yet high in later childhood; children who showed a
ogressive retardation of developmental rate after being "normal" for
e first few weeks; children who showed a temporary developmental
rest and then developed normally; and children who were advanced
infancy and merely average in later years. It is particularly import-
it to draw attention to the occasional slow starter—the child who is
ther backward at first and later does very well. Such exceptions are
re but always have to be remembered.

Gesell drew particular attention to the various factors which

* *Psychology of Early Growth*, p. 224.

affect the course of development. These are discussed below. He wro¹
that in some cases presenting unusual patterns, or with physical defec
which alter the course of development, prognosis should be complete
withheld. In others the prognosis can only be built up cautious.
after repeated examinations. To use his words, "Diagnostic pruden¹
is required at every turn."*

Elsewhere[3] he wrote: "So utterly unforeseen are the vicissitud¹
of life that common sense will deter one from attempting to foreca
too precisely the developmental career even of a mediocre child."

Gesell considered that the prediction of mental superiority is
matter of considerable difficulty. One would have thought, in vie
of the retardation which occurs in all fields of development in mental
defective infants, that there would be corresponding acceleration abov
the average in children who are going to be mentally superior. Suc
in fact is not often the case. Gesell[2] wrote that such speeding up ma
be present in early infancy, presumably having begun *in utero*, an
that the whole cycle of development is accelerated. Much more ofter
however, the scorable end products are not far in advance of the a²
norms in early infancy, the child's superior quality being manifeste
in the manner of the performance of the tests, in his alertness, in tⁱ
intensification and diversification of behaviour, in the vividness an
vitality of his reactions. "He exploits his physical surroundings in
more varied manner. He is more sensitive and responsive to his soci¹
environment." Elsewhere[4] he described the superior infant as beir
"poised, self-contained, discriminating, mature. The total output ¹
behaviour for a day is more abundant, more complex, more subtle tha¹
that of a mediocre child."† He said that the acceleration becom¹
much more obvious in the second and third years, with the developme¹
of speech, comprehension and judgment. Gesell, like many others, sai
that consistent language acceleration before 2 years is one of the mo
frequent signs of superior intelligence. General motor ability an
neuromuscular maturity are not nearly as often advanced. Some ¹
these exceptional cases are described in detail in his *Biographies*
Child Development.[3]

After the period of infancy, the gifted child may show unusu²
imagination, notable powers of concentration, wide interests, a retentiⁱ
memory, precocity in speech and rapid learning. He may show a¹
unusual ability in describing things which he has seen, and in recoun
ing incidents and events. He may show striking creative ability in h²
drawings. Many such children learn to read at the age of 3 or .
Twenty per cent. of the gifted children in Terman's study[11, 12] learned ¹

* *Psychology of Early Growth*, p. 224.
† *Developmental Diagnosis*, p. 312.

:ad before 5; 6 per cent. learned before 4, and 2 per cent. before years of age.

'ivergent Views

There have been many studies concerning the predictive value of evelopmental tests, and the findings have differed widely. I have :viewed these in detail elsewhere.[6] Many workers, and especially 3ychologists, have concluded that developmental tests are of no value.)thers, and especially pædiatricians, have found that their value is onsiderable. I feel that the main reasons for the divergent views are s follows:

1. Psychologists have usually studied selected children with a ood level of intelligence, and have excluded mentally subnormal nes. Having found little correlation between test scores in infancy nd tests in later childhood, they have generalized and concluded that evelopmental tests on the whole range of levels of intelligence are of o value. Such generalization is impermissible.

2. Psychologists have almost always depended on purely objective :sts, in an effort to be really scientific. Pædiatricians, on the other and, have based their assessments on the whole child, and have taken ito consideration the previous history of the rate of development, and articularly of factors which might have affected the course of develop-1ent. They have paid great attention to important aspects of develop-1ent which it has proved impossible to translate into figures or scores— he child's responsiveness, alertness, concentration and interest in his urroundings. They have formed a clinical impression of these which as guided them in forming their conclusion. Psychologists have ended to rely on the readily scorable items, mainly involving motor evelopment. Unfortunately many of the most readily scorable items re the least important ones for developmental prediction, while those vhich cannot be scored at all are the most important. Arnold Gesell epeatedly emphasized the importance of these unscorable items.

Vhat We Can Do

The main value of developmental testing in infancy is the detection f mental subnormality and of neurological conditions such as cerebral 1alsy. Few pædiatricians, I imagine, would doubt that mental sub-1ormality can be diagnosed without much difficulty in the first few 1onths of life.

At the Children's Hospital, Sheffield, I followed up 135 children vho had been thought in their first year to be mentally subnormal. 3retins, mongols and hydrocephalics were excluded. They were ollowed up by school medical officers at school age. Thirty-four had lied, and in all 10 in which autopsy examinations were carried out,

gross defects of the brain were found. Of the 101 survivors, 59 were i
the ineducable class (IQ below 50), 24 had an IQ of 50 to 75, 13 had a
IQ of 76 to 94, and 5 had an IQ score of 100 or more. Three of thes
were known to be normal long before the first birthday, but they ha
to be included because the diagnosis of mental subnormality had bee
made. These figures supply good evidence that mental subnormalit
can be diagnosed satisfactorily in the first 2 years. Of those diagnose
in the first 6 months, 3 of the survivors had an IQ of 100 or more
these 3 are included in the 5 mentioned above.

In a different group of 230 infants at Sheffield, assessments fo
suitability for adoption were made, in the first year, mainly at the ag
of 6 months. They were graded when first seen into the following
categories.

(A) Possibly above average.
(B) Average.
(C) Doubtful.
(D) Retarded.

At school age IQ tests were carried out by psychologists who wer
unaware of my grading.

The table shows the mean IQ for each group at school in relatior
to the score in the first year.

| | Grade in First Year | | | |
	A	B	C	D
Total	69	92	54	15
Mean IQ at School	111·8	108·1	98·6	76·0

The table below shows the number of children with high or low IC
at school in relation to their grading in infancy.

Grade in First Year	A	B	C+D
IQ at School below 80	1 (1·5%)	1 (1·1%)	15 (21·7%)
over 120	14 (20·6%)	14 (15·2%)	1 (1·4%)

More important than the actual figures was the fact that only 2 c
161 children thought in the first year to be average or possibly bette

roved to have an IQ at school of less than 80. One of 69 children
iought to be doubtful or retarded fared better than expected, with an
Q of over 120.

I agree entirely with Ausubel's[1] comments that: "Developmental
orms are valuable because they provide a standard or frame of
ference for evaluating and interpreting the status or current behaviour
f an individual." Knobloch[7] wrote: "As clinicians we would feel that
n examination which would allow us to make the following statement
an eminently acceptable and useful tool. This infant has no neuro-
gic impairment, and his potential is within the healthy range:
epending on what his life experiences are between now and 6 years of
ge, he will at that time have a Stanford Binet IQ above 90, unless
ualitative changes in the central nervous system are caused by noxious
gents, or gross changes in milieu alter major variables of function."

Elsewhere[8] she wrote that "the main objective of the develop-
iental assessment is to identify the infant who has a significant neuro-
gic or intellectual deficit. It is *not* to identify the one who has function
ithin the normal range and will later be superior on the basis of an
nriched cultural environment. Mental subnormality due to patho-
gic conditions can be identified in infancy, the milder as well as the
rosser degrees of defect. The child with later sociocultural retardation
annot be so identified, since he is essentially normal in infancy."

I have no doubt myself that developmental tests in infancy are of
nmense value, if for no other reason than that they enable one to detect
iental subnormality, cerebral palsy and other neurological handicaps.

What We Cannot Do

We cannot assess a baby in the first month of life. We can detect
ertain abnormalities in that period: and we can detect cerebral palsy
f the spastic type if it is moderate or severe: but we cannot say whether
eurological signs in the new-born period will be permanent or not—
nless they are marked, in which case they are most unlikely to
isappear.

We cannot give an exact score for an infant's intelligence quotient.
nyone who does this reveals his ignorance of developmental testing.
ll we can do is to give a range into which the development fits.

We cannot predict, except occasionally from the family pattern
f development, that the child's development will accelerate, or that
eneral maturation is going to be slower than usual. To put it in another
ay, we cannot say in advance that the child is going to prove to have
een a slow starter.

We cannot usually predict environmental influences which will
etard a child's development.

We cannot predict illnesses and injuries which will retard develop ment. These include meningitis, encephalitis, hypoglycæmia and lea poisoning. We cannot usually predict development in a retarded chil who has fits.

We cannot predict the effect of opportunity, of bad health, or c personality, on the child's development. We cannot say what he wi do with the talents which he possesses.

We cannot usually diagnose mental superiority in infancy.

There are so many variables, and so many factors which affec a child's development, that the correlation between developmenta scores in infancy and future attainments never can be a high one That does not prove, however, that developmental tests are of no valu

The Prediction of Personality

It would be a matter of great interest if one could predict the futur personality of a child when he is yet an infant. One feels that one ca predict in infancy that a child will have average intelligence. But ther remains the serious possibility, as a result of the bad family backgroun which inevitably pertains in many children for whom adoption desired, that he may have a particularly unpleasant character, for is now almost universally accepted that personality and character ar products partly of heredity and partly of environment. Very fe agree with the "Behaviourists," who consider that character is entirel engendered by environment. Watson[13] wrote: "Give me a doze healthy infants, well formed, and my own specified world to bring the up in and I'll guarantee to take any one at random and train him t become any type of specialist I might select—doctor, lawyer, artis merchant, chief, and yes, even beggar man and thief, regardless of h talents, peculiarities, tendencies, abilities, vocations and race of h ancestors. There is no such thing as an inheritance of capacity, talent temperament, mental constitution and character." It is undeniabl that environment has a profound effect on character formatio but there can be no doubt that much of a child's basic character inherited from his parents.

In view of the profound effect of environment on character forma tion it seems almost inevitable that character prediction durin infancy is practically doomed to failure, though one might think tha some of the basic personality patterns might be present in infancy an persist into later life, even though moulded and modified by late environment. The obvious personality characteristics in infancy a discussed elsewhere. It is another matter to decide whether suc personality patterns persist into later life in spite of the impact c environment. Glover,[5] in the Foreword to Middlemore's book o

The Nursing Couple, wrote: "We have every reason to assume that within a week or so of birth infants manifest in a primitive form all the various types of response which form the basis of adult characterology. The book gives the strongest support to the view that what happens at the breast can really affect the infant all through his life." Shirley[9] found individual differences in behaviour in the 25 babies studied in the first 24 hours of their life. She wrote: "Each baby exhibits a characteristic pattern of personality trends that changes little with age."

The difficulty of furnishing scientific proof that personality traits can be predicted in infancy is obvious. The greatest difficulty of all is the fact that personality traits are largely unscorable. It is not surprising that the number of studies on the subject which are worth quoting is extremely small. Arnold Gesell[3] attempted to assess 15 character traits in the first year of life and to determine whether there would be any correlation with an independent assessment by another observer at the age of 5 years. The traits which were recorded were energy output, motor demeanour, self-dependence, social responsiveness, family attachment, communicativeness, adaptivity, exploitation of environment, humour sense, emotional maladjustment, emotional expressiveness, reaction to success, reaction to restriction, readiness of smiling and readiness of crying. There was a high degree of correlation. Shirley[10] wrote three volumes of detailed observations on 25 children who were observed by her from birth until the second birthday. Neilon[9] saw 15 of these at the age of 17, 15 years after Shirley's description had been written. She prepared new character sketches without reference to the original ones. Independent judges were then asked to try to match Neilon's 15 sketches with 19 sketches by Shirley. Ten sketches of boys were successfully matched by 5 judges, and 5 sketches of girls were matched by 10 judges. It was therefore proved that some of the important personality traits manifest in the first 2 years were also manifest in adolescent life.

It is obvious that the accurate prediction of character from the personality traits in infancy is of great difficulty. It is true that most intelligent parents of more than one child have little doubt that they could detect differences in the first few weeks of life in the personality of the second child from that of the first-born and that their original impressions were confirmed in later years. But it is one thing for parents with intimate knowledge of their own children to have an impression—which incidentally is probably correct—and another thing for an outside examiner with less knowledge of the child in question to furnish statistical proof that such prediction is possible. The most that one can hope to do is to predict the continuance into later life, whatever the

environment, of certain outstanding inborn character traits, such a'
independence of character, determination, placidity, ready smiling and
social responsiveness. One might certainly be guided by a study of the
character of the parents, but it is likely to be very difficult to forecas'
which traits the child has inherited from each parent, unless botl
parents have in common certain outstanding personality characteristics

For some reasons it is a good thing that personality prediction is so
difficult. From the point of view of adoption it would be a grea
pity if such prediction were possible. Parents who have been unable
to have children themselves certainly have a right to want to know
whether the child whom they are thinking of adopting is of norma
intelligence or not, but they must not expect to know in detail wha'
his personality will be like. All parents take a risk in having children
and do not even know whether they will be mentally normal or not
Those who are about to adopt children have to take a risk in the form
of the child's future character. If they are not willing to take that
risk they should not consider adoption. It is a serious tragedy for a
child to be considered unsuitable for adoption, for it means that he
is condemned to institutional life and the deprivation of a normal home
life, with all that that means to his future. It is a good thing that he
cannot be considered unsuitable for adoption on account of some
possible future personality traits.

References

1. AUSUBEL, D. P. (1958). *Theory and Problems of Child Development*. New York.
   Grune and Stratten.
2. GESELL, A. (1929). *Infancy and Human Growth*. New York. Macmillan.
3. GESELL, A., AMATRUDA, C. S., CASTNER, B. M., THOMPSON, H. (1930). *Biographies
   of Child Development*. London. Hamish Hamilton.
4. GESELL, A., AMATRUDA, C. S. (1947). *Developmental Diagnosis*. New York.
   Hoeber.
5. GLOVER, E., in Middlemore, M. P. (1941). *The Nursing Couple*. London. Hamish
   Hamilton.
6. ILLINGWORTH, R. S. (1966). *Development of the Infant and Young Child, Normal
   and Abnormal*. 3rd Edn. Edinburgh. Livingstone.
7. KNOBLOCH, H. (1959). "Pneumoencephalography and Clinical Behaviour."
   Pediatrics, **23**, 175.
8. KNOBLOCH, H., PASAMANICK, B. (1963). "Predicting Intellectual Potential in
   Infancy." *Am. J. Dis. Childh.*, **106**, 43.
9. NEILON, P. (1948). "Shirley's Babies after 15 Years. A Personality Study." *J.
   genet. Psychol.*, **73**, 175.
10. SHIRLEY, M. M. (1931). *The First Two Years of Life*. Minneapolis. Univ. of
    Minnesota Press.
11. TERMAN, L. M. (1926). *Genetic Studies of Genius*. London. George Harrap.
12. TERMAN, L. M., ODEN, M. H. (1947). *The Gifted Child Grows Up*. Stanford.
    Stanford University Press.
13. WATSON, J. B. (1925). *Behaviourism*. London. Kegan Paul.

CHAPTER 13

THE NORMAL COURSE OF DEVELOPMENT

The following is a brief account of the normal course of development in the first 3 years. It is inevitably based largely on the books and papers of Arnold Gesell, supplemented by those of Shirley,[17] Bühler[3,4] and others, and by my own experience. For further information the reader should consult these works, and particularly Arnold Gesell's books, *Developmental Diagnosis*,[10] *The First Five Years of Life*,[8] *Infant and Child in the Culture of To-day*,[9] *Feeding Behaviour of Infants*[7] and *Biographies of Child Development*.[6]

The Principles of Development

The chief principles of development may be summarized as follows:

(1) Development is a continuous process from conception to maturity. Development must not be thought of in terms of mere milestones. Before any "milestone" is reached a child has to go through many preceding stages of development, and in developmental diagnosis one has to be thoroughly conversant with all these stages. Diagnosis does not consist so much of observing *what* a child does but *how* he does it. For example, in a 7-month-old child one has to observe not whether he can sit, but how he sits, and with what degree of maturity he does it. Statistical studies almost invariably miss this. They record the fact that a child can sit, but fail to record the maturity which he has reached.

(2) Development depends on the maturation and myelination of the nervous system. Until that has occurred no amount of practice can make a child learn the relevant skill. When practice is denied, the ability to perform the skill lies dormant, but the skill is rapidly learnt as soon as an opportunity is given.

(3) The *sequence* of development is the same for all children, but the *rate* of development varies from child to child. For example, a child has to learn to sit before he can walk, but the age at which children learn to sit and walk varies considerably.

(4) Certain primitive reflexes anticipate corresponding voluntary movement and have to be lost before the voluntary movement develops. Examples are the walking reflex and the grasp reflex of the new-born

period. Another is the reciprocal kick—the rhythmic kicking of the legs, which disappears when walking begins. In mentally defective children these primitive reflexes are likely to persist beyond the usual age. It is common, for instance, to see a 2-year-old mentally defective child demonstrating the reciprocal kick.

(5) The direction of development is cephalocaudal. The first step in the development of locomotion, for instance, is the acquisition of head control, involving the neck muscles. Later the spinal muscles develop co-ordination so that the child is able to sit up with a straight back instead of a round one. The child can do much with his hands before he can use his legs. He can crawl, pulling himself forward with his arms, the legs trailing behind, before he can creep, a movement which involves the use of the legs.

(6) Generalized mass activity gives way to specific individual responses. The young baby, for example, shows pleasure by a massive general response. His eyes widen, his respirations increase, his legs kick and his arms move vigorously. The older child or adult shows his pleasure simply by facial expression or by appropriate words. The aimless movement of the arms and legs of the first 6 months are replaced by the specific movements of locomotion and manipulation.

The New-born Baby at Birth

For our knowledge of the neurological features and examination of the new-born baby, we are indebted particularly to Albrecht Peiper,[16] Heinz Prechtl,[16a] and André Thomas.[19] I have described the features more fully elsewhere.[12]

The full-term baby in the new-born period sleeps for the greater part of the 24 hours. He yawns, hiccoughs, sneezes, coughs, stretches and salivates. He can suck and swallow, and can smell, taste and hear. He lies on his side with his arms and legs flexed. In the prone position he lies with his knees drawn up under the abdomen with the pelvis high. His head is turned to one side. When held in ventral suspension (with one's hand under his abdomen), the head hangs down. There is some flexion of the elbows and knees.

He shows a variety of primitive reflexes. The important ones are as follows:

(1) The Moro reflex. This is seen when the baby is suddenly moved. Any sudden movement of the neck initiates the reflex. It consists of a rapid abduction and extension of the arms, with opening of the hands. The arms then come together, as in an embrace.

The reflex is of clinical importance, because the nature of the reflex gives an indication of muscle tone. The response may be asymmetrical, if muscle tone is unequal on the two sides, or if there is weakness of an arm or an injury to the humerus or clavicle. The reflex normally disappears in 2 or 3 months.

(2) The grasp reflex. When the baby's palm is stimulated, the hand closes. He can be lifted off the couch by one's finger which has been slipped into his palm. There is a corresponding plantar grasp reflex. It disappears in about 2 months in normal children.

(3) The crossed extension reflex. When one leg is held extended at the knee, and the sole of the foot on the same side is firmly stroked, the free leg flexes, adducts and then extends. It is not normally obtained after the first month.[23]

(4) The walking reflex. When the sole of the foot is pressed against the couch, the baby walks. This disappears in 3 or 4 weeks. It can be elicited for a good many more weeks, however, if the head is extended by the application of upward pressure under the chin.[15]

(5) The limb placement reflex. When the front of the leg below the knee, or the arm below the elbow, is brought into contact with the edge of the table, the child lifts the limb over the edge. Zapella[22] studied the reflex in 350 infants, and found it present on the first day in all infants weighing over 1800 g. In those under 1600 g., it appeared 5 to 50 days after birth. He could not elicit the reflex in mentally defective children with a mental age of less than 3 or 4 months.

(6) The asymmetrical tonic neck reflex. When the baby is at rest and not crying, he lies at intervals with his head to one side, the arm extended to the same side, and often with flexion of the contralateral knee. The reflex normally disappears after 2 or 3 months.

(7) Galant's reflex (trunk incurvation). When a stimulus is applied to the lumbar region, the trunk flexes towards the side stimulated.

(8) Cardinal points. There is a variety of mouth and lip reflexes. Gesell used the term "Rooting Reflex" for the baby's "rooting" for milk when his cheek contacts the mother's breast. When the corner of the mouth is touched, the lower lip is lowered on the same side and the tongue moves towards the point stimulated. When the finger slides away, the head turns to follow it. When the centre of the upper lip is stimulated, the lip elevates.

(9) Blink reflexes. Various stimuli provoke blinking whether the child is awake or asleep.

(10) The doll's eye reflex. When the head is rapidly rotated, there is delay in the following by the eyes. The reflex only lasts for a few days after birth.

When the examiner holding the baby spins round rapidly two or three times, the eyes deviate in the direction of the rotation; when the rotation stops, they deviate in the opposite direction and coarse nystagmoid movements occur.

The pupils react to light.

(11) Plantar response. This is extensor in the first 8 days. The response may be obtained by stimulation as high as T3. From the age of 5 to 20 weeks stimulation anywhere from the sole to the thigh causes an extensor response. After 21 weeks the receptive field shrinks: and the extensor response becomes less definite. After the age of 8 months the response is usually limited to the side stimulated. In the second year of life the response is usually flexor.

(12) The tendon reflexes. These are present in the neonate. They are of great value for the diagnosis of cerebral palsy.

(13) The abdominal reflexes. These are present in 78 per cent. of new-born babies.

The Landau reflex will be mentioned here, though it is confined to the older infant from the age of 3 months. It is seen in most babies in the second 6 months, but is not usually seen after the first birthday. It consists of elevation of the head and arching of the back with the concavity upwards when the child is supported in ventral suspension. There is also partial extension of the hip and knees.

The Development of Locomotion

The first step towards the development of locomotion is the development of head control—the ability to support the head in all positions of the body. The steps in this are observed in three situations: in ventral suspension, the prone position and in the supine position (*Figs. 21–35*). Another essential to the development of locomotion is the reciprocal kick—the rhythmic kicking of the legs, which disappears before walking begins. Other stages in the development of locomotion can be observed in the sitting and standing positions. For the sake of continuity these positions are described separately. An attempt has been made to tabulate the more important milestones of development in Table IX (p. 174). The table enumerates the various new skills which are acquired at different ages.

Ventral Suspension

When the new-born baby is held above the couch in the prone position with the hand under the chest or abdomen (ventral suspension) the head drops down. There may be a fleeting tensing of the neck muscles, but that is all. The elbows and knees flex, and there is some extension at the hip. By about 4 weeks of age the momentary tensing of the neck muscles is more obvious and the baby is able to lift the head up a little for brief moments. By the age of 6 weeks he is able momentarily to hold the head in line with the plane of the body. By 8 weeks he can momentarily lift the head up beyond that plane, and by 12 weeks he can maintain that position. After this age there is no further point in testing a child's head control in this position. The position of ventral suspension is the most sensitive one for the testing of head control in the first 3 months.

Pulling the Child to the Sitting Position

An essential test for head control consists of placing the child in the supine position on a firm surface and then pulling him to the sitting position. When supported sitting, the position and movements of the head are noted, together with the degree of roundness or straightness of the back. When the new-born baby is pulled to the sitting position there is complete head lag. In the sitting position there is uniform rounding of the back because of lack of strength in the spinal muscles and the head droops forward, though he lifts it up for a short distance momentarily. By 6 weeks of age the head lag is clearly not complete, for he lifts the head up in the last part of the movement when being pulled up. By 8 weeks the head lag is less. The head still droops forward when he is held in the sitting position, but he can lift it up for seconds at a time. By 12 weeks the head lag is only slight. By 16 weeks there is only slight head lag, in the very first part of the movement of pulling him up, and when supported in the sitting position he holds the head up for prolonged periods and looks round actively. When the trunk is swayed gently by the examiner the head sways with it or plunges forward, whereas by 20 weeks this is inhibited. By 16 weeks the curvature of the back is seen only in the lumbar region. By 20 weeks head control is almost complete. There is no head lag when he is pulled to the sitting position. At 24 weeks he lifts his head off the couch in the supine position as the examiner is about to pull him up, and he holds his arms out to the examiner to help him. He likes to be propped up in his pram and he can sit for a few minutes with a cushion for support in his high chair. He holds his trunk erect. By 28 weeks he spontaneously lifts his head off the couch as if asking to be pulled up, and he can sit with his hands forward for support. From this age onwards there is no point in using the test of pulling the child up to the sitting position unless he is retarded. One must observe, however, the maturity with which he sits. At 32 weeks he can sit for a few seconds without support, but it is not till 36 weeks that he can sit for 10 minutes unsupported. At this age he is still apt to overbalance by falling backwards or sideways when trying to reach for an object at his side. It is not till 40 weeks that he can pull himself up from the supine to the sitting position. He can go forward from the sitting to the prone position, and thence back to sitting. By 46 weeks he can lean over sideways and recover his balance, and by 48 weeks he can twist well round to pick up an object without overbalancing. By about 15 months he can seat himself in a chair, often by the process of facing it, climbing on to it, standing up on it, turning round and then sitting down. By 18 or 21 months he can sit in it in the adult fashion.

The Prone Position

The new-born baby lies with his head turned to one side, with the pelvis high. He kneels, with the knees drawn up under his abdomen. By the age of 4 weeks he momentarily lifts his chin off the couch. The knees are not drawn up under the abdomen as much as before and the legs are intermittently kicked into extension. At 6 weeks he readily lifts his chin off the couch so that the plane of the face is at an angle of 45 degrees to it. By 8 weeks the child no longer kneels, for the legs are partly extended. At 10 weeks he frequently lifts the chin off the couch so that the plane of the face is at an angle of 45–90 degrees to the couch. At 12 weeks he holds his chin and shoulders off the couch for a long time, bearing the weight on the forearms. The legs are fully extended. At 16 weeks he often arches his back so that his weight rests on his abdomen and lower chest, the arms and legs being lifted off the couch. He holds his head and chest off the couch so that the plane of the face is at 90 degrees to it. At 24 weeks he bears his weight on his hands with extended arms, the chest and upper part of the abdomen being off the couch. He may roll from prone to supine. (It is usually a month later before he can roll from supine to prone.) He may assume the "frog" position, with the legs extended symmetrically in abduction, with the feet everted. At 28 weeks he bears the weight on one hand while he looks round for a toy. From 30 to 40 weeks he makes increasing efforts to crawl. He often progresses backwards in the process. He may progress across the room by rolling. At 40 weeks he is able to move forward, pulling himself by his hands. He lies on his abdomen and the legs trail behind. His legs begin to help, and at 44 weeks he creeps with the abdomen off the couch. From time to time one foot may be seen to be flat on the couch, in the form of a primitive step. At 1 year he may walk on hands and feet like a bear. Creeping may persist long after this date, but at any time from now onwards he may discard the creep position and walk.

Though most children creep before they walk, not all go through this stage. I suspect that most of those children who miss the creeping stage have not often been placed in the prone position for exercise.

The Standing Position

In the first five or six weeks or so his back is rounded when held in the standing position, and his head falls forward. By 8 weeks he holds his head up momentarily, but at 12 weeks for a long time. At 20 weeks he bears some weight on the legs, and at 24 weeks a large fraction of his weight, if his mother gives him a chance to try. He sags at knee and hip. At 28 weeks he can maintain full extension of knees and hip when supported, and he bounces in delight. Much depends on whether his mother gives him a chance to stand. Many mothers deliberately prevent their children from bearing weight on the legs for fear they will become bow-legged. At 36 weeks he stands holding on to furniture, but he has to be helped into that position. By 40 weeks he can pull himself up to the standing postion. At first his feet get into the wrong position and he has many slips and falls in his efforts. He is likely to be unable to let himself down, and falls down with a bump or cries for help. At 44 weeks, while standing holding on to furniture, he lifts and replaces one foot. He finds it extremely difficult to pick up a toy from the floor in this position. At 48 weeks he walks sideways holding on to furniture ("cruising") and walks with two hands held.

By one year of age he walks with one hand held. He may continue to demand this support for as long as 5 or 6 months. The age at which he decides to walk without support now depends in part on his confidence and his dislike of spills. The average age at which children walk without support is about 15 months. Many workers give an earlier age (e.g. 13 months). Walking is delayed by an aberrant form of progression called shuffling or hitching on one buttock and one hand. At 13 months he is likely to stand alone for a few seconds. When he eventually walks without help he progresses on a wide base, with a high-stepping gait, with steps of varying length and in varying directions. He falls repeatedly. He tends to keep his elbows flexed, with his arms abducted from the shoulder. He can creep upstairs, but has no idea of the importance of gravity and is likely to lean back into space when halfway up. At 15 months he can get into the standing position without support, but he cannot throw a ball without falling and he cannot stop or go round corners. He falls suddenly on to his buttocks. By 16 or 18 months he can walk backwards as well as forwards. He can walk upstairs, two feet per step, holding on to the rail. He can run and pull a toy as he walks. He can throw a ball without falling. By 21 months he can pick an object up from the floor without falling. At 2 years he can go up and down stairs alone with two feet per step. He can kick a ball without falling. At 2½ he can walk on tip-toe and jump, but he cannot stand on one foot. At 3 he can walk upstairs with a foot to each step, but when coming down he places both feet on the same stair. He jumps off the bottom step. He can now stand for a few seconds only on one leg, but he cannot skip. Even at 3 he has much to learn and the development of locomotion is still incomplete.

Manipulation

The primitive grasp reflex disappears before true voluntary grasping begins. Before voluntary grasping can occur the tightly closed hands of the new-born have to open, and the eyes have to become co-ordinated with the hands. The grasp reflex disappears by about 3 months of age, and often little trace of it can be seen at 8 weeks. At about 12 weeks, and sometimes sooner, the baby begins to pull at his dress with his hands, and when a rattle is placed in his hand he retains it for several moments. When a brightly coloured toy is placed in front of him, he shows his obvious desire to get it and excites, with rapid movements of the arms and legs and increased respiration rate. Gradually and imperceptibly, as he grows older, it will be noticed that his hands are beginning to go forward to reach the object. At first he grossly misjudges the distance, trying to get an object which is quite out of reach or overshooting the mark. He plays longer and longer with a rattle placed in his hand. He eventually touches a larger toy but cannot grasp it. From 12 to 16 weeks he characteristically watches his hands as he lies on his back. At 16 weeks his hands come together into the midline and he plays with them. He pulls his dress over his face. By 20 weeks he can grasp an object near his hand. He is ataxic in his approach, still overshooting the mark, but eventually he gets what he wants. He soon grasps everything within reach: his mother's hair, clothes, brooch, spoon, paper and anything else he sees. He takes everything to his mouth, for the mouth is at this time the chief organ of "manipulation." He is able in the supine position to get his legs into full extension and he plays with his toes. He loves to splash in the bath and he crumples paper. His approach to objects is two-handed. He can only grasp large objects. When he holds a cube in the hand it is held in the palm, not between the fingers. In the early stages of development it is held on the ulnar side of the hand, and later on the radial side. It is not until about 40 weeks of age or more that he can hold it between finger and thumb. At 28 weeks he characteristically begins to transfer objects from one hand to the other. It is now noted that he is beginning to go for objects with one hand instead of two. He can feed himself well with a biscuit and he helps to hold the spoon when eating. Whereas at 24 weeks he drops a cube from his hand if another is offered, at 28 weeks he retains the first when the second cube is presented. At 36 weeks he brings the two cubes together, as if comparing the size, and bangs them on the table. As manipulation increases mouthing decreases, so that by a year few things are taken to the mouth. He can easily lean forward now to pick objects up. At 40 weeks he can bring his finger and thumb together and so pick up small objects, such as a piece of string. His index finger protrudes as he goes for it. Release of objects begins at about this age. Up to this time he was able to grasp objects but he could not deliberately let them go. He soon discovers the joy of deliberately letting one thing after another drop on to the floor, particularly if there is someone to pick them up for him. At 44 weeks he will hold an object out to his mother and even put it into her hand, but he will not let it go. By 48 weeks he will release it into her hand, and soon thoroughly enjoys the give-and-take game. He also loves to put one object into another, and spends a happy half-hour merely putting one cube after another into a basket and taking them out again. He particularly enjoys this repetitive game and continues to do so for the next 2 years. At 13 months he can hold two 1-in. cubes in one hand. His release is so accurate that he can build a tower of two cubes, but it is 21 months before he can build a tower of five or six cubes, and 3 years before he can build a tower of nine or ten cubes. At 12 months, when feeding himself, he rotates the spoon when it is near his mouth, spilling the contents, but by 15–18 months he gets it into his mouth before the contents are dropped. At 18 months he can feed himself completely, managing a cup with only occasional slight spilling. He turns two or three pages of a book at a time, but by 24 months he can turn them over singly. From 15 or 18 months he has tried to put his gloves, socks or shoes on but not succeeded. At 24 months he can put them on. He can now pronate and supinate the wrist sufficiently to turn an easy door handle or unscrew a lid. He begins to draw with pencils. At 2½ he can take his pants off and put them on and thread beads. He begins to fasten easily-placed buttons. At 3 he can dress and undress himself completely with some help with back buttons, and he can buckle his shoes. Many children can draw quite well at this age and can cut paper fairly accurately with scissors. They can paint quite well over a suitable design.

The Use of the Eyes and Ears

The new-born baby is capable of visual fixation and following from the day he is born.[2] He will turn his head and eyes towards diffuse light when it falls on one side of his face. He blinks and his pupil responds when light is cast on to his eye, and opticokinetic nystagmus can be demonstrated when a suitable moving drum rotates in front of his eyes, an indication of vision. By 3 or 4 weeks he watches his mother's face intently as she speaks to him, and he will watch a toy which is brought into his line of vision, following it from one side nearly to the midline. At 6 weeks he is beginning to follow moving persons with his eyes. At 8 weeks he will follow a moving toy from the side to a point past the midline, and at 12 weeks he will follow it well over to the other side. At 8 weeks the eyes show convergence and focusing. His eye becomes quicker and quicker at catching sight of objects in front of him. By 12 weeks he turns his head in the direction of sound. He excites when he sees toys in front of him and from now on shows increasing efforts to grasp toys, until eventually at about 20 weeks his eyes and hands are sufficiently co-ordinated for him to grasp them voluntarily. Up to 16 weeks very small objects failed to catch his eye, but he can see them now though he cannot touch them. He watches his hands from 12 to 16 weeks as he lies on his back. He shows considerable excitement when he sees his feed being prepared and shows obvious interest in a strange room. At 6 months he adjusts his position to see objects—craning his neck, bending back or crouching to see what he wants to see. He cannot follow a rapidly moving object until he is nearly a year old. By 2 years he can see everything which the adult can see.

According to Peiper[16] it is possible to rule out all forms of colour blindness by the start of the third year.

It can be shown that most new-born babies can hear if properly tested when awake and not actively feeding or crying. The reactions to sound include quieting, blinking, crying, inhibition of sucking, the startle reflex, and a momentary catch in the respirations. The fact that the infant has heard can be demonstrated by the E.E.G., the E.M.G., the cardiotachometer (recording the heart rate), and the establishment of a conditioned reflex.

It is now known that it is incorrect to suppose that the vocalizations of a deaf baby in his first 7 or 8 months are reduced.[14] Tape recordings and other methods have shown that until the factor of imitation enters (sometime after 7 or 8 months), the vocalizations of the deaf child are the same as those of hearing infants.

By 3 or 4 months the baby turns his head towards the source of sound. At 32 weeks he responds to his name, and at 36 weeks he may

In the following illustrations Figures 17, 18, 21, 23, 26, 28, 29, 32, 33, 34, 37, 41 are repro-
ꞓced from *Diseases of Children* by courtesy of Edward Arnold Ltd., and Figures 19, 20, 22,
ꞓ, 25, 27, 30, 31, 35, 36, 38, 39, 40, 42–52 inclusive from *Development of the Infant and Young
ꞓild* by kind permission of Messrs. E. & S. Livingstone Ltd.

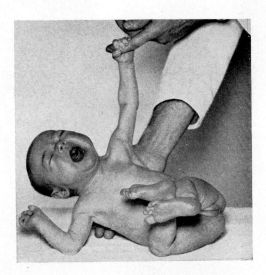

FIG. 17. Grasp reflex.

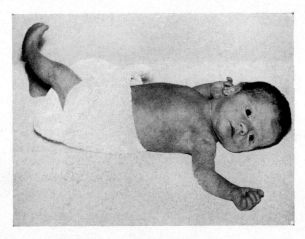

FIG. 18. Asymmetrical tonic neck reflex.

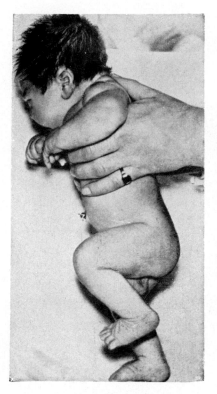

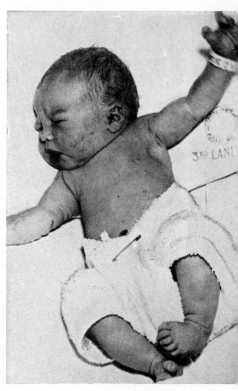

Fig. 19. Walking reflex.

Fig. 20. Moro reflex.

Fig. 21. Ventral suspension.
2 to 3 weeks.
Considerable head lag.

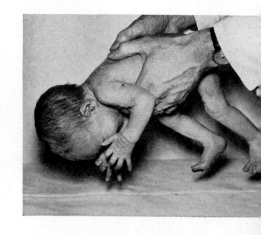

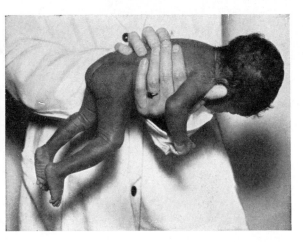

FIG. 22. Ventral sus-
pension. 6 weeks.
Head held in same
plane as rest of body.

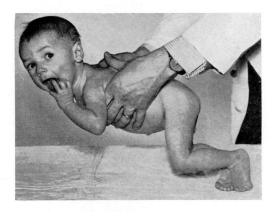

FIG. 23. Ventral suspension.
8 to 10 weeks.
Head held well beyond plane
of rest of body.

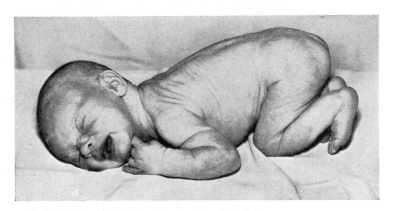

FIG. 24. Prone. Newborn baby.
Pelvis high, knees drawn up under abdomen.

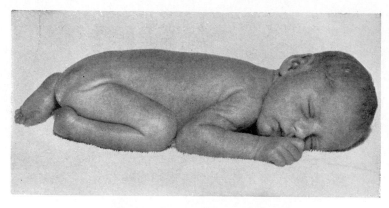

FIG. 25. Prone. Premature baby.

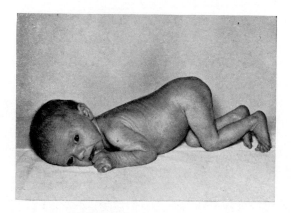

FIG. 26. Prone. 3 to 4 weeks.
Pelvis high, some extension of hip and knees.

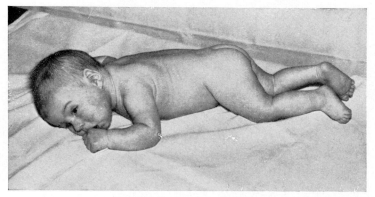

FIG. 27. Prone. 6 to 8 weeks.
Pelvis low. Legs extended.

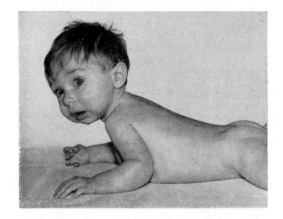

FIG. 28. Prone. 4 months. Weight on forearms.

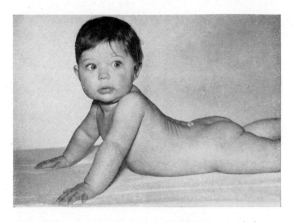

FIG. 29. Prone. 5 to 6 months. Weight on extended arms.

FIG. 30

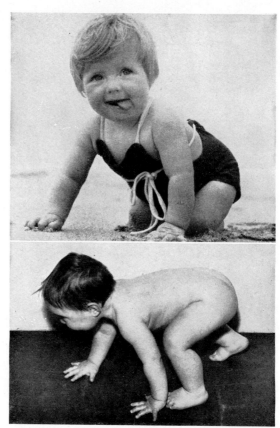

FIG. 31

FIG. 30. Prone. 44 weeks—creep.
FIG. 31. Prone. 52 weeks—walking like a bear.

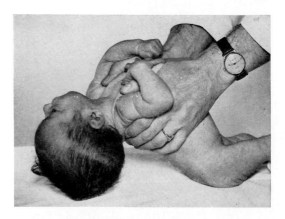

FIG. 32. Pulling to sitting position. Newborn.
Complete head lag.

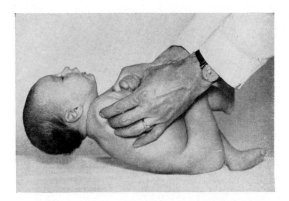

FIG. 33. Pulling to sitting position. 3 months. Much less head lag.

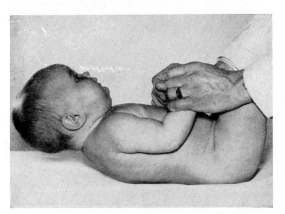

FIG. 34. Pulling to sitting position. 5 months.
Head raised when about to be pulled up.

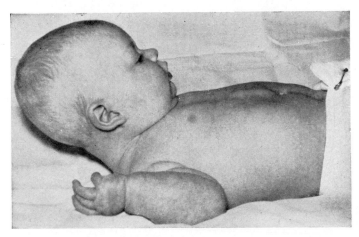

FIG. 35. Supine. 6 months. Head raised spontaneously.

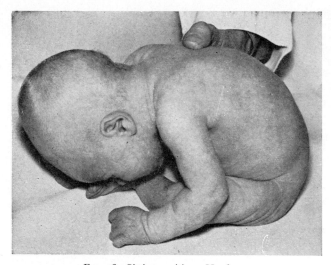

FIG. 36. Sitting position. Newborn.

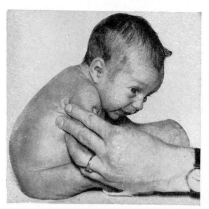

FIG. 37. Sitting position. 1 month.
Head held up slightly.

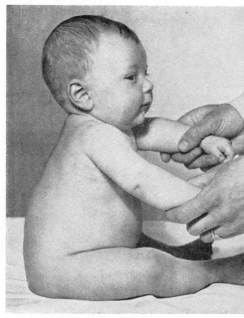

FIG. 38. Sitting position. 16 weeks.
Back much more straight.

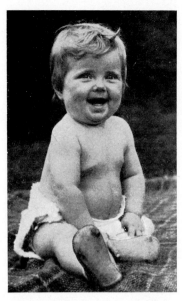

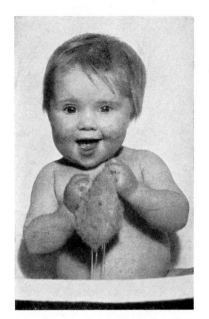

FIG. 39. Sitting position. 6 months.
Hands used for support.

FIG. 40. Sitting position. 7 months.
Sitting unsupported momentarily.

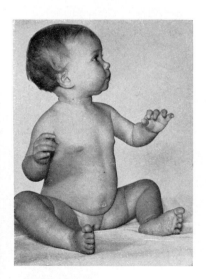

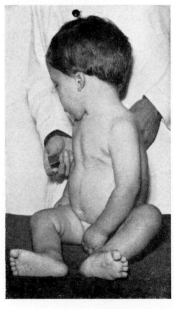

FIG. 41. Sitting position. 9 months.
Sitting unsupported, securely.

FIG. 42. Sitting position. 11 months.
Pivoting.

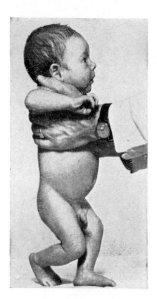

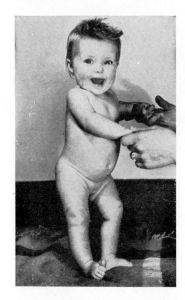

Fig. 43. Standing position. 12 weeks. Some weight on legs.

Fig. 44. Standing position. 24 weeks. Large part of weight on legs.

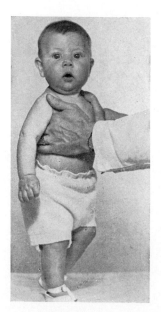

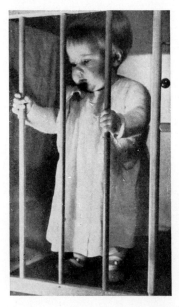

Fig. 45. Standing position. 28 weeks. Full weight on legs.

Fig. 46. Standing position. 40 weeks. Standing, holding on to furniture.

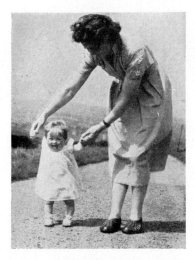

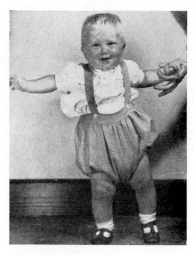

FIG. 47. Walking position. 48 weeks.
Walking, two hands held.

FIG. 48. Walking position. 52 weeks.
Walking, one hand held.

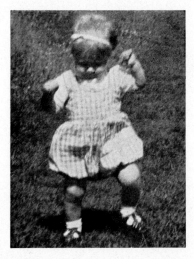

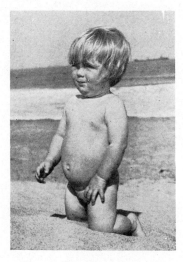

FIG. 49. Walking position. 13 months.
Walking without support.

FIG. 50. Kneeling. 15 months.

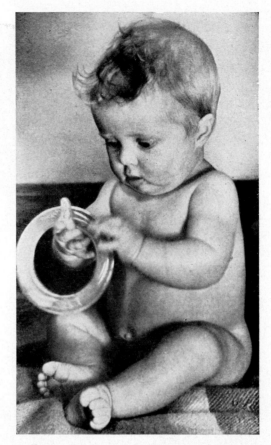

FIG. 51. Manipulation at 6 months. Transfer.

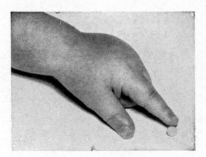

FIG. 52. Index finger approach. 40 weeks.

imitate sounds made by his mother. Between 9 and 12 months he understands the meaning of several words, such as names of members of the family.

General Understanding

The whole of a child's development is so intimately bound up with the development of his understanding and with his intelligence that it is difficult to discuss the development of understanding separately.

Probably the first sign of the dawn of understanding in a baby is seen when his mother talks to him at the age of 3 or 4 weeks. He quiets, watches her intently, opening and closing his mouth, often bobbing his head backwards and forwards, obviously enjoying the conversation. By about 6 weeks he begins to smile, at first only once or twice a day, when his mother speaks to him, but more and more frequently and to more and more different stimuli as he grows older. In a further 2 or 3 weeks he vocalizes his pleasure when spoken to. By 10 weeks he has considerable interest in his surroundings, following moving persons with his eyes. At 12 weeks he may be quite reluctant to be left outside, much preferring to be in the kitchen where he can see some activity. His interest and excitement when he sees a brightly-coloured toy is an index of his understanding. He recognizes his mother at this age. He turns his head towards a sound. He may resist the nose swab of cotton wool by turning his head away when he sees it approach. (The reaction to cotton wool swabs from the age of 2–10 months is used by Charlotte Bühler in her developmental tests.) At 16 weeks he shows his understanding by opening his mouth for the feeding bottle or breast. He cries when his mother departs. His interest in his surroundings has increased and he shows obvious interest in a strange room. He tries hard to grasp objects. At 20 weeks he smiles at his own mirror image, and when he drops his rattle he looks to see where it has gone to. At 24 weeks in the supine position he stretches his arms out when he sees that his mother is about to pull him into the sitting position. When he drops his rattle he not only follows it with his eyes but tries to recover it. He smiles and vocalizes at his mirror image, and at 28 weeks he pats it. Any time after the age of 5 months he may begin to imitate such acts as chewing or protrusion of the tongue. From the age of about 24 weeks he shows his memory of foodstuffs by his strong reaction of like or dislike when he sees them. His interest in his surroundings is partly related to his personality, but most babies of this age are intensely interested in their surroundings and they bend their necks and twist round to see what is happening. He may try to establish contact with a stranger by coughing or making other noises. He enjoys the game of peep-bo

7

with a towel or napkin over his head or over his mother's head. He responds to his name. At 32 weeks he reacts to the cotton wool swab by grasping his mother's hand and pushing it away. He reaches persistently for toys out of reach. He responds to "No." At 36 weeks he tries to prevent his mother washing his face by putting his arm in front of it. The degree of concentration on his toys should be particularly noted from this age. Some children can only concentrate for a minute or two on a toy, while others play for prolonged periods with them. Such prolonged concentration and determination to reach a toy is a good sign of intelligence. At 40 weeks he may pull the clothes of a person to attract his attention. He learns to clap his hands and to wave bye-bye, laughing as he does it. He learns to repeat any performance laughed at, and if he finds that his audience laughs when he drops spoonfuls of food on to the carpet or smears it over his hair, he will repeat the act. He is beginning to release objects, and greatly enjoys the game of dropping bricks or other objects from his high chair for someone else to pick up. Any time after 9 months he will perform simple acts on request, such as sitting down or standing up. He enjoys the frequent repetition of nursery rhymes and may anticipate certain actions in the rhyme by bodily movement, thus well revealing his developing memory. He begins to co-operate in dressing by holding his arm out for the sleeve of his coat, or the foot up for his shoe. At 44 weeks he will hand a toy to his mother, but at first he refuses to let it go when it has reached her hand. He soon learns to kiss on request. He shows considerable interest in the colour masses in pictures in his books, particularly when his mother describes them. He shows that he is beginning to understand quite a number of words, such as foot, shoe, sock, though he may be unable to say any. At 11 months, he enjoys the peep-bo game and now covers his own face up with a towel. He laughs at his mother when she pulls faces at him or puts some strange object on her head. He will go on a simple errand such as fetching his sock from the other end of the room. Speech has been developing in the last 3 months and he may now be able to say three or four words with meaning, though he understands the meaning of many more.

The development of understanding in the first year has been discussed in some detail, because it is in the first year that developmental diagnosis is regarded by many as particularly difficult. The various manifestations of understanding, and especially the baby's powers of concentration, persistence and interest in surroundings, are particularly important in such diagnosis. Further signs of developing intelligence after the first birthday are briefly summarized below.

In the second year his increasing understanding is shown by his

reater and greater understanding of what is said to him and his
bility to execute simple requests. It is shown by his increasing
nterest in books and his ability to point out objects in them on request.
t is shown by his imitation of his mother in sweeping, washing and
oing odd jobs about the house. The girl's play with her doll is well
orth observing. The play becomes more and more complex as she
rows older. From 18 months to 2 years it is apt to be fairly simple
nd include "potting," napkin changing and washing. From $2\frac{1}{2}$ to 3
ears it is much more complex and her imaginativeness should be noted.
t is observed in her play with boxes, bricks and other toys. The child
ay arrange complicated situations with her dolls and spend long
eriods dressing them and undressing them.

The tests commonly used for the investigation of a child's intelli-
ence between the ages of 1 and 3 years are tabulated in Table IX,
nd there is no need to repeat them all here. From 18 months onwards
he child enjoys playing with pencil and paper, and his memory is well
hown by his ability to draw, though other factors play a part. By
$\frac{1}{2}$ years he can tackle simple jigsaw puzzles (e.g. those made of four or
ive pieces) and enjoys matching wools of various colours, and cards
ith pictures on them. His ability to match such cards and pictures
s a good index of his intelligence. His memory is tested by his ability
o repeat digits. He knows his full name by $2\frac{1}{4}$, and at this age he is
irst likely to note anatomical differences between the sexes. By 3 he
s constantly asking questions, shows great interest in his surroundings
nd knows various nursery rhymes.

Pleasure and Displeasure

The first sign of pleasure is the quieting of the new-born baby when
e is placed in a warm bath or when he is cuddled by his mother.
When he is fed, his crying stops, and he shows his pleasure by the
playing of his toes and their alternate flexion and extension. As he
grows older he shows more and more pleasure at being picked up by his
mother and at being spoken to. By 6 weeks he smiles at her as she
peaks to him, and in 1 or 2 weeks vocalizes his pleasure. In the third
month he emits squeals of delight. By about 16 weeks he shows his
delight by a massive general response—by his rapid panting respira-
ions, widening of the palpebral fissure and rapid movements of the
rms and legs. He laughs aloud. He thoroughly enjoys playing with
he rattle which is placed in his hand and soon he is able to grasp objects
imself (by 20 or 24 weeks). Thereafter he takes particular pleasure in
he newly-acquired skills—manipulation, sitting, standing and walking.
After 20 weeks he is constantly using his hands, banging bricks, grasping
verything which comes within his reach. He smiles when pulled to

the sitting position and dislikes lying down. When he is able to stan
he enjoys standing and dislikes sitting. When he is able to walk h
wants to be helped to walk all day long. After 5 months he enjoy
simple games such as peep-bo (see section above on General Under
standing), and from now onwards he takes increasing pleasure i
any simple game. At 4 or 5 months he becomes ticklish, and soo
he laughs at the mere prospect of being tickled when the finger i
approaching. At 6 months he smiles when he sees a dog or anothe
baby, and often smiles at every stranger he sees. After a year h
delights still more in his newly found skills of manipulation and h
enjoys domestic mimicry, imitating his mother in her housework. H
enjoys his books, toys and his friends. Much can be learnt from th
simple observation of a child's behaviour with his toys and from hi
response to various stimuli. In general the nature of the stimuli which
produce pleasure depends on his developmental level.

A baby can show his displeasure before he can show his pleasure
but as he matures he shows less displeasure and more pleasure. Th
causes of crying are discussed elsewhere and will not be discussed here

Feeding Behaviour

For details of the development of feeding behaviour in childre
the reader is referred to the book by Gesell and Ilg.[9] The new-bor
baby frequently gags and chokes. He hiccoughs when his stomac
is distended by a good feed. He cannot usually approximate his lip
tightly to the areola of the breast, so that milk leaks out as he suck
and he swallows air. As he grows older he approximates his lips much
more tightly, so that there is no leakage and practically no air swallow
ing. The older baby therefore has much less trouble with wind tha
the younger one. He cannot take solids at this age, for they initiat
sucking movements with elevation of the posterior part of the tongue
so that the food is ejected. He begins to chew at about 6 months and s
can manage true solids. At this age he can approximate his lips well t
the rim of a cup, and his eyes are so well co-ordinated with his hand
that he can feed himself with a biscuit or crust. From the age of
months almost everything which the baby picks up is taken to th
mouth and this persists until he is really adept with his hands, whe
mouthing largely ceases.

Most babies make some attempt to help to feed themselves at abou
6 months by helping to hold the bottle, cup or spoon. This should b
encouraged. They can manage a biscuit, crust or toast at this age
and by 9–12 months they can manage by one means or another largel
to feed themselves. They are apt to put their fingers into the food an
to play with the food with their hands. They tend deliberately to dro

tems of food from the high chair on to the floor, particularly if this
auses laughter. They smear it over their faces and often into the
air. They may even invert the dish on to the head. Anna Freud
wrote: "It is an error to ascribe this messing of the young child to lack
f skill. The child's actions in this respect are deliberate and inten-
ional. They are motivated by the pleasure of smearing an anal-
rotic activity transferred from the excrements to the foodstuffs which
re similar to the former in consistency, colour and temperature."
  prefer to regard the messing as a sign of the child's inco-ordination,
vith a natural desire to feel the consistency of foods, together with a
lesire for attention. He is much more likely to make a mess with food
vhich he does not like than with that which he enjoys. When he is
irst given the cup without help he is apt to let go as soon as he has
lrunk what he wants. Later he tends to bang it down on to the table.
The age at which children learn to manage a cup with practically no
pilling varies tremendously. It is greatly influenced by the factor of
practice. If he is given a chance early he is likely to manage it early.
Gesell and Ilg[9] said that the typical age at which self-management of
a cup occurs is 65 weeks. Some need help to the end of the second year.
There is no doubt, however, that many children manage a cup well
by 12 months. Similar remarks apply to the age at which a child learns
o use a spoon. Gesell said that spilling from a spoon is marked at 15
months, moderate at 18 months and tends to disappear by the close of
he second year. Without statistical study, I feel that most children who
re given a chance early can manage a spoon with a minimum of spilling
by 15–18 months. Earlier than this they are apt to rotate the spoon
ust before it reaches the mouth, spilling the contents. This rotation
may persist as a habit, and has to be checked accordingly. By the age of
$2\frac{1}{2}$–3 years most children can manage a knife and fork with help in cut-
ing such hard articles of food as toast. It is a good thing to let the child
ise a knife and fork as soon as he is developmentally ready, instead
f a spoon. At about this age he should be encouraged to use an
rdinary plate instead of a child's plate with a high rim.
  Many make the mistake of expecting perfect table manners in the
2- or 3-year-old. It is a mistake to be too strict at mealtimes and to
nake mealtimes a misery. Gentle loving advice is altogether desirable,
but constant remonstrances do nothing but harm. The child will
lowly but surely learn by imitating his parents. The parents should
ee that their own manners leave nothing to be desired.
  The frequency of demands for food decreases with age. Between
he fourth and ninth day many babies demand up to twelve or thirteen
eeds in the 24 hours, including two at night. Aldrich and Hewitt
howed that at 1 month of age 61 per cent. of a large number of babies

observed by them at Rochester preferred a three-hourly feed, an
26 per cent. a four-hourly feed. By 7–9 months the majority of babie
want four feeds a day. By the age of 1 year 91 per cent. wante
three meals a day. Some babies as early as 2 or 3 months, howeve
only demand three feeds in the 24 hours. The great majority of babie
drop the night feed by the age of 10 weeks.

Speech

The earliest manifestations of developing speech are the throat
sounds of the 4-week-old baby and the vowel sounds—ah, eh, uh–
of the 8-week-old child. By the age of 12–16 weeks a baby will hav
a long conversation in his own way with the mother, responding t
her overtures by prolonged "speech." At about 20 weeks he begins t
use guttural sounds and say "Ah goo." At 28 weeks he says "Ba,
"Da," "Ka" and sounds like "mm" when he is crying. At 32 week
he begins to combine syllables, saying "Baba," "Dada," "Kaka,
Not until about 44 weeks does he say one word with meaning, sayin
"Dada" more in his father's presence than when he is not there. Th
average child says about three words with meaning by about a year
Between 15 and 18 months jargoning begins, the child speaking in
language of his own. By 21–24 months children put two or three word
together into sentences. At 24 months they use pronouns—I, me, you
By the age of 3 the child has an extensive vocabulary and talks in
cessantly throughout the day.

Karelitz and Rosenfeld[13] have carried out an interesting an
important study of infants' vocalizations by means of tape recording
They described the cry of the young infant as short, staccato an
repetitive, building up to a crescendo when the stimulus is applie
and diminishing as the stimulus is removed. As the baby grows, th
cry lengthens, and becomes disyllabic. The pitch begins to vary and b
about 6 months the inflections become more plaintive and meaningfu
Later still syllables of real words can be heard as part of the cry.

Handedness

In many children handedness is not finally established until th
age of 4 years. Gesell thought that the direction of the asymmetrica
tonic neck reflex was a pointer to ultimate handedness.[11] During th
first year there are commonly shifts in handedness.

It is thought that handedness is partly genetic but largely environ
mental, and the result of imitation and instruction. There are probabl
other factors, which are not fully understood. Left handedness is mor
common in uniovular twins than in singletons. It is also more commo
in genius and in criminals.

There seems to be some association between left handedness or ambidexterity and speech and reading difficulties, but the nature of the association and its importance is not clear.[20],[21]

Left handedness is not simply the converse of right handedness. Right handedness is usually constant, while most left handed children also on occasion use the right hand ("mixed handers"). Mixed handers are more likely to have delayed speech than "fixed" handers.

The subject of handedness is a complex one. It has been well reviewed by Barsley,[1] Clark[4] and Zangwill.[20],[21]

In the older child laterality can be tested in the hand by getting him to draw, cut paper with scissors, wind a clock, place an object in a tin; in the foot, by kicking a ball: in the ear, by holding a watch in the midline in front of him and asking him to listen to it: and in the eye by making a hollow roll from a piece of firm paper and asking him to look at an object through it.

Sphincter Control

The development of sphincter control and other aspects of psychological development are discussed elsewhere.

Method of Examination

I have described elsewhere the method of conducting the developmental examination,[12] with the difficulties of developmental assessment, and an account of the pitfalls which await the unwary.

Summary

Table IX gives a summary of the principal milestones of development.

For convenience the table has been divided into six columns. This is in many ways purely artificial, for there is inevitably some overlapping. Some skills which are included in the column entitled "Manipulation" could well be included under the column entitled "General Understanding," and vice versa, largely because general understanding is required for so many manipulative feats.

The table does not set out to give a list of all the child's skills at the various ages listed. This would involve a great deal of repetition. The age at which a child learns to smile, for instance, is given as 6 weeks, but this is not mentioned under all the subsequent age headings, it being assumed that all "normal" children over the age of 6 weeks are able to smile. The table is intended solely to give the ages at which average children first acquire the skills described. In using the table in the assessment of an individual child of a given age, therefore, one has to determine how far he has developed in comparison with average

Age*	Gross Motor	Manipulation
4 weeks	Held in sitting position—may hold head up momentarily. Held in prone position with hand under abdomen, momentary tensing of neck muscles should be noted. Prone—momentarily holds chin off couch. Pull to sit—almost complete head lag.	
6 weeks	Held in prone position with hand under abdomen—the head is held momentarily in line with the body. Prone—readily lifts chin off couch so that plane of face is at angle of 45 degrees to couch. Pull to sit from supine—head lag not quite complete.	
8 weeks	Held in sitting position—head is held up but recurrently bobs forward. Held in prone position with hand under abdomen—holds head up so that its plane is in line with that of the body. Prone—head no longer mainly turned to one side as in earlier weeks. Recurrently lifts chin off couch so that plane of face is at angle of 45 degrees to couch. Held in standing position—is able to hold head up more than momentarily.	
12 weeks	Prone—holds chin and shoulders off couch prolongedly, so that plane of face is at angle of 45–90 degrees from couch. Bears weight on forearms. Pull to sit from supine—only moderate head lag. Held in prone position with hand under abdomen—holds head up so that its plane is beyond that of the body.	Pulls at his dress. No more grasp reflex. Holds rattle voluntarily when it is placed in hand; retains it more than a moment. Hands no longer tightly closed as in previou weeks, but mostly open. Desire to grasp objects seen (see next column).
16 weeks	Held in sitting position—holds head well up constantly. He looks actively around, but head still wobbles if examiner causes sudden movement of trunk. Curvature of back now only in lumbar region as compared with rounded back of earlier weeks. Prone—holds head and chest off couch so that plane of face is at 90 degrees to couch. Weight still on forearms. Pull to sit—only slight head lag in beginning of movement. Supine—head no longer rotated to one side as in earlier weeks.	Hands come together and he plays with his han⟨ He pulls his dress over his face in play. Approaches object with hands, but overshoots ⟨ mark and fails to reach it. Plays with rattle prolongedly when it is placed his hand, and he shakes it.
20 weeks	Full head control. Held in sitting position—head stable when body is mildly rocked by examiner. Pull to sit—no head lag.	Now able to grasp objects deliberately. He plays with his toys, splashes in the bath a crumples paper. (From this time onwards one must note ⟨ maturity of the grasp, the ease with which is able to secure objects, the security w⟨ which he holds them and the size of the obj⟨ which he is able to grasp. He cannot br⟨ finger and thumb together to grasp a sm⟨ object of the size of a thin piece of string he is about 9 months old.)
24 weeks	Prone—weight borne on hands with extended arms, the chest and upper part of abdomen therefore being off the couch. Pull to sit—head lifted off couch when about to be pulled up. Hands are held out to be lifted. Sits (supported) in high chair for a few minutes. Rolls from prone to supine. Held in standing position—bears large fraction of weight.	He grasps his feet. Holds bottle. Supine—may take toes to mouth. If he has one cube in hand he drops it when seco⟨ one is offered.

* For mature babies; due allow⟨

General Understanding	Speech	Sphincter Control	Miscellaneous
:ches the mother when she talks to him. •pens and closes mouth as she speaks, bobs his •ad, quiets. (In next two weeks or so, before •ailing begins, note the duration and intensity ' this reaction in assessing a child.) •ine position—regards dangling toy when it is •ought into his line of vision and will follow it, •t less than 90 degrees.			
•les momentarily when talked to by mother. •miling henceforward becomes more and more •equent. The frequency of smiling and the •se with which it is elicited should be noted.) •ine—looks at dangling toy when it is in •idline; follows it to midline when it is moved •om the side. •nning to follow moving persons with eyes.			
•ine—follows dangling toy from side to point •st midline. (Always note the promptness •ith which child sees the ring. At this age he •es not usually see it immediately.)			Eyes show fixation, convergence, focusing.
•ne—follows dangling toy from one side to •e other (180 degrees). Catches sight of it •mediately. •only smiles when spoken to but vocalizes with •easure. Squeals of pleasure heard. •m now onwards it is essential to note the •ild's interest in what he sees. One must •so note the obvious desire to grasp objects. •his desire can be observed long before he can •luntarily go for them and get them. In •other month his hands go forward for the •ject, but he misjudges the distance. By 5 •onths he can get the object.			Supine — characteristically watches movements of own hands.
•eral understanding becoming much more •vious. Excites when he sees toys. Shows •nsiderable interest when he sees breast or •ttle. Shows interest in strange room. •ghs aloud. Vocalizes pleasure when pulled to •tting position. •s to be propped up in sitting position. •ns head towards a sound.			
•les at image of self in mirror. When he drops •s rattle he looks to see where it has gone to.			
•es and vocalizes at his mirror image. •n he drops the rattle he tries to recover it. •"blow bubbles" or protrude tongue in •itation of adult. •show fear of strangers and be "coy." •ghs when head is hidden in towel in peep-bo •me. •nning to show likes and dislikes of foods.			

•e made for prematurity.

Age*	Gross Motor	Manipulation
28 weeks .	Prone—bears weight on one hand. Sits with hands forward for support. Rolls from supine to prone. Standing position—can maintain extension of hip and knees for short period when supported. He bounces with pleasure. (Previously he sagged at hip and knees.) Supine—spontaneously lifts head off couch.	If he has one cube in hand he retains it wh second cube is offered. Transfers objects from one hand to the other. Bangs objects on the table. Now goes for objects with one hand instead two, as he did previously. Takes all objects to mouth. Feeds self with biscuit. Loves to play with paper.
32 weeks .	Readily bears whole weight on legs when supported. Sits for a few moments unsupported.	
36 weeks .	Stands holding on to furniture. Sits steadily for 10 minutes. Leans forward and recovers balance. (Cannot lean sideways.) Prone—in trying to crawl may progress backwards. May progress by rolling.	Can pick up small object such as currant betwe finger and thumb. When he has two cubes he brings them togeth as if making visual comparison between them
40 weeks .	Pulls self to standing position. Pulls self to sitting position. Goes forward from sitting to prone, and from prone to sitting. Sits steadily without risk of falling over (except for occasional accident). Crawls, pulling self forward with hands, abdomen on couch.	Goes for objects with index finger. Beginning to release objects, letting them deliberately instead of accidentally as before.
44 weeks .	Prone—creeps (abdomen off couch). When standing holding on he lifts and replaces one foot. Sitting—can lean over sideways.	Will place object into examiner's hand on reque but will not release it.
48 weeks .	Walks sideways, holding on to furniture. Walks with two hands held. Sitting—can turn round to pick up object.	Rolls ball towards examiner. Gives and takes toy in play, releasing object i examiner's hand.
1 year .	Walks with one hand held. Prone—walks on hands and feet like a bear. May shuffle on buttocks and hand.	
13 months .	Stands alone for a moment.	Can hold two cubes in one hand. Makes line or marks with pencil.
15 months .	Can get into standing position without support. Creeps upstairs. Walks without help with broad-base, high-stepping gait and steps of unequal length and direction. (The maturity of the gait must be noted from now onwards.)	Builds tower of two cubes. (This requires so accuracy in release.) Constantly throwing objects on to floor. Takes off shoes.

* For mature babies; due allow

General Understanding	Speech	Sphincter Control	Miscellaneous
ts image of self in mirror. sponds to name. ies to establish contact with person by cough or other noise. ay imitate movement, such as tongue protrusion.	Says "Da," "Ba," "Ka."		Feeds well from cup. Chews and so can take solids.
aches persistently for toys out of reach. sponds to "No."	Combines syllables, "Da-da," "Ba-ba."		
ts arms in front of face to try to prevent mother washing his face. rom this age onwards note excitement when certain liked foodstuffs are seen. Note particularly degree and maintenance of concentration in getting objects and in playing with toys.)			
ay pull clothes of another to attract attention. ays "Patacake" (clapping hands). aves bye-bye. ts the doll. olds arm out for sleeve or holds foot up for sock in dressing. rom this age the understanding of words should be observed. The child can understand the meaning of perhaps a dozen words by the age of a year, though he is only able to say two or three words at that age. At 9 months he may respond to such questions as "Where is Daddy?" "Where is the cow?")			Slobbering and mouthing beginning to decrease.
vers own face with towel in peep-bo game. ops objects deliberately in order that they will be picked up. ginning to put objects in and out of containers. he maturity of the release behaviour and the manipulative skill must be noted as he plays with his toys.)	Says one word with meaning.		
peats performance laughed at. w likes repetitive play, putting one cube after another into basket, etc. ticipates with bodily movement when nursery hyme being told. ows interest when shown simple pictures in book. (This interest should be carefully noted rom now onwards.)			
ay understand meaning of "Where is your book?" "Where is your shoe?" ay kiss on request. ich evidence of developing memory is important and must be noted.)	Says two or three words with meaning.		Apt to be shy. Very little mouthing of objects. Little slobbering except during concentration on an especially interesting toy.
y kiss mirror image.			
ks for objects by pointing. ts pictures and may kiss pictures of animals. gativism beginning. eds self, managing cup.	Jargon.	Tells mother that he has wet pants. (First sign of sphincter control.)	

be made for prematurity.

Summary of Normal Developm

Age*	Gross Motor	Manipulation
18 months .	Climbs stairs unaided, holding rail. Runs. Seldom falls. Jumps. No longer broad-base and high-stepping gait when walking. Seats self in chair, often by process of climbing up, standing, turning round and sitting down. Pulls toy as he walks. Throws ball without falling, as previously.	Builds tower of three cubes. Manages spoon without rotating it near mouth previously. Turns pages of book two or three at a time. Scribbles spontaneously. Takes off gloves, socks. Unzips fasteners.
21 months .	Walks backwards in imitation. Picks up object from floor without falling. Walks upstairs, two feet per step.	Builds tower of five or six cubes.
2 years .	Goes up and down stairs alone, two feet per step.	Builds tower of six or seven cubes. Turns pages of book singly. Turns door knobs, unscrews lid. Puts on shoes, socks, pants. Washes and dries hands.
2½ years .	Jumps with both feet. Walks on tiptoe when asked.	Builds tower of eight cubes. Holds pencil in hand instead of in fist.
3 years .	Goes upstairs one foot per step, and downstairs two feet per step. (Goes downstairs with one foot per step at 4 years.) Jumps off bottom step. Stands on one foot for a few seconds. Rides tricycle.	Builds tower of nine cubes. Dresses and undresses self if helped with buttor and advised occasionally about back and fro and the right foot for the shoe. Unbuttons front buttons. Can be trusted to carry china and so to help to s the table.

* For mature babies; due allowance to be made for prematurity.
† Two cards, showing dog, cup, house, shoe, flag, clock, star, leaf, basket, book.
‡ Penny, shoe, pencil, knife, ball.
§ "Take it to mother," "Put it on the chair," "Bring it to me," "Put it on the tab
‖ Copying a circle implies copying a representation of a circle on a card given by

General Understanding	Speech	Sphincter Control	Miscellaneous
...ts to picture of car or dog in book. ...ure Card.† Points correctly to one when ...sked "Where is the . . .?" ...ple objects.‡ Names one. ...ts to nose, eye, hair on request. ...ies mother in her domestic work—e.g. sweep-...ng the floor, dusting. ...ries out two simple orders.§		Clean and dry with only occasional accident.	Dawdling in feeding.
...ls people to show them objects. ...ows four parts of the body. ...ure Card.† Points correctly to two when ...sked "Where is the . . .?" ...ple orders.§ Obeys three.	Joins two words together. Repeats things said. Asks for drink, toilet, food.		Sleeping difficulties common. Sleep rituals beginning.
...tates train with cubes, without adding chimney. ...tates vertical stroke with pencil. ...ows two common objects.‡ ...eys four simple orders.§ ...allel play—watches others play and plays near ...hem, without playing with them. ...ture Cards.† Names three when asked ...What is this?" Identifies five when asked ...Where is the . . .?" ...uch can be learnt by noting the maturity of the ...lay and the imaginativeness shown.)	Uses words: I, me, you. Talks incessantly.	Dry at night if lifted out late in evening.	
...tates train with cubes, adding chimney. ...tates vertical and horizontal stroke with ...encil. ...eats two digits (one out of three trials)—e.g. ...sked to say "Eight—six." ...ure Cards.† Names five objects when asked ...What is this?" Identifies seven when asked ...Where is the . . .?" ...mmon objects.‡ Names three. ...inning to take interest in sex organs. ...k of negativism. ...es full name. ...ps to put things away.		Attends to toilet without help, except for wiping. Climbs on to lavatory seat.	Colour sense beginning.
...ies circle with pencil,‖ imitates cross (copies ...ross at 3½, square at 4, diamond at 5.) ...nstantly asking questions. ...ows own sex. ...ure Card.† Names eight when asked "What ...s this . . .?" (Names ten at 3½ years.) ...eats three digits (one out of three trials). ...Repeats four digits in one out of three trials ...t 4½.) ...eys two requests when asked "Put the ball ...nder the chair, at the side of the chair, behind ...he chair, on the chair." (Obeys four at 4 ...ears.) ...ows some nursery rhymes. ...y count up to 10. ...w joins children in play. ...sses and undresses doll. ...inning to draw objects spontaneously (e.g. a ...lan), or on request. ...ies. Imitates building bridge of three cubes.			

...miner. When a child "imitates" a circle he draws one after seeing the examiner do it.

children. In other words it may be found that a 40-week-old infant has only developed as far as the average 28-week-old child.

The sequence of development in locomotion and manipulation is shown in Table IX. These milestones were chosen partly because they are patterns which are readily observed by anyone and partly because of their importance as being particularly characteristic for the age.

Most children will reach these milestones sooner or later then the ages given. The ages are only useful for helping to form a picture of the development as a whole.

References

1. BARSLEY, M. (1966). *The Left Handed Book.* London. Souvenir Press.
2. BRAZLETON, T. R., SCHOLL, M. L., ROBEY, J. S. (1966). "Visual Responses in the Newborn." *Pediatrics*, **37**, 284.
3. BÜHLER, C. (1930). *The First Year of Life.* New York. John Day & Co.
4. BÜHLER, C. (1935). *From Birth to Maturity.* London. Kegan Paul.
5. CLARK, M. M. (1957). *Left-Handedness.* London. Univ. of London Press.
6. GESELL, A., AMATRUDA, C. S., CASTNER, B. M., THOMPSON, H. (1930). *Biographies of Child Development.* London. Hamilton.
7. GESELL, A., ILG, F. L. (1937). *Feeding Behaviour of Infants.* Philadelphia. Lippincott.
8. GESELL, A., HALVERSON, H. M., THOMPSON, H., ILG, F. L., CASTNER, B. M., AMES, L. B., AMATRUDA, C. S. (1940). *The First Five Years of Life.* London. Harper.
9. GESELL, A., ILG, F. L. (1943). *Infant and Child in the Culture of Today.* New York. Harper.
10. GESELL, A., AMATRUDA, C. S. (1947). *Developmental Diagnosis.* New York. Harper.
11. GESELL, A. (1948). *Studies in Child Development.* New York. Harper.
12. ILLINGWORTH, R. S. (1970). *Development of the Infant and Young Child. Normal and Abnormal.* 4th Edn. Edinburgh. Livingstone.
13. KARELITZ, S., KARELITZ, R. E., ROSENFELD, L. S. (1960). In Bowman, P. W., Mautner, H. V. *Mental Retardation.* New York. Grune and Stratten.
14. LENNEBERG, E. H., REBELSKY, F. G., NICHOLS, I. A. (1965). "The Vocalisation of Infants Born Deaf and Hearing Patients." *Human Development*, **8**, 23.
15. MACKEITH, R. C. (1965). "The Placing Response and Primary Walking." *Guy's Hosp. Rep.*, **79**, 394.
16. PEIPER, A. (1963). *Cerebral Function in Infancy and Childhood.* London. Pitman.
17. SHIRLEY, M. M. (1931). *The First Two Years of Life.* Minneapolis. Univ. of Minnesota Press.
18. THOMAS, A., CHESNI, Y., DARGASSIES SAINT ANNE (1960). "The Neurological Examination of the Newborn." *Little Club Clinics in Dev. Med.*
19. ZANGWILL, O. (1960). *Cerebral Dominance and its Relation to Psychological Function.* London. Oliver and Boyd.
20. ZANGWILL, O. L. (1968). *In Language and Language Disorders.* Ed. Dorfman A., "Child Care in Health and Disease." Chicago. Year Book Pub.
21. ZAPELLA, M. (1966a). "Placing Reactions in the First Year of Life." *Develop. Med. Child Neurol.*, **8**, 393.
22. ZAPELLA, M., SIMOPOULOS, A. (1966b). "Crossed Extension Reflex in the Newborn." *Ann. Pæd. Fenn.*, **12**, 30.

CHAPTER 14

GENERAL FACTORS WHICH AFFECT THE COURSE OF DEVELOPMENT

The factor which affects the rate of development more than any other is the intelligence of the child. This has already been discussed. The following additional factors have always to be borne in mind when an assessment of a child is being made:

Premature Delivery

It is obvious that if a baby is born prematurely, due allowance must be made in comparing his development with that of average children. If, for instance, he was born 2 months prematurely he has missed 2 months' development *in utero*, and so he must be expected to achieve various skills 2 months later than full-term infants. A corresponding allowance has to be made in the case of post-mature infants.

Factors which increase the Risk of Mental Subnormality

I have discussed elsewhere the prenatal factors which increase the risk that a child will be mentally subnormal.[4] They include in particular prematurity, especially if extreme: multiple pregnancy: antepartum hæmorrhage: and severe toxæmia. There are many studies of prematurity, indicating that the smallest premature babies have a considerably increased risk of mental and physical handicaps.

The Environment

Development depends on the maturation of the nervous system. It cannot be accelerated by training and practice until the nervous system is ready, and then the acceleration is only slight. It can be considerably retarded by lack of practice when the nervous system is ready for a particular skill. Owing to the fact that the nervous system continues to mature throughout the period of deprivation of practice, there is a rapid progress as soon as practice is allowed, so that in a short time the child catches up to the average.

The Dennises performed a particularly cruel experiment on a pair of twin girls whom they obtained at the age of 5 weeks. They reared them with an absolute minimum of stimulation and of practice until the age of 14 months. The children were not allowed to see each other. They were removed from the crib only for the purpose of feeding or washing. No one spoke to the twins or made any kind of overture to them. They were given no opportunity to sit, stand or practise other skills. Neither twin was able to sit alone at a year of age and neither could bear any weight on the legs, but after 4 days of practice they could sit and bear their weight on the legs.

Gesell,[3] Bowlby[1] and many others have discussed the profound effect which institutional life has on the rate of development. Children who are brought up from earliest infancy in institutions are frequently not given opportunities to sit when they are ready for it, to stand holding on when they are ready to do so and to walk with help when they have reached that stage, simply because no one really has time to give to them. As a result they are retarded in sitting, walking and other skills. There is also retardation in physical, intellectual and social development. Even by the age of 2 or 3 months babies in such institutions are found to vocalize less than normal babies. By 4 months there is considerable retardation. Bowlby wrote that the developmental quotient falls from about 65 for those who have been in institutions for 2–6 months to 50 for those who have been in them for over a year. The retardation is least marked in locomotion and most marked in speech. Sphincter control is acquired late, because there is no in-dividualization of training, all children, irrespective of their needs merely being taken to the toilet at set times. Bowlby therefore empha-sized the importance of early adoption, before the harmful effects of institutional life are fully experienced. The progressive nature of the retardation is important in the assessment of suitability for adop-tion, for when one finds that a child so separated from his mother is retarded, it is wrong to ask to see the child again for assessment after a further period in the institution, for in that case further re-tardation will have occurred. The correct line to take is to try to have the child placed into a good foster-home as soon as possible and then assess him after 2 or 3 months in such a home. If his retardation was merely due to institutional life and emotional deprivation, it may rapidly disappear as soon as he gets into a good home. If there is still significant retardation after such a trial period, the prognosis for future intelligence is poor. Every effort is now being made to reduce the damaging effect of institutional life on the child's development.

Minor degrees of emotional deprivation and of restriction of opportunities to learn commonly occur in the home. Some mothers seem to be unable to hear the cries of their baby in the pram outside the house. He cries for hours on account of sheer boredom and inability

to see what is going on and to practise his new skills. Full-time employment by the mother is apt to lead to this neglect of children when they
most need their mothers. Some mothers deliberately keep their
children off their feet for fear that they will develop knock-knee or
rickets. They prevent them from sitting for fear that the spine will be
weakened. Severe illnesses have a similarly retarding effect. It must
be remembered that when practice is given, the recovery is rapid.
It is inevitable that a child who is never given a chance to learn to
feed himself or to dress himself will be late in learning those skills.
A child who is given no chance to use a toilet when he asks to do
so will inevitably be late in acquiring sphincter control. One commonly
sees a 6- or 7-year-old child in an out-patient clinic who is dressed and
undressed by his mother, and has never been given the opportunity to do
it himself.

The same kind of deprivation may be responsible for lateness in
speaking. Some mothers fail to talk to their children. They fail to
point out the names of objects and to show them pictures in books.
As a result their children are late in learning the meaning of words,
and so they are later than others in learning to speak.

The factor of practice is of vital importance in development. Due
allowance must always be made for it in the assessment of a child.
It affects almost all fields of development, and failure to allow for it
may lead to considerable errors.

It should not be thought that the effect of the environment is
purely a negative one. It is in fact most important to note that a
really good loving environment, which stimulates the child to achieve
his best, may well raise the child's performance well above the average
level. Only a good environment will help the child's potential skills to
emerge.

Familial Factors

It is well known that intelligence is in large part genetically determined. Bowlby[1] went so far as to say that the intelligence of the
parents is probably the best guide to the intelligence of the child,
though he admits that this is only a rough guide. One difficulty is
that there is a tendency for the intelligence of children from one
generation to another to revert to the average. Terman and Oden,[6]
in a long-term follow up of 1,528 children with an IQ of 140 or more,
found that the mean IQ of 384 offspring was 127·7. Nevertheless
the number of offspring with an IQ of 150 or more was 28 times
greater than that of unselected children. On the other hand, Skodak[5]
tested the intelligence of 16 children whose mothers were feeble-minded,
with an average IQ of 66·4. The average IQ of the children was

116·4, ranging from 95 to 131, and therefore within normal limits. Fairbank made a similar observation with a much larger number of children. In each case there is a tendency for the level of intelligence to revert to the average.

The familial factor is often prominent in individual fields of development. In some families the development of locomotion, speech or sphincter control may be unusually early or unusually late, the development in all the other fields of development being average.

Sex

Girls tend to learn to walk, speak and to acquire sphincter control earlier than boys.

Variations in Maturation

There are great normal variations in the rate of development. These variations concern primarily individual fields of development, though the rare abnormal patterns of development, such as that of the slow starter, have been mentioned elsewhere. Particular emphasis has been placed on the fact that most children will pass the various "milestones" of development earlier or later than the average figures given. It is impossible to give the range of "normality" because it is impossible to define "normality" in development. As a rough guide, however, I have set down below some of the variations in the ages at which various milestones are passed by children who turn out to be perfectly "normal" in later years. It would be wrong to suggest that any child who fell outside these ranges (on the wrong side of them) was mentally defective or otherwise abnormal, but it stands to reason that the further away from the average a child's development is the less likely it is to be "normal."

Smiling. The earliest age at which I have myself seen a child smile in response to social overture was 3 days. From that day onwards the smiling in this child became more and more frequent. Very few normal full-term babies have reached 8 weeks of age without having begun to smile.

Grasping. Voluntary grasping may occur as early as 3½ months. It is commonly not seen till the age of 6 months.

Locomotion. Few normal children are unable to sit without help by the age of 8 months. I have, however, seen a child who was unable to sit without help until 19 months, or to walk without help till 30 months. He had no detectable physical disability, and he was followed up till the age of 5 years, when his IQ was 110. It is quite common to see a normal child who cannot walk without help until the age of

17 or 18 months. On the other hand, I have seen children sitting without support on the floor at 5 months. I saw a child roll from supine to prone at the age of 18 weeks, creep at 22 weeks, pull himself to the standing position at 25 weeks, walk holding on to furniture at 6 months, and walk well with two hands held at the same age. He walked unaided at $8\frac{1}{2}$ months. He was in no way advanced in any other field of development, and at the age of 5 his IQ was 88.

Speech. The normal variations in speech are considerable. Gesell and his co-workers[3] wrote that the first word is usually spoken with meaning any time between 9 and 15 months. They found that the normal 2-year-old may have only a few words in his vocabulary or well over 2,000. Speech in some is acquired unusually early and there are many recorded instances of precocious speech. Barlow, for instance,[1] described a child who could talk perfectly at 4 months and read at 1 year. It is recorded that Thomas Carlyle, hitherto unable to say a single word, at the age of 10 months heard a fellow baby crying and suddenly said, "What ails thee, Jock?" and from that time onward spoke in sentences. Retardation in speech is extremely common; some of the causes of this are discussed on p. 190, but in many children there is no discoverable cause. It is common for no word to be spoken till the age of 15 months, and for a child normal in every other respect to be saying nothing but single words at the age of $2\frac{1}{2}$ years. One has certainly heard of otherwise normal children who could not be said to be able to "talk" till the age of 4 or 5 years, but such children should always be fully investigated for the various factors mentioned and especially for high-tone deafness.

Sphincter Control. There are great individual variations in the age at which this is acquired. In many children the early "conditioning" may be replaced gradually and unnoticeably by voluntary control, so that they are dry by day from 6 months or so onwards without anything but an occasional accident. Apart altogether from mismanagement, which is discussed on p. 288, some children do not acquire control by day till $2\frac{1}{2}$ or 3 years and are still unreliable by night at the age of $3\frac{1}{2}$ years. In all other respects they are normal.

It is worth emphasizing again that no child is mentally retarded who is backward in a single field of development and normal in all other fields. The mentally retarded child is backward in all fields of development, except sometimes in sitting and walking. As far as I know the only exception to this rule is the child who acquires the mental defect as the result of encephalitis, a vascular catastrophe or a demyelinating disease, after a period of normal development. It is obvious that in such a child the milestones may have been passed at the ordinary times. Other exceptions to the rule are excessively rare and can for practical purposes be ignored.

Personality

The personality of a child may have a considerable bearing on the age at which he learns various skills. Some babies are much more independent than others, and therefore more determined to practise new skills such as feeding themselves or attending to their own toilet needs. Lack of confidence will retard walking. Some children have a greater desire than others to speak, and the age at which speech is acquired is therefore influenced by this.

The great part played by personality in the later progress of the child is responsible for the comparative failure of many efforts to predict a child's future progress. Developmental tests may with reasonable certainty enable one to predict average intelligence, but the prediction of personality is a matter of extreme difficulty. A man with only moderate intelligence but the right sort of personality is quite likely to do better in life, given equal opportunities, than a man with a high degree of intelligence with an unpleasant personality. The personality factor is the source of the greatest difficulty in the assessment of a child for the purposes of adoption. It is inevitable that a child will have inherited personality characteristics from his parents, and it is almost impossible, particularly without knowledge of the parents, to know how these will affect his future.

Physical Handicaps

Cerebral palsy may affect almost all fields of development and cause severe general retardation. Other handicaps such as deafness and blindness have a considerable influence on the rate of development. This is not the place to discuss the early diagnosis of these conditions. They were discussed in detail by Gesell and Amatruda.[3]

Lulls and Spurts

When one skill is being actively learned another skill tends to go into abeyance. When for instance, a child is actively learning to grasp objects, vocalization may decrease. It then reappears, only to decrease when sitting is being perfected. There is often a lull in the development of speech at the time when a child is learning to walk. He seems to make no progress at all for some months, and then suddenly, for no apparent reason he makes rapid headway. I have seen a child who at 15 months was well below the average in speech, while at 18 months he was far above the average. It seems as if in some children two major skills cannot be learnt at the same time. During the decreased activity in the one skill, however, the nervous system is maturing, and when the activity reappears it is found that surprsingly extensive progress is suddenly made.

References

1. BOWLBY, J. (1951). "Maternal Care and Mental Health." *Bull. Wld Hlth Org.*, **3**, 355.
2. DENNIS, W. (1941). "Infant Development Under Conditions of Restricted Practice and of Minimum Social Stimulation." *Genetic, Psychol. Monogr.*, **23**, 143.
3. GESELL, A., AMATRUDA, C. S. (1947). *Developmental Diagnosis.* New York. Hoebner.
4. ILLINGWORTH, R. S. (1970). *The Development of the Infant and Young Child; Normal and Abnormal.* 4th Edn. Edinburgh. Churchill Livingstone.
5. SKODAK, M. (1938). "The Mental Development of Adopted Children whose True Mothers are Feeble Minded." *Child Development*, **9**, 303.
6. TERMAN, L. M. (1926). *Genetic Studies of Genius.* London. Harrap.

CHAPTER 15

RETARDATION IN SINGLE FIELDS OF DEVELOPMENT AND FACTORS RESPONSIBLE

The Use of the Eyes and Ears

Just as some children are later than others of the same level o intelligence in learning to sit, walk, talk and control the bladder, som are late in appearing to see and hear. I described two otherwise norma children with "delayed visual maturation".[5] Gordon[4] has also writte about it. Others have described delayed auditory maturation.

Both of these conditions are rare. By far the commonest cause o delay in responding to sight and sound is mental subnormality. Defec tive vision and defective hearing are less common.

Sitting

The age at which a child learns to sit is affected by all the genera factors mentioned in the preceding chapter. The role of practice i particularly important. If a mother has kept the baby lying flat a day he will inevitably be retarded in learning to sit. Hypotonia for an reason, such as rickets, postpones the date at which the child is abl to sit alone. Due allowance must always be made for prematur delivery.

It is interesting to note that children who are brought up in insti tutions sometimes learn to creep before they learn to sit. This i presumably because they are able to creep without help, but they nee help in learning to sit and there is little time for the attendants to hel them in this way.

Walking

Any of the general factors already mentioned may delay walking Anything which keeps a child off his feet, whether illness, mismanage ment or institutional life, will retard walking. Some babies become s adept at creeping that they do not bother to learn to walk. Man babies learn an aberrant form of progression called shuffling or hitching progressing by means of buttock and hand, often at considerable speed This retards walking, largely because the movements involved i shuffling do not naturally lead to walking.

The personality of the child has an important bearing on the ag at which a child walks without help. Some babies are cautious an are unwilling to walk without support when ready for it, even though that support consists only of the mother's finger. It is not unusual to see a child who has been walking with one hand held for 4 or 5 months because of such lack of confidence. When he does walk without support he walks well, because his nervous system has been maturing throughout, and within a day or two of first taking off without support he is walking a great deal with only an occasional fall. A cautious child like this is apt to be badly disturbed by falls, and he may refuse to try to walk for several days after a bad bump. Falls are apt to occur as a result of slipperiness of the soles of shoes, and for this reason the soles of shoes for children of this age should have a non-skid surface.

Walking is severely delayed by hypotonia, due to rickets, pink disease and other conditions, and by hypertonia due to cerebral palsy. Congenital dislocation of the hip does not delay walking. Familial factors are important. In some families children walk particularly early, at 8 or 9 months of age, while in others they walk later than the average, at 17 or 18 months, and yet the children are "normal" in every other respect. It is likely that there is a genetic factor which governs the rate of myelination of parts of the nervous system, and so the age at which the relevant skills are learned. Obesity probably does not delay walking.

Sphincter Control

Sphincter control may be seriously delayed by mismanagement of "training" in the form of compelling the child to sit on the toilet when he is trying to get off, and punishing him for "accidents." It is delayed in children in institutions which are apt to have rigid routines that involve placing all the children on the toilet at definite times every day. This inevitably fails to take into account the needs of the individual, and control is likely to be months later in such children than in others. A similar failure to help children when they are learning to control the sphincters is found in some homes. In private homes, however, excessive attempts to "train children" are far commoner than neglect to "train" them at all.

In more than half of all cases of serious delay in the acquisition of control of the bladder, there is a family history of the same complaint.

The single passage of a hard stool which causes pain may lead to withholding of stools, and so to constipation with diarrhœa and incontinence. Structural changes in the urethra may delay the acquisition of control of the bladder for years. Personality factors operate here as in other fields of development. Some children acquire control with little emotional disturbance. Others, particularly the more sensitive and determined types, are apt to experience phases of resistance and so are delayed in the acquisition of control.

Manipulation

The way in which children are delayed in learning to feed and dress themselves has already been described.

Play behaviour is greatly modified by the parental management. Some parents fail to give their children toys suitable for their age, and in particular they fail to give them constructive toys at a time when they are ready for them and enjoy them. It is inevitable that such children will be less advanced than others who have had more opportunities to use their fingers.

Speech

By lateness in the development of speech I do not mean lateness in learning to speak distinctly. Dyslalia, or the substitution of letters, leading to indistinctness of speech, though it often occurs in children who have learnt to speak late, by no means always does so. By lateness in developing speech I mean lateness in beginning to say single words with meaning, and subsequently in putting two or three words together.

The commonest cause of lateness in the development of speech is a low level of intelligence. A mentally backward child is late in all fields of development (except occasionally in locomotion and sphincter control), and he is usually more retarded in speech than in motor and manipulative development. It is essential to reiterate, however, that one should never even suspect mental retardation in a child who is late merely in one field of development, like speech, and who is normal in other fields. The understanding of words is of much greater importance in assessing a child's intelligence than his ability to say them. I saw a 15-month-old child who could readily point out 200 common objects in picture books, when asked "Where is the . . . ?" (drum, cup, soldier, etc.), though he could only say four or five words himself. Einstein caused considerable anxiety in his parents because he was unable to speak at the age of 4. Many other highly intelligent children have been late in learning to talk. The factors responsible are obscure.

Familial factors are commonly concerned with speech development. When a child is late in learning to speak, and yet there are other indications that his intelligence is normal, one more often than not finds that there is a family history of similar lateness in speech development. Speech like other skills may depend on myelination of the appropriate part of the nervous system, and that is related to familial factors.

Deafness is a most important condition which must always be borne in mind in these children. The child who is deaf in both ears in infancy does not learn to speak without special training. When a child is partially deaf in both ears, he may learn the sounds which he can see made—b, f, w but not the g, l, r. He tends to substitute other letters—d for g, y for l, w for r.

High frequency deafness is an important cause of lateness in speaking. The defect in hearing involves pitches which are used in human speech, normally those between 512 and 2,048 double vibrations per second, while the child may be able to distinguish sounds of the 256 or 512 double-vibration tuning forks, responding to the low-frequency whispers, clicks and clapping of the hands that are commonly used as hearing tests. He can hear the passing car and banging door and will listen to the radio, so that his parents are loth to consider the possibility that he is deaf. Such children are either late in learning to speak, or more commonly speak badly owing to the omission of certain high-pitched sounds such as consonants, and particularly the s and f, which they do not hear in the speech of others.

Simple tests for hearing have been described by Sheridan[7] and Fisch.[3] They include the response to the sound of the crumpling of paper, ringing a bell, a rattle, and a tinkle of a cup and spoon. In the first few weeks the baby responds by reduction of motor activity or quietening of respirations especially if he is crying. Alternatively he may cry, blink his eyes or show a startle reflex. By about 3 or 4 months of age he should respond by turning his head to the source of sound. It is important in testing not to let the child *see* the test. An important paper on the subject was that of Dix and Hallpike.[1]

Attention has already been drawn to the fact that the development of speech, including vocalization, goes into abeyance when other skills, such as walking, are being learnt. A child may appear to make no progress at all in speech for some weeks or months, and then quite suddenly speak a great deal.

Speech tends to be learnt later in twins than in singletons. The reason for this is not clear. It may well be due to the fact that the mother of twins has less time to talk to and read to the children than the mother of a singleton. The first child in the family tends to speak earlier than subsequent children. Girls tend to speak earlier than boys.

It has been said that delay in the establishment of handedness is associated with delay in learning to speak, but I am doubtful whether this is true. I am also uncertain whether the so-called "congenital word deafness" ("congenital auditory imperception") exists or not.

When a child is brought up in an institution, he may not be given opportunities to learn speech because attendants have not sufficient time to talk to him. It is fashionable to say that some children are late in learning to speak because their parents do not talk to them sufficiently, or because they do everything for them so that they do not bother to speak. I do not believe that there is any truth in these ideas. I do not believe that any child fails to speak because he is "lazy." It is wrong to instruct a parent of a late speaker not to do things for the child unless he speaks, on the grounds that he is being lazy. I have seen this cause the most troublesome behaviour problems. The child does not speak because he cannot, and it is sheer cruelty to refuse to attend to his needs in an effort to make him talk.

The psychological background of late speakers was fully reviewed by Eisenson.[2] He concluded that there is a higher incidence of maladjustment in the parents of late speakers than there is in parents of children who speak at the usual time. There was a greater emotional instability in those parents, more perfectionism, restrictiveness and over-protectiveness. The home environment tended to be characterized by confusion, tension and lack of organization. Obviously this did not apply to all cases: but it did apply to the group of late speakers as a whole.

Eisenson suggested that parental rejection, taking the form of continuous disapproval and criticism of speech as well as of other forms of behaviour, may cause a child to stop talking or to talk less. He wrote that a child's speech may regress when a new sibling arrives. In my opinion the idea that jealousy is a common cause of lateness in speech is overdone. I have never seen such a case. All children are jealous, and lateness in speech is common. It is not easy to relate one to the other. Lateness in speech is never due to tongue tie. In cerebral palsy lateness in speech is common; it may be due to one or more of the following factors—a low level of intelligence, incoordination or spasticity of the muscles of the tongue, partial deafness, or to the cortical defect. A rare cause of delayed speech is infantile autism.

It must be admitted that in many cases the reason for lateness in speech is not clear.

Dyslalia. The commonest form of dyslalia is the lisp, due to protrusion of the tongue between the teeth when the letter s is being used. In the great majority of children it disappears without treatment. Dyslalia should only be treated by a speech therapist if it persists past the fourth birthday. It should be treated then, so that the child's speech will be normal by the time he starts school.

Every child with dyslalia should have his hearing tested. If this is not done, high tone deafness will be missed.

"Nasal speech," involving the substitution of b for m, may be due to postnasal obstruction by adenoids. The speech returns to normal a few weeks after their removal. The distinctness of speech is often temporarily disturbed by coryza.

Tongue tie may cause difficulty in the pronunciation of certain letters (p. 92). Severe malocclusion may be a cause of indistinct speech. As speech is learnt by imitation, it is obvious that defective speech may be learnt from others.

The problem of stuttering is discussed elsewhere (p. 334).

Conclusion

It will be seen that there are many factors other than the intelligence of the child which affect the course of development. Some of those factors affect practically all fields of development, while others affect isolated skills only. All these factors must be considered in the assessment of every child. *Developmental diagnosis is a personal individual problem, in that no prediction can be made until all the various factors which may have affected the development and which may affect it in the future are duly assessed.* It is for this reason that some large-scale statistical studies have failed to demonstrate correlation between observations in infancy and subsequent intelligence tests. They were impersonal, failing to consider the children as individuals.

No diagnosis of mental deficiency must ever be made or suspected on account of retardation in a single field of development. If such a diagnosis is made, it will be wrong.

The Treatment of Isolated Retardation

When a child is retarded in a single field of development, such as locomotion, speech or sphincter control, there is usually nothing to be done about it, unless there is an underlying cause which is treatable, such as lack of practice in the case of locomotion, deafness in the case of speech or parental mismanagement in the case of sphincter control. It has already been explained that development depends on the maturation of the nervous sytem, and that no amount of practice and teaching will enable a child to learn skills unless the nervous system is ready for them. The physiotherapist cannot help to make a child walk unless there is an associated mechanical difficulty, such as hypotonia or spasticity. The speech therapist cannot help in teaching a child to talk unless there is an underlying cause of the retardation, such as deafness, and the nervous system is otherwise ready for the acquisition of speech.

References

1. Dix, M. R., Hallpike, C. S. (1952). "Diagnosis of Deafness in Young Children." *Birt. Med. J.*, **1**, 235.
2. Eisenson, J. (1956). In *Psychology of Exceptional Children and Youth*, by Cruickshank, W. M. London, Staples.

3. FISCH, L. (1963). "Early Detection and Management of Deafness in Children." *Brit. J. clin Practice*, **17**, 179.
4. Gordon N. (1968). "Visual Agnosia in Childhood." *Develop. Med. Child Neurol.*, **10**, 377.
5. ILLINGWORTH R. S. (1961). "Delayed Visual Maturation." *Arch. Dis Childh.*, **36**, 407.
6. ILLINGWORTH, R. S. (1970). *Development of the Infant and Young Child. Normal and Abnormal.* 4th Edn. Edinburgh. Livingstone.
7. SHERIDAN, M. (1958). "Simple Hearing Tests for Very Young or Mentally Retarded Children." *Brit. Med. J.*, **2**, 999.

CHAPTER 16

DEVELOPMENTAL DIAGNOSIS

The Developmental History

It is often said that it is a waste of time to take a history of past development because it is so unreliable. I disagree strongly with this opinion. It is obvious when they are questioned, that some parents know little about the skills which their children have developed and when they developed them. Of all the hundreds of parents whom I have interrogated concerning their children's development, probably the least knowledgeable were a doctor and his medically-qualified wife. Many parents are not only non-observant but have a bad memory, and therefore cannot remember when skills were learned. This is particularly liable to be the case in large families. Nevertheless it is always the task of a doctor in taking a history to assess the story which he is given. In taking a developmental history the doctor assesses the mother's veracity and memory. He decides by the way she replies whether the answer was made up on the spur of the moment or whether it was likely to be a true one. When in doubt he comes back to the point at issue and asks the question in a different way in order to see whether the replies tally. He knows quite well that parents of a retarded child are often unwilling to allow themselves to believe what they know is the truth—that the child is backward. They try to make themselves believe that his development and his understanding are normal. It is the duty of the examiner to observe this attitude and so to assess the weight which can be placed on the story given. Many mothers, having forgotten when their child acquired various skills, fabricate their replies, basing their answers on the age at which they know these skills are usually acquired instead of on what they can remember of their own child. It is the duty of the examiner to read the mother's mind and decide how much reliance can be placed on her story.

The developmental history is of particular importance if the child, on examination, is unco-operative on account of shyness or for other reasons. Objective examination of the child is always necessary, but in some children such an examination can be difficult. It must also be borne in mind that even when a child is fully co-operative, it is likely to be impossible even for the most skilful of examiners to obtain a full picture of the child's behaviour and achievements. An observant mother sees much more of her child's skills by living with him and watching his day-to-day progress than an examiner who only sees him for half an hour in the strange surroundings of a consulting room on perhaps two or three occasions, or even less. In my opinion a full, careful developmental history is of vital importance in the establishment of a developmental diagnosis.

The first essential in taking the history is to ensure that the parents and the examiner each know exactly what the other means. For this reason it is impossible for the examiner to take a developmental history of any value unless he is thoroughly conversant with the normal development of infants. Below are some important examples of milestones which show the importance of accuracy in history taking for their correct interpretation.

Smiling. Some mothers interpret facial grimaces due to wind as smiling. It is always necessary when a mother refers to the age at which smiling began, to ask her what it was that made the child smile. The first smiles are always in response to social overture, when the mother talks to her baby. If the mother says that the smiles were in response to other stimuli or not in response to any stimulus at all, the story should be disregarded.

It is extremely difficult to say when a child first smiles. Smiling is not a thing which suddenly happens for the first time. There is a gradual, almost imperceptible advance from the intent regard and mouthing of the 4-week-old baby to his smile when he is 6 weeks old.

"Taking notice." This is also difficult to define, and unless a definition is made it is of little value to ask a mother when her baby first began to "take notice." A child of 2 or 3 weeks often "takes notice" in the sense that when the mother talks to him, when he is in a good temper, he watches her face intently. From that age onwards he takes more and more notice until at about 12 weeks he is seen to turn his head from side to side to follow his mother about the room, and at about 16 weeks he turns his head towards a sound.

"Holding the head up." It is common to read in a "scientific" paper that a baby "held his head up" at such and such an age. Without accurate definition such a statement means nothing. At 2 weeks of age a baby, when held in the sitting position or in ventral suspension (with the hand under the abdomen), may momentarily hold the head up. It is obvious that the further a child is propped up the easier it is for him to "hold the head up." It is not until the age of 28 weeks that the average child can lift his head off the couch when he is lying supine.

Grasping. Every new-born baby shows the grasp reflex, and this must be distinguished from the voluntary grasp of later weeks. At

2 weeks or sooner a baby will hold a rattle when it is placed in his
and, but this achievement precedes by 8 weeks or more the age at
hich he can go for an object and grasp it when it is placed near his
and, and probably by 3 or 4 weeks more the age at which he can
rasp an object placed within reach at a distance from his hand. It
; 9 months before a child can pick up a small object of the size of a
urrant between finger and thumb. It is of little value to ask a mother
vhen the child was "able to grasp objects" without being more precise
1 one's question.

Sitting. A child can be held in the sitting position immediately
fter birth. By about 5 months he can sit up well in a pram when
ropped up, but it is not until about 6 months that he can sit for a few
econds in the pram without support, and 7 months that he can sit
nsupported for a few seconds on a hard surface. At about 6 months
e can probably sit with his hands forward for support. It is not until
bout 9 months that he is reasonably secure in the sitting position. It
; not enough merely to ask a mother when her child was first able to sit.

Self-feeding. Whereas a child of 6 months can hold a biscuit and
ed himself with it, it is not until 15–18 months that an average
hild can feed himself with a spoon and manage a cup without help.
Ie has to go through numerous intervening stages of trying to load
he spoon, of succeeding in loading the spoon but not getting it any
vhere near his mouth, and later of getting it near the mouth but
otating it and therefore spilling the contents just before it enters the
nouth. With the cup he has to go through the stages of helping to
old it, of suddenly letting go when he is drinking or has had what
e wants, of spilling most of the contents, until finally he can pick it
p, drink and replace it with only occasional accidents. It would
e futile merely to ask a mother "when he was able to feed himself"
vithout more accurate definition.

Speech. It is still regrettably common to find in a medical journal
hat a child "first spoke at 12 months." This means in itself practically
othing. It is common to be told by a mother that her child began
o say words at 6 months. On further questioning it is found that
he child was making the sounds "mm," "mum" when crying or
nnoyed. Later on the proud father hears the baby combine syl-
ables—"baba," "da-da-da"—at about 32 weeks and calls this a
vord. All children go through this stage. It is not till about a year
f age that the average baby begins to say one word *with meaning*. In
he case of "da-da" he shows that he means "daddy" by saying it
nore when his father is present than when he is not there. By the age
1–24 months the average child combines two words for the first time.
It is difficult to decide when a child says his first word and to decide

how many words he can say at a given age, chiefly because of the difficulty in defining what is meant by a word. It is not usually the case that a child one day is unable to say a word, while he can on the next day. The evolution of speech is a more gradual process. The baby may say "g," denoting "girl" a few weeks before he says "gir" and finally "girl." He may "moo" when he sees a cow and make primitive barking noises when he sees a dog, or else on seeing the dog he says "g," and later "og," before finally he can say "dog." He may make a sound like "tebba," meaning "teddy bear," months before he can say "teddy bear" properly. It is a hopeless undertaking to count the number of "words" he really can say. Of much greater importance than the number of words he is able to say is the number of words which he can understand.

Walking. There are still many papers which make the bald statement that a child first "walked" at a given age. Without accurate definition this is of little value. The child of 8 or 9 months may walk after a fashion with two hands held, but it is not till 13 months or so that he can walk without support for a few steps. It has already been pointed out that a cautious child may walk with one finger held for some months before daring to walk without support. This can be elicited by careful history taking.

Helping to Dress. The first sign of helping to dress is holding the arm out for the armhole or holding the foot out for a sock.

Sphincter Control. This, like all other skills, is learnt gradually and it is essential to be precise in one's questions. Points of value are the age at which a child first begins to point out the fact that he has wet his napkin, the age at which he begins to tell the mother that he is about to pass urine and the age at which he can first do without a napkin by day, and later by night, with only an occasional "accident." It is not enough to ask when a child was first "clean."

It is essential in taking the developmental history to cover, as far as possible, all fields of development—locomotion, manipulation, play and social behaviour, memory, the mode of display of pleasure and displeasure, feeding behaviour, sphincter control and speech. The history should include the general understanding, the degree of concentration shown on toys and books, the response to such stimuli as the repetition of nursery rhymes, the appearance of food, the methods of drawing attention and the other items listed in the table which need not be repeated here.

It is also useful to ask the mother how the child in question compares with his siblings or with neighbours' children in the various fields of development. A simple question about the progress of these children in school gives an idea whether they are likely to be reasonably normal

It is important to ask about the various factors which are
nown to affect the course of development, such as the amount of
ractice which the mother has given the child, the sort of toys he
as, the history of illnesses and other factors. Some of the relevant
articulars about the child's personality should also be elicited.

In my opinion the developmental history is an essential part of the
evelopmental diagnosis. It enables the doctor to assess the rate of
evelopment and to determine whether there has been any change in
ie rate, such as that which occurs with the advent of a degenerative
isease of the nervous system, or with a sudden spurt of development
rhich is seen when a child is taken out of an institution and placed in
good foster-home. It enables him to determine whether there are
ny environmental or other factors which may affect his development.
t enables him to obtain the family history. If the developmental
istory tallies with the findings on examination it helps to confirm the
ccuracy of one's findings. If it does not tally, one has to decide
vhether the mother's story is correct, or whether for some reason the
hild's true abilities have not been revealed by the examination. In
ither case it would be essential to see the child again in order to check
ne's findings.

he Assessment of Gestational Age

There are many methods of assessing the gestational age of a baby
i utero or after birth, without relying on the date of the mother's last
ienstrual period. They include quickening, the size of the uterus,
aginal cytology, examination of the cells, creatinine and bilirubin in
he amniotic fluid, and x-ray methods. Parkin reviewed those and
iethods of assessing the maturity of the baby at birth. External features
iclude the amount of vernix, the texture of abdominal skin folds, the
olour of the skin, the presence of œdema, lanugo, the length and
exture of the nails, the firmness of the ears, breast size, the localization
f the testes, the prominence of the labia minora and the firmness of the
kull. He picked out the following features:

Breast palpable	— gestational age unlikely to be less than 34 weeks.
Skin pink	— 36 weeks
Pinnæ firm	— 36 weeks
Testes fully descended	— 36 weeks
Areas of baldness	— 37 weeks
All vernix off	— 39 weeks
Skin pale	— 40 weeks

8

He concluded that assessment by a combination of signs was mucl more likely to be accurate than reliance on single signs.

In Sheffield Dubowitz and his colleagues[2] elaborated a scorin method which combined the external criteria—œdema, skin texture colour and opacity, lanugo, plantar creases, nipple formation, breas size, ear form and firmness, and the appearance of the genitals, wit the infant's posture, wrist flexion, foot dorsiflexion, arm and leg recoi popliteal angle on extending the knee with the hip flexed, heel to ea and scarf signs, the head lag when he is pulled to the sitting positior and the posture in ventral suspension. They emphasized that by thi combination of signs a much more accurate diagnosis could be mad than by the use of single criteria. They found that the duration c gestation, using this method, could be assessed to within a week. Thos interested should refer to their paper for details.

The Developmental Examination

For research purposes the examination must be performed i exactly the manner prescribed by the originators of the tests, with th exact equipment specified, for otherwise the norms laid down are nc strictly applicable. The nearer one adheres to the method of examina tion described by the authors of the tests the more accurate will be th results. For details of these methods the reader should consult th works of Arnold Gesell (particularly his *Developmental Diagnosis* an *The First Five Years of Life*). Charlotte Bühler described further tes in her book, *The First Year of Life*, along with other tests based o those of Gesell. Cattell's tests are also based on those of Gesell. He book has the merit of giving good simple descriptions of the tests, bu they do not sufficiently cover all fields of development. For ordinar purposes extreme accuracy is not needed, and hence in the sectio to follow no rigid methods of performing the tests are given. It is fo the specialist, to whom are referred the specially difficult cases. t employ accurate tests in order that valid comparisons can be made a subsequent examinations.

The first essential in the developmental examination is to secur the full co-operation of the child. At Gesell's clinic care was alway taken to determine beforehand the infant's normal playtime, and th developmental examination was timed accordingly. It is almos useless to test a small child when he is tired or hungry. I usually prefe to have the mother present during the examination, but she must b asked not to interfere with the tests by trying to "help." Much ca sometimes be learned of the mother's attitude to the child, and th hild, especially the toddler, is apt to be more co-operative when she present.

In the first 2 months the baby is best examined in the first place in is mother's arms. The mother should be asked to talk to him, so that 1e responsiveness, the intentness of his regard and, after the age of weeks, his smiling and even vocalizations can be noted. He is then eld in ventral suspension with the hand under the abdomen, so that ead control can be observed, and thereafter placed in the supine osition. Here his posture is watched. The younger child always lies rith the head turned to one side and at frequent intervals shows the symmetrical tonic neck reflex. The dangling ring or rattle is brought up) the midline about a foot away from his head and then moved 1to his line of vision. When he catches sight of it, it is moved slowly)wards the midline or beyond in order to observe how far he will)llow it with his eyes. During this test the hand is observed. In the ew-born the hand is clenched. It gradually opens as he grows lder. The baby is then pulled into the sitting position so that the xtent of the head lag can be seen. In the sitting position momentary levation of the head is noted. The position of the head as n index of head control is also seen in the supported standing osition.

Between 2 and 4 months it is again wise to observe the child first in is mother's arms. The interest which he shows in his surroundings, is smiling and his vocalizations are noted. By the age of 3-4 months e may show an obvious desire to grasp a toy when it is held in front f him: he excites, both arms move, he watches the toy intently, but 1 the earlier weeks of the period he does not go for it. Later he moves oth hands out for it but completely misjudges the distance and does ot contact it. This can readily be observed as he sits on his mother's nee. A rattle is placed in his hand. By about 3 months of age he ill hold it and soon wave it deliberately. He is then held in ventral uspension in order to observe head control, and then placed on his ack and tested with the rattle or dangling ring, so that his eye following an be estimated. In the latter part of the period his hands come)gether in the midline and he may pull at his dress. The hand egard, characteristic of the 12-18-week-old baby, should be looked)r. He is pulled to the sitting position in order to test for head lag, nd in the sitting position the degree of roundness of the back is noted. he head should be held well up at this age, but in the earlier weeks it ends to bob forwards. If it is held up by the baby, the trunk should e gently rocked so that one can observe whether the head is held teadily even if the baby is moved. Head control is also tested in the tanding position, in which he bears a small fraction of his weight. He

is placed in the prone position so that head control and the posture c
the lower limbs can be seen. From this age onwards it is particularl
important not to begin with the supine or prone position, because it 1
so often disliked by babies and crying then results.

From 4 to 8 months the interest shown by the baby, his alertnes
and responsiveness are noted before the examination proper begin:
He is offered a cube in the supported sitting position and the maturit
of the grasp is observed. In the latter part of the period he is offere
a second cube so that one can see whether he drops the first on seein
the second. He is offered a small pellet or a thin piece of string in th
latter part of the period, in order to test for finger-thumb appositior
Head control and the other necessary preliminaries to locomotion ar
tested in the sitting, prone and standing positions. In the supine an
prone positions the posture of his lower limbs should be noted. He :
allowed to see himself in a mirror so that the response can be seen. Afte
about 6 months of age he should transfer objects from one hand t
another, and the maturity of this act is assessed. After 6 months he goe
for objects with one hand instead of two. In the latter part c
the period he is likely to try hard to crawl without success. Th
maturity of his rolling is observed. His vocalizations are carefull
listened for.

From the age of 8 months to a year the child is first tested in th
sitting position, and then standing. Even at this age he may dislik
the prone position. The development of locomotion and manipulatio
is observed, particular emphasis throughout being placed on *how* th
acts are performed and with what degree of maturity he does then
The most careful observation is needed to observe such characteristi
behaviour as the nature of the grasp, the index finger approach t
objects, the beginning of release and the understanding of the meanin
of words.

After the age of a year it is particularly important to secure th
child's co-operation. When he first enters the room he should b
allowed to wander about as he wishes and to play with toys which hav
been placed there for the purpose. No apparent notice is taken c
him, but he is closely watched, for much can be observed from hi
behaviour. When he is old enough to understand, his confidence ca:
often quickly be gained by taking notice of his shoes and clothes an
by talking about his dolls or toys.

In this age group it is particularly important to maintain the child'
interests in the tests. They must be done rapidly and not repeated mor
than is absolutely necessary. There is not usually much difficulty i
testing the infant under a year, but it can be difficult to get a determine
child in the negativistic stage to co-operate. He is distractable, activ

nd easily bored. He is given a picture-book at the outset and much
an be learnt by the interest which he shows in the pictures and his
bility to point out familiar objects. In order to maintain interest it is as
ell to try roughly to alternate the more interesting tests with the less
iteresting ones. The former include the cubes and pictures. The less
iteresting ones include verbal tests, such as the repetition of digits.
.s soon as boredom seems to be impending a rapid change is made to
iore interesting tests. The method must be elastic so that changes like
iis can be made if necessary. The child is never told that he has
iade a mistake. The word "no" is never used. Nothing but en-
iuragement is given.

Fallacies and Difficulties in Developmental Diagnosis

A developmental diagnosis must never be made on clinical im-
ression. It can only be based on a careful history and thorough
:amination. Mental superiority is often wrongly diagnosed in a
- or 3-year-old child because of charm of manner, absence of shyness
nd good looks. An infant is apt to be called mentally defective
ecause of a peculiar facies, an unusually large or small head, or because
f asymmetry of the skull—all conditions which are perfectly com-
atible with normal mental development. Unusually bad behaviour
i a child may lead the unwary to diagnose mental deficiency. Shyness
nd failure to co-operate in tests for any reason must never lead one
) a wrong conclusion about a child's mental development. Some
iildren at about the age of 3 may regard some of the tests as
lly and so fail to co-operate. Failure to present the tests quickly
nough and to maintain interest in the tests will lead to a fallacious
:sult.

Many mistakes are made as a result of attaching too much im-
ortance to an unusual performance in one particular field. Mental
iperiority can never be diagnosed on the basis of advancement in one
articular field of development, with the sole possible exception of early
)eech. Mental deficiency can *never* be diagnosed on account of
:tardation in any one skill, such as locomotion, speech or sphincter
)ntrol. It can largely, however, be eliminated by the normal or
iusually early development of speech—provided that the mental
:tardation did not develop after speech had been learnt. It can
:rtainly not be eliminated by the early acquisition of sphincter
)ntrol, which is sometimes learnt relatively early in mentally defective
iildren—earlier, in some cases, than in some children of superior
itelligence.

It is easy to be misled by lulls which occur in some fields of

development. I once saw an intelligent child who at the age of 11 month
was thought to be rather backward compared with a sibling in feedir
himself. Suddenly one day he decided to use the spoon himself, and
was immediately noted that he was in fact considerably advanced in th
skill, for there was minimal rotation and spilling. It was clear tha
owing to progressive maturation of the nervous system, he was well ab
to manipulate a spoon although he had no practice. The common lul
which occur in speech development have been discussed elsewher
When a 12–18-month-old child is unable to walk without help it
essential to note the degree of maturity with which he walks whe
supported, in order that one can decide whether the factor which
preventing him from walking alone is merely his personality. It me
even be observed that although he cannot walk alone he can stand alor
and pick an object up from the floor without support, or that he can g
up into the standing position without holding on to anything-
performances which normally *follow* the ability to walk unaided instea
of preceding it. The factor concerned in this behaviour is merely lac
of confidence, which is not related to his intelligence.

It is always wrong to conduct a developmental examination in a
epileptic child when he is in a confusional state after a major convulsio
or when he is under the influence of sedative drugs.

In the actual performance of the test other mistakes can be mad
Head control cannot be properly tested when the child is sleepy
crying. One can easily be misled into thinking that there is excessi
head lag when one pulls the child into the sitting position from lying c
his back. In the prone position babies are often cross and may fail
lift the head up as far as they are able to do. A child may refuse to s
without support during the examination if he has a wet or soile
napkin while he is normally able to do so.

Serious mistakes are made in developmental diagnosis if the vario
factors which affect the course of development are not properly co
sidered, and if the normal variations which occur are not borne
mind. It is for these reasons that it is so rarely desirable to assess th
"intelligence quotient" in terms of a single figure in a pre-scho
child. Such a figure cannot take into account the various factors ar
variations which the trained observer knows to be of importance. Son
of the tests used, for instance, in the 2–3-year-old child depend c
the acquisition of speech. But a child may be of normal or superi
intelligence and yet be unusually late in learning to speak. Norms
development, used in the assessment of the developmental quotient (DC
will miss this and lead to the child being given an unduly low sco
simply because he cannot speak. Simple observation might well sho
that the child's understanding of words, as shown by his ability

dentify objects and to carry out simple acts on request, is considerably ιdvanced and indicates mental superiority. In the same way a child night be given a low score in other fields of development, such as sphincter control, while in fact his lateness in acquiring sphincter control was due to nothing more than parental mismanagement and ore no relationship to his intelligence. Serious fallacies, therefore, would arise if one were to attempt to calculate the DQ merely by converting each observation in the developmental examination into a igure, adding all the figures up, and taking the average.

Attention has already been drawn to the occasional slow starter, who is somewhat backward for some weeks or months in infancy und then shows a normal or superior performance later. The occasional occurrence of encephalitis, vascular catastrophes or demyelinating diseases must also be borne in mind. If their possibility is forgotten, undue reliance on previous milestones of development may lead one to make the mistake of saying that a child is mentally normal whereas actually he is mentally defective. In these cases his general behaviour, lestructiveness, lack of concentration, hyperkinesis and general disinterestedness in the surroundings reveal the underlying mental deficiency, even though in other fields of development he is within normal limits. *In any doubtful case with any unusual features the developmental examination should be repeated after an interval, an opinion being in the meantime withheld in order that the rate of development can be observed.*

The rate of the appearance of teeth and the closing of the fontanelle are of no value as milestones of development.

The great difficulty in developmental diagnosis lies in the fact that some of the most important items—the alertness, the rapidity with which acts are performed, the degree of concentration and of understanding, and the interest shown by the child—are unscorable. One can only form an impression of those features. Tests which are entirely sensorimotor, covering locomotion and manipulation only, inevitably miss important aspects of development. It is unfortunate that the least useful skills for the assessment of a child happen to be the easiest to study and to record.

Another difficulty is the fact that the tests do not include the personality of the child. Though one thinks that one can predict the child's intelligence with reasonable likelihood of being right, it is extremely difficult to predict his personality.

This is not the place to discuss the various physical handicaps, such as cerebral palsy, which retard development in children who are mentally normal. A good review of these conditions, under the name of "pseudo-feeblemindedness," was given by Bakwin.[1]

References

1. BAKWIN, H. (1950). "Feeblemindedness and Pseudo-Feeblemindedness." *J. Pediat.*, **37**, 271.
2. DUBOWITZ, L. M. S., DUBOWITZ, V., GOLDBERG, C. (1970). "Clinical assessmen of Gestational age in the Newborn Infant." *J. Pediat.*, **77**, 1.
3. PARKIN, J. M. (1969) "The Assessment of Gestational Age." M.D. Thesis University of Newcastle-upon-Tyne.

CHAPTER 17

THE BASIS OF BEHAVIOUR

All children have behaviour problems. All parents have behaviour problems. All teachers have behaviour problems. Behaviour problems in a child represent a conflict between his developing personality and that of his parents, teachers and siblings, and with other children with whom he comes into contact. In order to understand the reasons for this conflict it is important to consider something of the basis of behaviour in general.

Preconceptional Factors

Behaviour problems have their origin before birth, and often before conception. They date back to the parents' childhood and personality, to the sort of family life which they had, to the amount of love and security which they experienced. There is good evidence that a child brought up from birth without affection may grow up to be unable to give or receive affection himself. Whenever one is faced with a child who is rejected and unloved by his parents, one nearly always finds that his mother or father had an unhappy childhood. Rejection, unhappiness and lack of love in a child's life may well affect the next generation.

As Leo Kanner remarked, the attitudes of parents are the crystallization of their whole life experiences. Their personality, like that of the child, was partly inherited and partly the product of their environment. Their personality was moulded by their home life and by their subsequent experiences in life. A parent who was regularly beaten and chastised by *his* parents may grow up to apply the same treatment to his children.

The parents were affected by the social class in which they were brought up; by the personality and attitudes of *their* parents; and by the love and security or lack of it which they experienced in childhood.

Other preconceptional factors include the age of the parents, the intensity of their desire for a child, or for a child of a particular sex. The duration of married life before conception may be highly relevant to the personality of the child—not just because of their age, itself a relevant factor. When a child was referred to me with innumerable symptoms, none of them amounting to disease, it was clear that the diagnosis lay in the fact that the parents had been married for 17 years before they had been able to conceive this, their only child. The over-anxiety and over-protection were tremendous—and the child was becoming a hypochondriac as a result.

A forced marriage may stamp the life of the children of the marriage in that the parents are not really a match for each other, and domestic conflict may result.

Everyone knows of the unwanted child, whose conception was never intended. If he were illegitimate, he will not suffer, if he is placed for adoption in the new-born period; but he may suffer a great deal if adoption is delayed, or worse still, if he spends his childhood in an institution.

Children are considerably affected by the spacing of births, and by the number of siblings. In general, the smaller the gap between births, the greater the likelihood of jealousy between the children. The youngest of a large family has a different childhood from the only child. The second only child (to use the expression coined by the late Dr. Cedric Harvey), the child who is born as an "accident," years after the next oldest in the family, is apt to be spoilt and petted not only by his parents, but by his grown-up siblings.

It is easy to imagine that the attitude of the parents to the child may be considerably influenced by his sex, if they were particularly anxious to have a child of a particular sex. If the first four or five children in the family were girls, and they had a special desire to have a boy, one can well imagine that if the next child to be borne is another girl, she may be at least partly rejected, and that if the child is a boy he may be the subject of favouritism and overprotection—with undesirable effects on his developing personality.

It need hardly be added that genetic problems are an important pre-conceptional factor which are going to have a considerable effect on the child to be born. The child unlucky enough to be born with any of the scores of serious genetic diseases, such as hæmophilia, is going to have to face many psychological and physical difficulties as the months and years go by.

It has been shown by several workers,[4] that a high proportion of criminal mental defectives have an extra Y chromosome. Inmates of Scottish Borstals and similar institutions, especially men who were tall, had been troublesome at school, and had been the black sheep of a respectable family, had the XYY arrangement. Others, with a lower level of intelligence, but a variety of behaviour problems, had the XXYY chromosomes. This observation opens up a new field for research into behaviour.

Other Prenatal Factors

This is not the place to discuss the innumerable prenatal factors, operating during pregnancy, which have such a profound effect on the child's life and health.

A variety of behaviour problems, such as over-activity, defective concentration, tics, and emotional lability have been found to correlate with the occurrence of toxæmia, hypertension, hyperemesis in pregnancy, or with anoxia at birth.[20]

There is increasing interest in the relationship between pregnancy experiences and their effect on the child's behaviour. Stott[16] in a series of papers has attempted to show that psychological stress during pregnancy may predispose the child to react in an undesirable way to a subsequent adverse environment, and so predispose to behaviour problems, and in particular to juvenile delinquency. He showed, for instance, that there is an association between delinquency and birth during the early war years. Drillien,[5, 6] confirmed some of Stott's findings. She showed that behaviour disturbance at school was significantly associated with low birth weight and with complications of pregnancy and delivery.

Gunther[7] studied the pregnancy of 20 married mothers who had a premature delivery without known physical cause, and 20 controls. She found that there was a significant association between premature delivery and psychosomatic symptoms and crises during pregnancy. It should be noted that psychological stress may lead to uterine dysfunction and so to difficulties in delivery.

Taft and Goldfarb[17] carried out a retrospective study of 29 children aged 6 to 11 with schizophrenia, 39 siblings of affected children, and 34 public school children. They found that in the case of schizophrenic children, there had been far more prenatal and perinatal complications, such as hyperemesis, toxæmia and abnormal delivery. Others[11] have found the same association. When a mother has a really difficult time during pregnancy, with hyperemesis, toxæmia or other ailments, or subsequently a troublesome delivery, one could imagine that her attitude to the child may be different from that of a mother who had a completely normal and uneventful pregnancy. The former might well feel a subconscious resentment against the child who caused her so much discomfort.

There is abundant evidence that the offspring of animals exposed to experimental stress behave in an abnormal manner.[18]

Natal and Postnatal Factors

I have several times seen complete rejection of a child at birth. The rejection was either because he was not of the desired sex, or because there was a physical defect, in particular a hare lip, the Sturge Weber syndrome or mongolism. Some animals, on finding that their offspring is abnormal, leave it to die. Prechtl[12] found that mothers who have given birth to babies who are unduly drowsy or overactive in the new-born period are more protective and dominant in their attitude to them in later years. A baby who is really difficult in his first few days, crying excessively and refusing to suck on the breast, not only causes the mother a great deal of anxiety at a time when she is least able to tolerate it, but later may be the object of some degree of resentment. This is difficult or impossible to prove; it is a clinical impression.

The study of the behaviour of animals (ethology) has given us a new insight into the behaviour of the infant and child.[8,13] For instance, if rats are separated from their mother for the first two to four days after delivery, and then returned to the mother, she rejects them; when they grow up, they themselves are poor mothers, and there is a high death rate in their pups. Sheep, goats and other animals have a strong motivation to lick their offspring at birth; if the lamb or kid is separated from the mother for two to five hours after birth and then returned, they are rejected by their mothers. Lambs and puppies separated from their mothers in this way, and then returned, behave abnormally, and when they grow up are poor mothers. Similar experiments have been carried out with monkeys, cats, rabbits and other animals, with the same results. It will be noted that the effect is a double one—the mother rejects, and the offspring develops abnormally.

We cannot say how far these observations are relevant to human beings. We do know that some mothers feel that it is important to them psychologically to be fully conscious at the moment of delivery, and that some mothers feel the urge to put the baby to the breast immediately he is born. Nurses in the obstetric hospital have told me that mothers who put the baby to the breast immediately are more likely to feed their babies successfully on the breast than others. We know from the work of Drillien and others[5,6] that prematurely born babies are more likely than others to have certain troublesome behaviour problems at school. It could be that one causative factor is the separation of the premature baby from his mother for the first days or weeks of his life. Some feel that it may be important for mothers to handle their premature babies,[1a] and we encourage this at the Jessop Maternity Hospital, Sheffield.

Despite opinions expressed by psychiatrists, there is no scientific evidence that breast feeding, as compared with artificial feeding, has any special psychological value to the child.[3] There are so many variables that it would be impossible to prove this, one way or the other. For instance, the sort of mother who wants to breast feed may be a different sort of mother from one who refuses to feed the baby on the breast; and in this country there is a higher incidence of breast feeding in the upper social classes than in the lower ones. There are many other variables which would make a study of the psychological value of breast feeding an unrewarding one.

The relevance of the sensitive or critical period to the behaviour and mental development of children is attracting increased attention. I reviewed some aspects of this matter with a surgical colleague.[9] By the term "*sensitive period*" one denotes that particular period of development at which the appropriate stimulus for a particular behaviour pattern is best applied. By the term "*critical period*" one refers to that period of development beyond which a stimulus will no longer elicit the relevant behaviour pattern. For instance, a wolf can be domesticated only if it is removed from the mother before its eyes open; a squirrel who is deprived of nuts to crack in the early part of its life will never learn to crack nuts if given them after the "*critical period*". There are numerous papers on the sensitive or critical period in birds and animals of many kinds. In our paper we pointed out that if a child is not given solids to chew at a time when he has recently learned to chew (normally 6 to 7 months), he is likely to refuse to take solids and will vomit them. It has long been known that if a congenital cataract is not removed soon enough, the child may never see, and that if a cleft palate is not re- paired soon enough, the child may never learn to speak normally. A deaf child who has not been allowed to hear sounds until the age of 3, is slow in learning to recognize new sounds, and if he has not heard them by 7, it is almost impossible to teach him the sounds. Madame Montessori applied the concept of the sensitive period to the teaching of young children, and so developed her teaching method. She claimed that there were certain sensitive periods in which children were ready and anxious to learn certain skills, and it was then that they should be taught them; subsequently it would be too late.[15] Bloom[2] indicated that the pattern of learning at school is set in the preschool years, and that the preschool home environment is essential for his subsequent learning ability. In our book *Lessons from Childhood*, concerning the early child- hood of famous men and women, we gave examples of the possible result of early teaching of the preschool child.[10] The concept of the sensitive or critical period may well prove to be of great importance for the teaching and behaviour patterns in childhood. It is thought that babies deprived of appropriate sensory stimuli in the early weeks may later be found to have troublesome perceptual problems.

The maturation of the nervous system, and in particular of the brain, is of the greatest importance in the study of child development. No child can learn to walk until myelination of the spinal cord will permit him to walk. It is probable that the acquisition of sphincter control depends to a large part on the maturation of the nervous system. There is clearly some relationship between maturation and intelligence, for it is obvious that the mentally defective infant is late in all aspects of development (except occasionally in walking). It is obvious that the child's level of intelligence has a profound effect on his behaviour. For instance, a low level of intelligence in one of twins may cause jealousy and unhappiness.

The conditioning process is an important one in the study of behaviour. For instance, the child who at mealtimes is coerced, threatened, bullied and smacked, in an effort to get him to eat, may well come to associate eating with discomfort, and develop a poor appetite (Ch. 21). A child who is compelled to sit on the pottie when he is struggling to get off it, or who is smacked for not using it in the appropriate way, becomes conditioned against the pottie, associating it with tears and discomfort, and then refuses to have anything to do with it.

The physical build of the child, and physical handicaps, may be intimately related to his behaviour. An unduly small child, and especially a dwarf, such as the child with achondroplasia, may feel inferior to his fellows, and respond accordingly by manifestations of insecurity, by cowardice and other problems. The child of small build is likely to eat less than the large child, and occasion much worry in his anxious mother, who then tries to make him eat more— with all the usual consequences. A high proportion of juvenile delinquents have a physical handicap.[16]

We are slowly learning more about the relationship between structural changes in the brain and behaviour, and between biochemical abnormalities and behaviour. For instance, the crying and irritability of the child with phenylketonuria rapidly responds to a reduction of the level of the serum phenylalanine by diet. The effect of hypoglycæmia on behaviour is well known. The psychological features of the child with thyroid deficiency, with Cushing's syndrome and other endocrinological conditions, is another example of the relationship of physical and structural changes to behaviour.

Physical handicaps, such as cerebral palsy, or visual or auditory difficulties, carry important psychological implications for the child. Handicapped children tend to be the cause of favouritism on the part of the parents and therefore jealousy on the part of the siblings.

Trevor-Roper[19] in his book on the effect of eye defects on art, discussed the personality of persons with myopia or hypermetropia. He wrote that children with myopia tend to be poor at games and sport, because of poor distant vision and to be disinterested in the theatre or cinema, but show more interest in reading, tending to be "know-alls," pleasing their teachers but losing their friends, and achieving greater academic success than their fellows; while long sighted children tend to be much more interested in sport and other outdoor activities, to be more masculine, aggressive, popular and extroverts, getting into trouble at school for truancy and inattentiveness because of poor near vision.

Other Aspects of Postnatal Environment

A child's personality is partly inherited and partly the product of his environment—the effect of his parents' and teachers' personality and attitudes, and the personality and behaviour of his siblings. It is unfortunate that difficult parents do not have easy placid children. They are much more likely to have difficult impatient children with whom they will come into conflict. The placid easy-going parent, who can cope with anything, is unlikely to have a really difficult child. To my mind the term "maladjusted child" is a silly one. He is reacting normally and predictably to a difficult environment. I have similar feelings about the term "child guidance clinic." It is not the child who needs the guidance, but the parents. The child is profoundly influenced by his parents' own experiences, their happiness or unhappiness, and by domestic conflict.

The child's whole life is moulded by the environment in his first few years—especially in the first 3 or 4 years. If his basic needs are met in the early weeks and months, his needs for food, love and comfort, he is much more likely to grow up to be a happy person than if he was thwarted and unhappy in these early months.

It is now widely believed that the psychological problems of the adult—the anxiety state, the aggressiveness, the marital unhappiness—have their origin in early life. The seeds of personality disorders and of social problems, of juvenile delinquency, divorce, illegitimacy, selfishness, dishonesty and war, are sown in the first 3 or 4 years of life.

The factors which culminate in a particular problem are usually multiple and complex. For instance, a child has asthma, with a strong psychological component. His mother had an unhappy childhood, because of the personalities and problems of *her* parents. She had a difficult pregnancy, with toxaemia, and the child was prematurely born. This was one factor in causing her to overprotect him. She has constant friction with her mother-in-law, and this is another factor in causing her to overprotect the boy. He has asthma, and she worries excessively about his every wheeze—with the result that the boy himself worries and responds by more wheezing. The mother then worries all the more. He becomes a hypochondriac, and is constantly worried about his health. His father is rejecting, regarding him as a weakling, and the boy knows this, feeling unwanted, and wheezes as a result.

Behaviour problems are rarely single matters: they are the end result of a concatenation of factors, and the doctor, in attempting to unravel and treat them, has to consider the family as a whole, not just the child and his symptoms.

Advice to the Parents

It happens far too often that the parents are given advice which is manifestly unsound, in that it completely ignores the child's fundamental needs, which are the cause of the problem. I was asked to see an older child on account of disobedience. A fortnight previously the mother had taken her to see a psychiatrist. His advice, given in the girl's presence, was that she should be thrashed into obedience. The girl, as one would expect, was a very great deal worse when the advice was carried into effect and was then brought to me. The psychiatrist had completely failed to recognize the fact that the cause of the disobedience was insecurity and a great yearning for love, which the mother had never given her. The mother herself had had an unhappy childhood and had been handed over as an infant to a relative to be brought up. A child of 7 was referred to me because of fæcal incontinence with gross constipation of 5 years' duration. The boy had been repeatedly taken to his doctor, who had always reassured the mother by saying, "It's just his nerves. He will grow out of it." A child of 3 was brought up on account of food refusal. A doctor had told the mother to lock her out of the house if she refused to eat her dinner. Such stories could be duplicated by every pædiatrician.

Problem children are children with problems. Problems are rarely isolated. If there is one behaviour problem, there is usually another. It is futile to attempt to treat the symptom—the thumbsucking, the aggressiveness, the lying—without treating the cause, which is so often insecurity and tension and lack of real love. It is the doctor's task to find out why he is insecure, and to do so he has to learn much about the parents' own life, about their attitude to their children, and about the family background. He has to take a full detailed history, and carry out a full detailed examination of the child, in order to eliminate organic disease in addition to the emotional problems, and then he has to use his common sense.

The tendency to blame the parents must at all times be avoided. The child's problems are not the *fault* of the parents. They have done their best, and it is no use criticizing them and condemning them for their mismanagement. They have their own personality problems, and have little help in coping with them. They receive conflicting advice from friends, doctors, magazines and books. Valuable books are those by Bakwin[1] and Spock.[14] What we should try to do is to help them to understand why the child is behaving as he does—so that they can find the answer to it themselves.

In conclusion, a child's behaviour is the end result of a wide variety of factors operating before pregnancy, during pregnancy, during delivery, and in his subsequent environment. His behaviour problems are the result of a conflict between the child's developing personality, and the personality and attitudes of his parents, teachers and peers; and physical factors have an important bearing on the child's reaction to conflict, on his behaviour, and on his learning.

Conclusion

A good practitioner cannot afford to be disinterested in the simple behaviour problems of childhood. He is in a better position than anyone to treat them, because he knows so much of the family background. It does not help the mother at all to tell her that "It's his nerves." "It is just naughtiness." "He just wants a good smacking." "He is just spoilt." "He will grow out of it." There is much more than that to the basis of behaviour.

References

1. BAKWIN, H., BAKWIN, R. M. (1966). *Behavior Disorders in Children*. Philadelphia. Saunders.
1a. BARNETT, C. R., LEIDERMAN, P. H., GROBSTEIN, R., KLAUS, M. (1970). "The Maternal Side of Interactional Deprivation." *Pediat.*, 45, 197.
2. BLOOM, B. S. (1964). *Stability and Change in Human Characteristics*. New York. Wiley.
3. CALDWELL, B. M. (1964). In Hoffman, M. L., Hoffman, L. W., *Child Development Research*. New York. Russell Sage Foundation.
4. COURT BROWN, W. M. (1966). "Medical Aspects of Criminal Behaviour." *Brit. med. J.*, 2, 1448.
5. DRILLIEN, C. M. (1963). "Obstetric Hazard, Mental Retardation and Behaviour Disturbance in Primary School." *Develop. Med. Child Neurol.*, 5, 3.
6. DRILLIEN, C. M., WILKINSON, E. M. (1964). "Emotional Stress and Mongoloid Births." *Develop. Med. Child Neurol.*, 6, 40.
7. GUNTHER, L. M. (1963). "Psychopathology and Stress in the Life Experience of Mothers of Premature Infants." *Am. J. Obst. and Gynec.*, 86, 333.
8. HINDE, R. A. (1966). *Animal Behaviour: A Synthesis of Ethology and Comparative Psychology*. McGraw-Hill.
9. ILLINGWORTH, R. S., LISTER, J. (1964). "The Critical or Sensitive Period, with Special Reference to Certain Feeding Problems in Infants and Children." *J. of Pediatrics*, 65, 839.
10. ILLINGWORTH, R. S., ILLINGWORTH, C. M. (1966). *Lessons from Childhood*. Edinburgh. Livingstone.
11. POLLACK, M., WOERNER, M. G. (1967). "Pre- and Perinatal Complications and Childhood Schizophrenia." *J. Child. Psychol. Psychiat.*, 7, 235.
12. PRECHTL, H. (1963), in Foss, *Determinants of Infan Behaviour*. London. Methuen.

13. RHEINGOLD, H. L. (1963). *Maternal Behaviour in Animals*. New York. Wiley.
14. SPOCK, B. (1946). *Baby and Child Care*. New York. Pocket Books Inc.
15. STANDING, E. M. (1957). *Maria Montessori*. London. Hollis and Carter.
16. STOTT, D. H. (1962). "Evidence for a Congenital Factor in Maladjustment and Delinquency." *Am. J. Psychiat.*, 118, 781.
17. TAFT, T. L., GOLDFARB, W. (1964). "Prenatal and Perinatal Factors in Childhood Schizophrenia." *Develop. Med. Child Neurol.*, 6, 32.
18. THOMPSON, W. R. (1957). "Influence of Prenatal Maternal Anxiety on Emotionality in Young Rats." *Science*, 125, 698.
19. TREVOR-ROPER, P. (1971). *The World Through Blunted Sight*. London. Thames and Hudson.
20. UCKO, L. E. (1960). "A Comparative Study of Asphyxiated and non Asphyxiated Boys from Birth to Five Years." *Develop. Med. Child Neurol.*, 7, 643.

CHAPTER 18

RELEVANT FEATURES OF THE PSYCHOLOGICAL DEVELOPMENT OF THE CHILD

The Need for Love and Security

It is not unusual to find that the crying of a day-old baby stops not when he is fed or when his napkin is changed, but when he is picked up and cuddled. From this day onwards there is an increasing demand for love and security. By 3 or 4 weeks of age the baby's manifestations of pleasure when he is picked up and talked to are obvious to all. His respirations slow, the mouth opens and closes, his head bobs backwards and forwards, while he watches his mother's face intently. Two or three weeks later he begins to smile, and shortly after to vocalize his pleasure. His demands to be picked up tend to increase as he grows older and he becomes reluctant to let the mother out of his sight. When he learns to sit and use his hands to play with toys he may become temporarily less demanding, and more willing to watch his mother depart without crying. At 9 months he may begin to fuss when he sees his mother picking up another baby or his older brother.

The child has an even greater need for love and security after the first year. He becomes increasingly dependent on his parents and increasingly demanding for their presence. He is learning things and seeing things which he has never seen before. He has nightmares and he is frightened by the unknown—by cars, dogs and noises, and he expects his parents to protect him. His demands for love and security are particularly great when he is ill, tired or in pain, as from a fall or from teething. He always needs to be assured of his parents' love. He constantly wants the feeling that he is wanted, that he is a person and has a place in the home. He needs love, above all, when he is cross, irritable or lachrymose, and when he is behaving badly and has been in trouble. He needs love most when he is least lovable.

As Vining wrote,[7] children appreciate love from the facial expression, the tone of voice, the patience, gentleness and understanding with which they are treated, from what the parents say to them and how they say it. To quote Vining: "In so far that the parents apply the forcing method in their endeavour to obtain obedience, and in so far that they make use of the heavy hand, the biting tongue and the frozen face, then so much the more does such a régime produce rebellion, negativism, unhappiness and a feeling of insecurity. I believe that if parents would cut out such words as 'naughty,' 'dirty,' 'disobedient,' 'bad,' 'I do not love you,' and in their place use 'good,' 'helpful,' 'brave,' 'I love you,' 'thank you,' even if the situation does not always deserve it, that the results would be the disappearance of many of these common behaviour problems. The more we give children courage, confidence, affection, and the more we lift them up and give them freedom, instead of keeping them down and suppressing them, the more they will respond. What children need more than anything, and what to a very large extent determines their behaviour and makes it easy and possible for parents to bring about normal behaviour, is love and affection." Unfortunately some parents seem to be unable to give this sort of love. Bowlby, in his excellent monograph on the effect of emotional deprivation in the first years of life, said that one of the outstanding consequences of such deprivation is the inability to give or receive love in later life. My colleague at Sheffield, Dr. Colin Woodmansey,[8] concluded an address on "Menta Illness in the Family," with the following words: "Though the psychopathology and the treatment of individual patients may be extremely complex, the principal aim of parent guidance is in principle very simple—it is just to help parents to be nice to their children."

Many parents think that love consists of giving the child everything he wants and buying him expensive presents. One often hears parents say: "We can't make it out. We have given him everything that he wanted, everything that money could buy." But they did not give him love. It takes a great deal more to make a child happy than to give "him everything that he wants." There is a big difference between feeling love and showing it.

English and Foster,[5] in their book *Fathers are Parents too*, wrote about the undesirability of giving children all that they want. They mentioned parents who, "because they themselves cannot bear to be denied anything, extend this privilege to their young." "Infants," they wrote, "are adept at driving a hard bargain with an appeasing parent by the time they are a few months old. By 2 or 3, the infant is a master at bullying. Appeasement is a peace at any price policy that brings no peace. Far from making them secure, it handicaps them severely, keeps them chronically dependent, and lays foundations for later neurosis. The child must have freedom and self expression, but he must learn to accept necessary frustrations and disappointments—to learn self control, self discipline, be thoughtful of others, to be a nicer person."

His feeling of security is disturbed by prolonged separation from either parent. He may be disturbed, for instance, when placed in a nursery every day so that his mother can work in industry, or when she consistently leaves him for a large part of the day so that she can go out and enjoy herself, or when she leaves the child in charge of a "nanny" because she cannot be bothered to bring him up herself or because she thinks that it is fashionable. No harm is done by an occasional short holiday away from the child. Repeated separations from the child cause insecurity. It is a mistake for parents to feel that they must never leave a child at all. Provided that he is looked after by someone he knows and loves, like a grandmother, he will come to no psychological harm, and it may help him. He has to be separated from his parents one day, and occasional short separations, during which he is looked after by a loving grandmother, help him, and certainly help his worn out mother. She comes back from a weekend away from him refreshed, more tolerant and better tempered.

The problem of the mother who wants to go out to work, or to keep up her professional career, is a difficult one. On the one hand it is desirable for the mother to be with her child at least for his first three years; on the other hand a professional woman may feel thwarted, bored and bad temperered if she abandons the career for which she is trained, and these feelings have a bad effect on her children. Yudkin and Holme[9] surveyed 1209 working mothers, and the factors which may adversely affect the child or leave him unharmed. They mentioned the age of the child when the mother first goes to work, the duration and frequency of the mother's hours away from him, the arrangements for the care of the child, the number and age of the siblings, the school hours, the previous separations and the physical conditions in the home. Douglas and Blomfield[4] also analysed the position, and concluded that children of working mothers were not normally at a disadvantage. Provided that the child can be left with someone who loves him and who the child loves, little harm is likely to be done. Each case must be decided on its merits.

Occasional short separation of the child from the mother, provided that he is being looked after by someone he loves, may possibly help in another way. He has to start on the road towards independence. Unless a baby monkey has frequent opportunities to leave and return to the mother in the first year, he may reach the point at which he refuses to leave her in adult life.

It is inevitable that children may be seriously disturbed by domestic friction, separation of the parents, or divorce.[2,3] The children are apt to have feelings of anxiety, sadness and guilt feelings. Boys separated from their fathers develop masculine traits more slowly. The mother may make matters worse by distorting the picture of the father and representing him as a monster. Such children are apt to respond by any of the manifestations of insecurity.

It goes without saying that a child may feel deserted and insecure when he loses one of his parents.[1] A child is gravely disturbed by stupid threats about exchanges—selling him if he is not a good boy, or of giving his baby sister away.

He is disturbed by removing from one house to another. He is upset by changes of "nannies." His feeling of security is disturbed when a new baby arrives, for then he fears the loss of the love which he has enjoyed so long without competition from another. Every effort should be made at this time to give him a constant feeling of certainty that he is wanted and loved just as much as he ever was.

He is upset by criticisms, disparagement, derogation and scoldings. I heard a father say to his boy, who was feeling shy: "Look intelligent. Close your mouth. Stop looking like a congenital idiot." A mother brought her 9-year-old child up on account of a behaviour problem, and said to me in front of her: "She is very backward compared with her sisters. She has always been a great disappointment to us." Another mother said in front of her problem child: "He will soon be going away to school, thank goodness." The child does not interpret this sort of remark as meaning that he is loved and wanted. In some homes every day is one long day of remonstrances. The child is in constant trouble over trivialities—about things which he does or says which are not wrong at all, and which are totally unimportant. Some parents hardly open their mouth except to criticize. Some well intentioned parents are determined that when their children grow up they will be perfect, and when the inevitable disillusionment comes they do not hesitate to make their disappointment obvious to their children—making them thoroughly insecure as a result. He needs to feel that his parents are not critical of him, that they love him for what he is, and that they are interested in what he says and does.

Every parent hopes that his child will grow up to love him. Lasting love is built up by hundreds of kindnesses, hundreds of occasions when tolerance and understanding have been shown; but children are liable to grow away from their parents in adolescence, and show little love for them, if there has been constant criticism and bickering in the home, constant scoldings and punishments, constant derogation, disapproval and disparagement.

It is always wrong to ridicule a child or to draw unfavourable comparisons between him and his siblings or friends. They are apt to promote bad feeling between child and child, and they lead to jealousy and insecurity. The devastating effect of favouritism is described elsewhere.

The Desire to Practise New Skills

Babies and small children take a great pride in practising the new skills which they have learnt or which they are in the process of learning. When a baby can sit, either propped up (at 2-6 months) or without support (from 7 months), he wants to sit, and dislikes lying down. When he is older, he delights in standing holding on to furniture (8-12 months), creeping (9 months), walking with two hands held (from 10 months) and then with one hand (at a year), and later without support (13-15 months). When he can grasp objects (5 months) he wants to have toys to play with, and soon to help in feeding himself by helping to hold the cup and spoon.

Meanwhile he takes great pride in other manipulative skills— playing with bricks (from 6 months), releasing objects into containers (from 10 or 11 months), threading beads and using blunt scissors (at about $2\frac{1}{2}$). He enjoys looking at books from about 9 months, beginning with linen or cardboard varieties. He learns to dress himself, beginning at 10-12 months, when he holds his arm out for a sleeve, and progressively improving until at 3 years he can dress and undress himself completely if he is helped with the back buttons and advised occasionally about putting the right shoe on the right foot and not putting clothes on back to front. The sight of a 2-year-old child being fed by his mother, or of a 5-7-year-old child being dressed and undressed by her, is all too common and a sad reflection on his upbringing.

The child takes pride in many other skills. They satisfy his ego and give him a feeling of responsibility and independence in the house. When he is learning sphincter control he should be given responsibility to look after himself as soon as he is ready for it. By the age of 2-3 years he is likely to be able to attend to his own needs, provided that he has some help with his pants and that he is wiped. Many mothers make the mistake of retaining entire responsibility for their children, so that they are delayed in learning to be clean.

An important principle of upbringing is the encouragement of a child to practise new skills when he enjoys doing so. He should be allowed to practise them even though he makes a mess or has an occasional accident, and even though it takes the mother twice as long to do a job with his "help" as without it. Probably the chief reason why children are not allowed to dress themselves at about the age of three is that they take a long time to do it and the mother can dress the child herself in half the time. Failure, however, to encourage him to learn new skills when he is ready and anxious to learn them leads to discouragement, dependence instead of independence and lack or initiative, and when the mother later decides that he is old enough to do things for himself he has lost interest and refuses.

The Ego and Negativism

The development of the ego and of resistance begins insidiously. The age at which its first manifestations appear depends largely on the intelligence and personality of the child. Many babies of 5 or 6 months have strong likes and dislikes and are quite firm in their refusal of disliked foods. Many of the common weaning problems are bound up with the development of the ego. One reason for advocating the early giving of solids is that the longer they are delayed the more difficult it becomes to persuade the baby to take them.

The baby's desire and determination to practise new skills may become obvious at 6 months. I have seen babies of 6–9 months who consistently refused all food and suffered a serious loss of weight because they were being denied the right of helping to hold the cup or spoon. As the baby grows older he insists more and more on being allowed to practise his new skills, and interference with this desirable trait is the cause of many tears.

From the age of 10 months or so he repeats performances which are laughed at. From this age onwards he shows an ever-increasing determination to be recognized as a person, and he adopts an ever-widening variety of methods of asserting himself. If he discovers any way of drawing attention to himself and putting himself in the centre of the stage, he will repeat the performance (see Attention-seeking Devices).

The child passes through a normal stage of aggressiveness in the transition from the dependence of infancy to the independence of later childhood. He becomes a domineering determined fellow. He wants his own way like his parents and sees no reason for being refused it. In the first 2 years at least he is utterly self-centred. It is only in the third and fourth years that the earliest signs of unselfishness appear. It takes him many months to realize that, important as he is, he is not the only one that matters. He talks incessantly to himself, makes a tremendous noise, and is completely oblivious to the feelings of others. It is wrong to try to break his character. His determination will stand him in good stead in later life. He will learn unselfishness in time. His love of praise, the assertion of his personality, is perfectly normal. It should be utilized in his training. Nothing helps him more than judicious praise and encouragement to be independent.

Negativism is a characteristic feature of the normal child from 18 months to 3 years or more. Children at this age are nonconformists. They seem to take a delight in doing the opposite of what they are asked to do. When the mother wants her child to go out he decides to stay in. When she wants to go upstairs he wants to go down. When she turns to the left he wants to turn to the right. If an attempt is made to make him hurry in eating, clearing his toys away or dressing, he will dawdle. If he discovers that his mother is most anxious for him to eat a particular food, and that his refusal will create a scene, he will certainly refuse it. If he finds that he can cause consternation by withholding a bowel movement or refusing to empty the bladder, he will hold it in, even though it causes him some discomfort to do so. If he finds that refusal to go to bed, to lie down or to sleep results in a fuss and enables him to get his own way and stay up longer, or cause his mother to stay in his bedroom and play games with him, then he will refuse and continue to be difficult until he finds that this method is no longer successful in giving him power over his environment. In short, he has emerged from the stage of being a little angel, and has become a little devil. His mother doesn't know what has got into him. It is because of the development of the ego and of negativism that it is always wrong to have a fight with a child over anything, for in a fight the child always wins. For the same reason any attempt to force him to do something against his will, unless it is really essential, is always undesirable. It is for the same reason that any display of anxiety over any habit or trick which he learns will almost certainly result in the continuance of the practice, for it enables him to assert his personality and to show his power.

There are other reasons for his resistance. Resistance is not always so much the child's revolt against authority as a desire to continue doing what he wants to do. He has no sense of time. A clock means nothing to him, except as a toy. He sees no reason why he should stop playing the game which he is enjoying so much, and he completely fails to see why his parents want him to stop. Often the parents themselves have an inadequate reason for their insistence. If they have a reason, if they want to take him out or if his meal is ready, he fails to understand why he should hurry.

It is difficult to draw the line between normal and abnormal negativism. It is greatly exaggerated by hunger, fatigue, insecurity and jealousy. It is exaggerated by excessive sternness, perfectionism, constant criticism, and by attempts to push him beyond his developmental level. It must be remembered that it is not all environmental in origin. It is developmental and some show it more than others, for it depends largely on the child's inherited personality.

Habit Formation

It is difficult to define a habit and to distinguish it from reflex action, association and conditioning. A child of 3 or 4 weeks may quieten when the bib is being tied on prior to the breast feed. From a month or two of age babies may be "conditioned" to pass urine in the pottie when regularly placed on it. It is uncertain whether any of these examples bear any relationship to the intelligence of the child.

Habit formation may arise as a result of evening colic in the first 3 months, which makes it necessary to pick the baby up and cuddle him at a time when he would otherwise have been in bed. Spock[10] drew attention to the sleep problems which may result, and I can confirm his observations. In a similar way the baby who is constantly being picked up when he is not in need comes to expect to be picked up whenever he is awake. As he grows older habit formation becomes more and more rapid. Any repeated departure from routine in the direction favoured by the child soon leads to habit formation. In an illness the mother may sleep in the child's room, or for the first time keep the light on throughout the night. On holiday the child may have to share a bedroom with the parents. Return to the original routine is difficult.

Habit formation is largely due to a desire to satisfy a primitive instinct. That instinct may be a desire for love or attention. If the result does not accord with the dictates of society, or with the mother's convenience or with her opinions as to what is best for the child, it is called a bad habit. The creation of good habits was the aim of the old rigid ideas of infant feeding, of bowel training and sleep management. The establishment of a routine of good habits is eminently desirable and rigid methods work well with many children, but not with all. In some children they have the opposite of the effect desired, for in children who have particularly well-marked primitive instincts of desire for love or desire for power they cause conflict between parent and child and lead to troublesome disturbances of behaviour. Attempts to break a bad habit cause similar conflict. If in the attempt to break the habit a great deal of anxiety is shown, if the child finds that by his behaviour he can attract attention, if he overhears his mother discussing his problems with her friends, the habit will continue as an attention-seeking device.

An important factor in habit formation is the child's natural imitativeness. Another is his intelligence and memory. It would be natural to assume that the highly intelligent child, who learns rapidly and has a greater understanding than others of his age, should develop habits good and bad quicker than the less intelligent ones.

Imitativeness

The earliest sign of imitativeness is seen at 5 or 6 months of age, when the baby may imitate the adult in putting out the tongue, chewing or making razzing noises. In the next 3 or 4 months the baby learns to imitate the mother in playing simple games—peep-bo, patacake—and in waving bye-bye. He learns to speak. Between 2 and 3 years domestic mimicry is a characteristic feature of development. The child copies the mother in sweeping the floor, washing and drying objects, in baking and in many other household occupations. A girl dresses and undresses her doll, places it on the pottie and changes the napkin. Between 18 months and 3 years children are especially apt to imitate the mannerisms and attention-seeking devices of their playmates.

It is inevitable that children should imitate their parents. The importance of example is obvious. Attempts to inculcate good manners, good habits and kindness to others are doomed to failure unless the parents set the example. If the parents fail to reply to their child when he speaks to them and if they constantly interrupt his conversations, if they are rude and impolite with him, they cannot expect him to be anything else. If they show bad temper and irritability, use bad language and are unloving, dishonest and selfish, they cannot expect their child to be different. When the divorce rate is 51,000 per year, what one might call the "friction rate"—the frequency with which the mother and father quarrel—must be a great deal higher. Domestic friction has a serious effect on the mind of the growing child.

The importance of example is in part related to his developing memory and understanding. At the age of a year the memory span may be one of several weeks. By the age of 3 it may be one of many months. Parents should not make the mistake of thinking that a child's memory is short-lived. His understanding is apt to be underestimated. It is far in advance of his powers of speech. They fail to understand this and so fail to realize the importance of a good example.

Sensitiveness to Atmosphere and Surroundings

The effect of maternal nervousness on the sucking of the new-born baby was described by Middlemore.[6] The baby of a thyrotoxic mother is liable to show feeding and sleeping problems as a result of the mother's nervousness. I have seen a baby burst into tears on several occasions between the age of 6 and 9 months when a mishap befell his sister or friends, or when he thought that his sister was being hurt by rough play. A child between 1 and 3 years of age readily cries when he sees his mother cry, without knowing what is troubling her. It is easy to understand that domestic friction, particularly if there is obvious resultant unhappiness or violence, may have a considerable psychological effect on the child.

At 4 or 5 months of age the baby may show interest in a room in which he has not been before, and he may refuse to sleep in a strange bedroom.

Imagination

Most children after the age of 15 months or so develop a vivid imagination. There are great individual differences. In general, the greater the intelligence the greater is the imagination. Between 15 and 18 months it begins to appear in his doll play. Between 2 and 3 he has imaginary playmates behind the sofa. He tells tall stories and plays highly imaginative games with his friends. He should not be discouraged or ridiculed for using his imagination; instead he should be encouraged. His imagination may lead to the development of fears— fear of the dark, of noises and of animals.

Suggestibility

Likes, dislikes and fears are readily suggested to a child. Dislike of certain foodstuffs is suggested by chance remarks made by adults. Fears of animals, motor cars and thunder are suggested in a similar way. In a child who is liable to travel sickness, vomiting is readily suggested by unwise conversation in front of him. Gruesome tales and stories about ghosts, giants, devils and suchlike may terrify the small child and lead to serious sleep disturbance.

Intelligence

Behaviour problems may arise in a child with a lower than average intelligence for a variety of reasons. He is likely to be a slow learner, and if his training is related to his age instead of to his level of development, too much will be expected of him, so that he becomes thwarted, negative and insecure. It is not easy to appeal to him, to explain to him what sort of behaviour is expected and to get him to understand the reason for restrictions which are necessary for him. Speech is late in developing and he feels thwarted by his inability to express himself.

Superior intelligence may be a problem in later years. It is probable that habit formation is quicker in the more intelligent child. He is likely to learn attention-seeking devices more quickly, because of his greater appreciation of the reaction of his parents. His greater imaginativeness may lead to fears of various kinds. Under-estimation of intelligence causes parents to be careless about speaking in front of him. It may lead them to be too slow in teaching him skills and responsibilities for which he is ready on account of his superior mental endowment.

Personality Differences

Full realization of the great differences in the personality of children is fundamental for an understanding of behaviour problems. Personality traits may be obvious in the new-born period. One baby takes the breast without difficulty. Another is irritable, sucks for a minute and screams and is difficult to manage. Some are much more intolerant of hunger than others. Some are much more active. The active babies, with rapid movements of the arms and legs, tend to posset excessively. The slow, placid babies present fewer feeding problems.

There are great differences in sleep requirements. Some babies even at 4 or 5 months of age are asleep for the major part of the day. Others at that age only have two or three short daytime naps. The active, determined baby discards the midday nap months or even years before his placid brother. Some are willing to lie outside in the pram all day long with no one to talk to and nothing to see. They have little interest in their surroundings. Others at 3 months, or even sooner, refuse to be left outside. They want to see what is going on, they are intensely curious and are perfectly content propped up in the pram in the kitchen, where the mother is busy with her household duties.

Some are placid, quiet babies who cry little even when they are tired. Others are active, determined ones who cry a great deal until given the attention which they demand, and are difficult to keep quiet when tired, hungry or bored.

Some babies present no problem at weaning time. They take what comes, with only mild likes and dislikes. They do not bother to try to feed themselves and would rather do without than have to help. Others have strong likes and dislikes; they spit the cod-liver oil out, they become greatly excited when they see a food which they like. They would rather starve than be denied the right of helping themselves.

There are great differences in social responsiveness. Some smile readily and are easily amused. Some love company, while others do not care so much. Some prefer cuddling to toys, others toys to cuddling. There are great differences in the demand for and giving of love.

After the first year the differences in the degree of determination, negativism and independence become more marked. Some will not tolerate the play pen for more than a week or two. For others it is a useful commodity for months. Some are willing to be wheeled about in a pram when they are 3 years old. Others will have nothing more to do with it when they are not yet two. Some are extremely insistent on practising their new skills and on "helping" the mother; others care much less and are more willing to have things done for them.

Children differ widely in the amount of caution which they show. Some show fear much more than others. They differ in imagination, sensitiveness to criticism, in concentration, in distractibility and in their demands for love and security. Some are born to lead, others to be led. Some boys are born to excel at rugger, others at the violin. Some girls are born to be nurses, some to be police women.

Rigid standardized methods of child management fail to take these individual differences into account. They work well for the average child but not for the child who is different from the average. It is for this reason, as well as for the differences in intelligence, that child management should be elastic and adaptable to the needs of the individual.

There is no doubt that differences in the personality of children are an important cause of behaviour problems. Trouble arises in a family when the first-born has a placid, easy-going disposition and the next is an active, determined independent child. The mother naturally tries to adopt the same methods of upbringing with the second child as those which she used successfully with the first, and it does not work. The child objects. Food-forcing, sleep-forcing and bowel-forcing methods are apt to result. It is most important that parents should understand that personality differences are almost inevitable in a family, and management should accordingly be elastic.

Annoying Characteristics of the Developing Child

Any parent could say a great deal about this subject, yet it is surprising how little sympathy many doctors show with mothers who are faced with behaviour problems. Mothers have to tolerate not only the dreadful social circumstances, such as overcrowding and poverty, in which they have to bring up their children, but they have to live with their children all through the day, with their annoying characteristics, which irritate and tire. They cannot get out in the evening. Holidays are out of the question. It is one thing for the father to see the children for an hour each evening, and another for the mother to have them for the whole of the day and never to be able to get away from them.

In the first 6 months, if the baby is of the active wide-awake type, his frequent demands for attention and his ready crying when the mother is tired and busy may get on top of her. After this age the baby should be learning to feed himself. He makes a dreadful mess with his food, dropping much of it on the floor and spilling milk on the carpet. He gets hold of some paper when her back is turned, tears it up into numerous pieces and eats some of it. After 9 months he is mobile and constantly creeping or walking into mischief. He has an insatiable desire to learn and wants to know what happens when he pulls the lamp flex or the table cover. The coal bucket and rubbish tin are fascinating. An open bookshelf or a cupboard carelessly left open keep him occupied for a long time. By the age of a year he may object to the play pen and refuse to stay in it. He may push it round the room or creep under it, the better to get into mischief. He possets on the new carpet.

His activity is greater after the first birthday. He gets into constant trouble, hitting the window with hard objects, playing with the coal bucket, pulling at the table cover or upsetting the clothes-horse. He loves casting games and throws one thing after another on to the floor. He is on the go all day long and will not sit still for a minute. He is constantly fighting his elder brother. He leaves a litter of toys all over the floor for the mother to fall over. He delights in noise and loves the drum which an unkind friend gave him, beating it for hours on end. He likes repetitive play, making the same noise, performing the same action over and over again till his mother is distraught. He never modulates his voice, and when he learns to talk he never stops talking for one minute. He constantly wants help in practising his new skills. He tends to cling to his mother instead of playing alone with his toys as she would like him to do. He totally fails to understand that she is tired, irritable, worried or feeling poorly.

By the age of 2 he is well into the resistant stage. He does the opposite of what he is asked to do, or else takes no notice of what she says and appears to be deaf. Of all the annoying tricks, dawdling can be one of the most trying. He takes a dreadful time to eat his dinner, to get ready for going out or to put his toys away, and any attempt to hurry him makes him worse. If sent to get ready or to fetch an item of clothing, he finds an interesting toy half-way to his destination and forgets what he has been sent for. He tries various attention-seeking devices—turning the gas tap on, constantly repeating the same noise which he finds gets on his mother's nerves, and even throws temper tantrums. She feels thwarted when she finds that she cannot make him do what she wants him to do. She cannot even obtain emotional release by smacking him, because it only makes him worse. When she finally gets him to bed he refuses to lie down. She cannot even leave him to cry it out because he has learnt to make himself sick if left to cry. She cannot reason with him because he is not old enough to understand. When she has a fight with him, he always wins. He sleeps badly and next day he is tired and even more resistive than usual. He wails and nothing pleases him. It rains all day; she cannot take him outside, and he is bored and intolerable. Where there is more than one child, the constant fighting, bickering, shouting and shrieking, aggravated by boredom, gets her down.

She wants to clean him up to take him out, but he runs away when she calls him, and the more angry she becomes the more difficult it is to catch him. When she has tidied him up she turns her back for two minutes to get dressed herself, and he gets into the coal bucket, vomits over his clothes or soils his pants. When they eventually reach her friends, before whom she wants to show him off, he is on his worst possible behaviour. She has friends into her house, and just before their arrival he empties the whole contents of his playbox with a crash on to the floor.

Between 2 and 3½ he begins to ask questions, and soon asks them all day long. She cannot answer many of them, but he insists on an answer. Each answer leads to another question. He asks: "Why is it to-day?" "When will it be to-morrow?" "Why is it not to-morrow now?" "What is a soul?" He asks her to "draw a difference," "draw an appetite," and repeatedly asks her why she cannot do it.

This picture is not exaggerated. Most mothers could add a great deal to it. The mother says that the child is getting on her nerves, has got right on top of her. She feels that she would love to run miles away. She becomes cross and irritable and tactless. The child then becomes worse. Many mothers have several small children; some of them have twins; and sometimes one of them is a mentally defective child of the hyperkinetic type.

Behaviour problems must be treated against this background. Far too little sympathy is shown with the mother. It is very easy to criticize her when she has lost her temper with the child. Ogden Nash* apparently knew something about it when he wrote the following lines:

> "Oh, sweet be his slumber and moist his middle.
> My dreams, I fear, are infanticiddle.
> A fig for embryo Lohengrins.
> I'll open all of his safety pins.
> I'll pepper his powder and salt his bottle,
> And give him readings from Aristotle.
> Sand for his spinach I'll gladly bring,
> And Tabasco sauce for his teething ring,
> And an elegant elegant alligator,
> To play with in his perambulator."

Friction in the Home

It has already been stated that behaviour problems usually represent a conflict between the developing personality of the child, and the personality and attitudes of his parents, teachers, siblings and other

* Ogden Nash (1943). "Song to be sung by the Father of Infant Female Children in *The Face is Familiar.*" London. J. M. Dent & Sons.

children. There is probably some friction in almost every home, if it is a normal home, but it is commonly excessive, worrying the parents and leading to insecurity in the child. Its origin, as in the case of other behaviour problems, are preconceptional, prenatal and environmental. Preconceptional and prenatal factors have already been discussed.

Relevant basic features of the developing child which cause conflict are his negativism, constant activity, noisiness, untidiness, aggressiveness, jealousy, selfishness, rudeness, and lack of consideration for the feelings of others, dawdling, dirtiness, carelessness with his clothes, or stuttering, his gormlessness when spoken to by strangers, his bad behaviour when visitors come to the house, his untruthfulness, or his lack of initiative. The parents, especially if they possess these personality traits themselves, as they usually do, are determined to make their child a model of virtue as soon as possible, not realizing how normal and almost universal these features of childhood are; they do not realize that with firm loving sympathetic understanding and discipline their children will learn to control the unpleasant features of their personality as they mature, and will probably grow out of their negativism, overactivity, noisiness and lack of consideration for others. Young children have no idea that their mother is tired, worried or in a hurry; they live in a world of self, until they grow older. Parents tend to forget that children, like adults, may become bad tempered when they are hungry, suffering from an infection, or bored, or when they have had a bad time at school at the hand of a bully, whether child or teacher. They then reprimand or punish him—and make him worse. The wise procedure to adopt when a child comes in from school in a bad temper is to give him a meal as soon as possible, and not to argue with him and try to teach discipline.

As children reach puberty, they are able much more to think for themselves. They no longer accept everything that their parents say as gospel. They want to know the reason why. Unfortunately parents dislike having their authority questioned, and reply to the child's queries with such expressions as "Don't argue." "I won't have any back-chat." "I won't have another word." The child is eventually reduced to furious sullen silence. Children as they grow older become less tolerant of such intolerance. When they were younger they had to accept the father's rudeness or threats of punishment; now they will no longer accept it, and they resent rudeness and unreasonableness, so that friction is the inevitable result.

Parents for their part have their own personality problems. When tired or hurried, they lose their sense of humour and become impatient and intolerant—or even deliberately provoke their children. The father may have a bad day at business, and the mother may be bored

9

and feel thwarted because she has to do the housework and has had to give up her professional career, so that the parents are bad tempered, and come into conflict with their children. Both parents may feel thwarted at being unable to control such problems in the child as annoying tics, overactivity and fidgeting, bed wetting, food or sleep refusal, bad temper, stealing, rudeness or jealousy—and lose their temper with the child—forgetting that none of these problems are under the child's voluntary control. The parents particularly resent personality traits in the child such as jealousy, which they possess themselves; they may envy the child for his freedom, for having meals prepared for him or for his youthfulness and subconsciously show their envy by directing anger towards him. Parents genuinely believe that the friction is entirely the child's fault. It never occurs to them that they might be responsible for it.

If the parents set a bad example of friction between each other, of rudeness, selfishness or bad temper towards each other or towards their children, their example will probably be followed—and the children will react in the same way.

Friction arises in innumerable other ways. There may be conflict about homework, about television programmes, about clothes or friends. One basic problem is the inability of each—parent and child—to understand the mind of the other.

When there is conflict, the parents should remember that when a child is behaving badly, is bad tempered and thoroughly unpleasant, it is then that he most needs loving; and that hostility, scoldings and punishment will do nothing more than make him worse. Furthermore, they must remember that his personality is partly inherited from them and partly the result of his upbringing; and that they, being more mature than the child, should be the ones who should be able to control their feelings and declare the cease fire. It is difficult for them to realize that the difficult troublesome youngster of today may well be the charming adult of tomorrow.

Why do They Annoy?

It is important to realize that small children are very annoying, and all parents could say a lot about that subject. Most parents would find it difficult, however, to say exactly why they feel annoyed at the doings of their children. It is the responsibility of the doctor to see both sides of the picture—the annoying ways of children, and the reasons why these ways annoy adults. If he does not see both sides, he cannot give adequate help to the parents, for behaviour problems are the result of an interaction of the child's developing personality and the personality of the parents. In the chapters to follow I shall say something

bout the parental attitudes which lead to conflict with the child, and
ae features of the parental personality which cause him to be easily
nnoyed and intolerant.

References

1. ARTHUR, B., KEMME, L. (1964). "Bereavement in Childhood." *J. Child. Psychol. Psychiat.*, **5**, 37.
2. BERNSTEIN, N. R., ROBEY, J. S. (1962). "The Detection and Management of Pediatric Difficulties Created by Divorce." *Pediatrics*, **30**, 950.
3. BRUN, G. (1964). "The Child of Divorce in Denmark." *Bull. Menninger Clinic*, **28**, 3.
4. DOUGLAS, J. W. B., BLOMFIELD, J. M. (1958). *Children under Five.* London. Allen and Unwin.
5. ENGLISH, O. S., FOSTER, C. J. (1953). *Fathers are Parents Too.* London. Allen & Unwin.
6. MIDDLEMORE, M. P. (1941). *The Nursing Couple.* London. Hamish Hamilton.
7. VINING, C. W. (1950). *Univ. of Leeds Med. Mag.*, **20**, 1.
8. WOODMANSEY, A. C. (1966). "Mental Illness in the Family and its Effect on the Child." *Proc. 22nd Child Guidance International Conference.* N. Association Mental Health.
9. YUDKIN, S., HOLME, A. (1963). *Working Mothers and their Children.* London. Michael Joseph.

CHAPTER 19

PARENTAL ATTITUDES AND MANAGEMENT

The Fear of Spoiling

Many mothers seem to be haunted by the fear of "spoiling" their children. It is a strange paradox that it is to these mothers that most spoilt children belong.

A child is not spoilt by being loved. A mother never harms her baby by giving him all the love that he demands. She should not hesitate to pick him up when he cries for company. His demands may be frequent at first, but if satisfied they usually soon decrease. If he cries because of colic, pain from teething, fatigue or other reasons, he should be picked up and loved. As Spock[3] wrote in his book, "A baby who gets extra attention when he is uncomfortable is usually perfectly willing to do without it when he feels well." A baby is spoilt more by a mother arguing with him than agreeing with him. It is surprising how many mothers turn a completely deaf ear to the crying of their child. They seem to be completely unperturbed by it. It may be convenient for the mother to leave the baby outside in the pram all day, however much he cries. It may well however, lead to behaviour problems later. According to Aldrich,[1] "Most spoiled children are those who as babies never had essential gratifications, owing to a mistaken attempt to fit them into a rigid régime. The spoiled child who has missed satisfaction as a baby adopts the efficient technique of whining and temper tantrums to get what he wants." He added: "The mechanism of spoiling is the neglect of needs rather than over-indulgence. Adults often present the behaviour problem instead of babies. It is negativism to fail to respond to a child's basic needs.

"Twenty-five years' experience has taught me that responsive adults breed responsive babies, and that rigid disciplinarians of babies at this age breed spoiled, unhappy children with no confidence in themselves or their parents."

Children certainly can be spoilt, and frequently are. The baby is spoilt by the mother who will never leave him alone when he is not wanting attention. Grandmothers are particularly liable to spoil their grandchildren in this way. After the first year a child is spoilt by over-protection, by never being allowed to do things for himself, by never being allowed out of his mother's sight. He is spoilt by lack of discipline because of fear of "repressing" him. He is spoilt by being

allowed to wreck the furniture, walk on the table, draw on the wall
and ride around the drawing-room on his tricycle. He is spoilt by
deprivation of love and affection and security. He is spoilt by determined efforts to avoid spoiling him.

Over-protection and Over-anxiety

The term "over-protection" signifies a great deal more than
excessive protection of a child against danger. It includes a failure to
allow him to grow up and look after himself. The mother continues to
feed him, dress him and attend to his eliminations long after a properly
treated child has learnt to take full responsibility for these functions
himself. It includes restriction of outdoor exercise in case he should
catch cold or get his feet wet. It includes over-indulgence with his toys
and play behaviour, with excessive domination in other ways. It
includes yielding to wishes and actions which no normal parent would
tolerate. It consists of preventing him playing with other children
because they are "rough." It consists of what Kanner called "smother
love" instead of "mother love." It convinces the child that he is in-
capable of looking after himself; he learns that he need not make any
effort himself, because his parents always rush to help him. When he is
at school they regularly help him with his homework. They support their
child whenever he criticizes other boys or his teachers. His mother goes
everywhere with him, taking him to school and bringing him back. He
is not allowed to choose the friends whom he wants to have into the home.
When there is a dispute, the older one is always rebuked—with the
result that the younger one deliberately annoys his older siblings in
order to get them into trouble. One of my patients had not been
allowed to mix with other children for fear she should pick up the local
accent. I saw two boys, whose father had died in their infancy, who
had their temperature taken by their mother every day for 15 years.

Over-protection is due to a variety of factors. It may occur when
the parents have had a long wait for the child, especially if on account
of age or other reasons it is not possible to have another. It is apt to
occur when there has been a succession of miscarriages, or a particularly
difficult labour. It occurs when parents, determined to have a girl,
eventually achieve their ambition after having a succession of boys.
It may arise when a child arrives many years after the last one, or
when a child returns home after a serious illness in hospital. It is likely
to be a feature of institutional care or of care by a nanny. It occurs
when a mother regards her child as delicate because of an illness,
physical disability or premature delivery. It may occur when a child
is adopted after a long period of sterility or when a previous child has

died. A mother who has had an unhappy childhood, or who is unhapp
in her married life, or who has been thwarted in her ambitions, ma
turn to her child to satisfy her own needs for affection. Psychologist
say that over-protection may be a mask to compensate for hostilit
or a rejecting attitude of which, as a rule, they are unaware.

Over-anxiety is due to the same causes as over-protection. Botl
are related in part to the mother's personality. It may be engendere
by doctors or nurses or by books on child care. It is often manifest a
soon as the baby is born. The mother is then apt to be worried abou
her ability to feed the baby, and is nervous and anxious when the bab
is put to the breast. If in addition the baby is irritable, lactation i
liable to fail. When she gets the baby home she weighs him daily, an
if the baby is breast fed she carries out test feeds every day. If he doe
not take as much as she thinks he ought to take, she tries to force hin
to take more, and food refusal occurs. She constantly goes in to se
him in the evenings, to see if he is still breathing, and keeps him in he
bedroom long after he ought to have moved into his own room. Sh
worries about his bowels and the amount of sleep he has, and so adopt
forcing methods and meets with bowel and sleep refusal. She neve
leaves him alone for a minute in the daytime, however quiet an
contented he is, always picking him up and playing with him. Sh
grossly overclothes him and keeps him out of the sun. She keeps hin
indoors if it is at all cold outside. She prevents him from sitting
standing or walking as long as she can, in case his back will be weakened
In the weaning period she becomes worried if he refuses a mouthfu
of food and tries to force him to take it, only to be met with furthe
refusal. She may even regard him as delicate and make him too fa
by overfeeding him. She constantly seeks advice from her mother, he
neighbours and from various doctors. She reads one book after anothe
about child management in an effort to find out how the child shoul
be brought up. She fails to let him feed himself in case he will choke
she will not allow him to go outside and play in case he hurts himself
when he plays with other children she constantly interferes with th
play in case he should be injured.

The result of over-protection is serious. The child's conduct i
immature. He remains utterly dependent on his mother and so i
late in learning various skills—in feeding himself, attending to th
toilet and in dressing himself. He is insecure. He does not play wel
with other children. He is afraid of getting hurt and he wants t
control the games himself. He is apt to be bullied by other children
He runs to his mother for protection and he is accident-prone. Late
on he fails to make friends. If the over-protection is associated witl
over-domination he is likely to be aggressive and boastful or submissive

timid and effeminate. In adolescent life and later he is unable to make any decision for himself without consulting his mother, for he fails to acquire normal independence. He does not take part in ordinary games with his fellows, preferring the shelter of home life. If the over-protection is associated with over-indulgence there are apt to be temper tantrums and other manifestations of aggressive behaviour. Obesity due to over-eating is sometimes a problem. Because of the excessive anxiety shown about his health, he becomes a hypochondriac.

Over-anxiety in the mother is a common picture familiar to all pædiatricians. In general, however, it is a diagnosis which is made far too frequently. It is easy to criticize a mother for being over-anxious, but it is not so easy for a parent to avoid over-anxiety, particularly when there has been a long wait for the child, or when he has been born prematurely or had some serious illness. One should always be sympathetic and understanding with such mothers, particularly when the child is her first one, constantly bearing in mind the fact that over-anxiety springs from love.

Favouritism and Rejection

Of all parental attitudes favouritism and rejection are probably the most harmful. Both of these are always vigorously denied by the parents, largely because they spring from the subconscious mind and are in no way deliberate or voluntary. The favouritism is obvious, however, to everyone else but the parents.

Favouritism arises from a variety of causes. If there has been a sequence of four boys and finally a much-wanted girl comes, she is apt to be treated as a favourite. The more intelligent bright child, or the child with the more pleasing and affectionate personality, or the child who is blessed with good looks, is apt to be favoured at the cost of her siblings. To a certain extent the causes of favouritism are the same as those of over-protection. When a child comes, for instance, several years after the previous one—especially when he was much wanted—he is apt to be favoured. It often happens that the mother's favourite is the boy, the father's is the girl, and the third is no one's favourite.

Favouritism is shown in scores of little ways, all mounting up to a great deal in the child's mind. The favourite one is not reprimanded as much as the other; he can do things which the unfavoured one is not allowed to do. He is given sweets, rides on the father's back and trips to the town, which are denied the unfavoured one. When the favoured one gets into trouble with one parent, the other parent defends him; when the unfavoured one gets into trouble, both parents attack him. The favoured one is given just a little more of the pudding or cake than the other. Grandparents are frequently guilty of marked favouritism.

When there is favouritism, the unfavoured child, in addition to the general signs of insecurity, may feel resentful against the parents. He shows little affection for them, and as a result a vicious circle is set up, the parents in turn responding by showing less affection for the child. He is secretive, and naturally will not confide in them. He is likely to be jealous of the brother or sister who is favoured by the parents and is liable to dislike them. The favoured child also suffers by being spoilt, by having all his own way, and by lacking discipline.

Parental rejection occurs for similar reasons. It may be due to the fact that the child was of the wrong sex. It may be due to his appearance or to the fact that he has a lower intelligence that that of his siblings. It may be due to the fact that he was not wanted, the pregnancy having been an accident. It may have been due to a difficult pregnancy or labour. It may be due to financial problems resulting from the child's birth. It is manifested by an excessively critical attitude to the child. The mother makes the most of his shortcomings, clearly exaggerating his bad behaviour and belittling his understanding and intelligence. She does not hestitate to make unfavourable comparisons between him and his siblings in his presence. She fails to give him the love which she gives to the others. At all times he is the unfavoured one. She is liable, if she can afford it, to hand the child over completely to a nanny to bring up. In the severest cases there is outright cruelty. The frequency with which a step-parent rejects a child is well known.

The result of rejection or of insecurity is considerable. Some of the reactions are merely exaggerations of features of every normal child: excessive fears, shyness, timidity, lacrimation, aggressiveness, quarrelsomeness, destructiveness, disobedience, jealousy, clinging to the mother, thumbsucking, masturbation, night terrors and attention-seeking devices. Other reactions include bedwetting, faecal incontinence, temper tantrums, tics, cruelty to animals, stuttering and head banging. Nearly all these arise through the subconscious, so that the child cannot help them. It follows that it is useless to try to treat the symptom; one has to treat the cause. A child may be neglected without being rejected—but it has the same consequences. Some parents are so fully occupied with charity, church work and various organizations that they neglect their own children.

Misjudgment of the Child's Developmental Level

The variations in intelligence and personality in children are so great that the only rational way of training them is to adapt the methods to the level of development reached. It is wrong, for instance, to instruct the mother to give her child solids as soon as he is 6 months old. She should give him solids when he can chew, which an average baby can do at 6 months, while others begin later. It is obvious that a child with a high intelligence quotient is ready to learn things long before an average child. In general the understanding of children tends to be under-estimated rather than over-estimated, partly because the mental processes are so far ahead of the powers of speech. If attempts are made to teach him before he is ready, he feels thwarted and insecure. One has seen children of 8 or 9 months smacked for taking an object to the mouth, a child of 15 months smacked for running alone across the road, and a child of the same age smacked for passing urine into his pants. One sees attempts being made to inculcate adult table manners in an 18-month-old child. Children of 2 are expected to be tidy. A child of nearly 3 can be taught the rudiments of tidiness by having to put toys away before a meal, but it should not be made an occasion for a fight and he should be helped in the task. A child of 2 is expected to have a conscience and to be unselfish, and he is scolded when he falls short of expectations. I saw a child of 3 being scolded for playing engines on a railway-station platform on the grounds that it was "silly."

Some parents cannot stop teaching their children. They are perfectionists and demand far too much for their level of development. They are often the sort of parents who want to show off their child in order to compensate for their own feelings of inferiority.

If, on the other hand, a child is not taught when he is developmentally ready and enjoys practising his new skills, he may lose interest and not want to learn later. It is common enough to see a child of 5 or 6 years who is unable to dress or undress himself, because he was never given a chance to do so at a time when he would have enjoyed learning, between 2 and 3 years. At 5 or 6 he is quite content to let his mother do it for him. He should be allowed to feed himself as soon as he is ready, in spite of the mess; he should be allowed to attend to his own eliminations as soon as he is developmentally ready, in spite of occasional accidents; he should be allowed to help to put the china away, in spite of occasional mishaps; he should be allowed to dress himself, in spite of the tremendous time it takes him to do it. He should be allowed at 2 years or so to have his own possessions, including books, and to assume responsibility for taking care of them.

Owing to the great differences in intelligence and personality in children there are wide variations in the ages at which children are ready to learn new skills. Rigid methods of training do not take these into account and so are apt to lead to unhappiness and insecurity.

Attitudes to Sex

The attitude to sex is of vital importance to the developing child. From the age of 15 months or so the child shows tremendous interest in the excreta. Parents must know that this is normal, and no notice should be taken of it. After the age of $2\frac{1}{2}$ children are likely to notice anatomical differences in the sexes. Their loud comments on such matters when in the grocer's shop may be embarrassing to the mother who has little sense of humour, but on no account should the child be reprimanded or laughed at for what he says. A simple question should be answered simply and truthfully in a way which he can understand. The parents may wrongly try to teach the child modesty at this age and by so doing suggest that nudity is evil and wrong. They do the child grievous harm. They should avoid being shocked when the first-born goes out of her way to peep at her young brother's genitals, and perhaps to handle them.

Sex play between small children is common and normal. They may handle each others genitals. Unfortunately many mothers are seriously disturbed when they see it happening. They should be reassured and advised not to show the least interest or anxiety in the matter. They should make no attempt to stop it. The most they can do is to distract the children, but that is not usually advisable. (See also masturbation, p. 325.)

Homosexuality

Features in the background of homosexuals are commonly a family history of the same condition, a domineering mother with a weak ineffective father; domestic friction, and unhappiness in childhood. Sometimes parents have been foolish enough to dress their boy as a girl. They commonly overprotect him and prevent him taking part in boys' sports and occupations. They may have ridiculed him when only very young for some playful experience with a little girl. There is often a background of puritanical attitudes to sex.

In a leading article in the British Medical Journal, the writer wrote as follows:

"Children reared in families which are incomplete, disturbed by distortions in personal relationships, or whose sexual attitudes are markedly clouded by repression or ignorance appear to be particularly vulnerable. Specific difficulties in relating to other people, lack of opportunity for satisfactory social contact with the opposite sex, or undue exposure to erotically stimulating contact with members of the same sex, such as may occur in single sex institutions or organisations, may result in the stirring of homosexual feelings in the adolescent." Significantly fewer lesbians regarded their childhood as happy. Boarding School experience was irrelevant.

References

1. ALDRICH, C. A., ALDRICH, M. M. (1938). *Babies are Human Beings.* New York. Macmillan.
2. *British Medical Journal.* (1969). "Female Homosexuality." Leading article. 1, 330.
3. SPOCK, B. (1946). *Baby and Baby Care.* New York. Pocket Books Inc.

CHAPTER 20

DISCIPLINE AND PUNISHMENT

Historical

In the Old Testament there are many references to punishment which today we would regard as somewhat excessive. In Proverbs XIII, 24, it is stated that "he who spares the rod hates his son, but he who loves him is diligent to discipline him". In Proverbs XXIII, 13, the following instruction is given "Do not withold discipline from a child. If you beat him with a rod he will not die". In the Second Book of Kings, 2:23 there is an example of excessive punishment, when Elisha dealt fiercely with some children who ridiculed him. "As he was going up by the way, there came forth little children, out of the city, and mocked him, and said unto him "go up, thou bald head, go up, thou bald head". And he turned back, and looked on them, and cursed them in the name of the Lord. And there came forth two she bears out of the wood, and tare forty and two children of them".

In Deuteronomy XXI, 18, the following appears:

"If a man have a stubborn and rebellious son, which will not obey the voice of his father, or the voice of his mother, and that, when they have chastened him, will not hearken unto them, then shall his father and mother lay hold on him and bring him unto the elders of his city and unto the gate of his place; and all the men of his city shall stone him with stones, that he die".

Amongst ancient laws there is the code of Hammourabi, in the second millenium B.C., which stated that "should a house collapse and kill the proprietor's child, the death punishment should be inflicted on the architect's child. Should a woman be stricken and death follows, the daughter of the aggressor should in turn be put to death".

There was a mosaic law called "Talion" whereby the penalty was matched to the offence—on the "eye for an eye, a tooth for a tooth" basis. (In 1384 a boy in Constance had his tongue torn out because of blasphemy).

In 19th century schools punishment in advance was an established method of social control; all the likely troublemakers were flogged at the beginning of the day to save time.[7]

Vicarious punishment was a feature of early times. A whipping boy was kept by Royalty (Henry VIII, the Dauphins of France), so that if the royal prince offended, the whipping boy received the punishment.

In 1801 a boy of 12 was hung at Tyburn Tree (Marble Arch) for the theft of a spoon from a dwelling house. Later the idea of expiation was substituted for vengence. Children had to expiate their sins by suffering so that they could repent.

Finally Lewis Carrol gave the following advice

"Speak roughly to your little boy
And beat him when he sneezes.
He only does it to annoy
Because he knows it teases".

The Need for Discipline

Every child must experience discipline. He has to learn to conform to custom, to behave in a manner acceptable to others, to be taught the limits of freedom and what is safe and unsafe. He must learn to accept a No, and he must be brought to realize that he cannot have all his own way. He has to learn respect for the property of others, and that others matter as well as he. He has to learn obedience.

All children as they mature, must be allowed to develop independence and self expression. They must, in time, be allowed to make mistakes, so that they learn from them. They must not, therefore, be over-protected.

The Bakwins[1] wrote that: "Proper child rearing requires a balance between encouragement for self-expression and freedom on the one hand and training for conformity on the other. He has his rights and privileges, but he has his duties and responsibilities as well. He needs increasing freedom as his legitimate needs and capacities grow, but his freedom must be limited by his ability to take responsibility. As he matures he may be told the reasons for restrictions and the consequences which might result from transgression. He should be encouraged to use his own judgment where possible, but this cannot be done without direction and guidance. Too few restrictions, like too many, are undesirable."

To use Stott's[8] words, "the best relationship between parent and child is one in which the child feels secure as long as he behaves himself, but knows that naughtiness will jeopardize that security." Authority which is firm, kind, reasonable and consistent gives the child that sense of security which is essential for his emotional development. He needs discipline so that he can learn self-discipline.

Lack of discipline is seriously harmful to the child and "spoils" him. It is practised largely by parents who have heard or read that firmness leads to repression, and by the ignorant, who as children themselves never learnt discipline. The result is the spoiled, insecure child, the child thought by all but the parents to be a horror, the child whom other parents do not want to mix with their own children because of the undesirable tricks which he teaches them.

He knows that he can get his own way by demanding it, if necessary with a temper tantrum. He is particularly difficult when taken out to friends, revealing his bad behaviour when faced with other children. He is apt to wreck the furniture, throw objects about the room, and generally to set a bad example to other children. He is aggressive to other children and apt to injure them by kicking them. He grows up to be an unpopular spoiled school child who does not fit in well with his fellows. Food fads and accident proneness are common.

Stott wrote that lack of discipline in the first years is a major factor in juvenile delinquency. It is also an important factor in accident proneness and in other undesirable traits in later life. To use the Bakwins' words: "The child reared without discipline has only a false freedom, for without the help of adult guidance and control he grows uncontrolled and unsure of himself, uncertain of what to do and what not to do, slow in making decisions and angry when he has made the wrong one." It seems to be a common belief that if there are children in a house, it is inevitable that the furniture and carpets will be ruined and that there will be pencil marks and scratches and stains on the walls. Accidents are always apt to occur, but with reasonable discipline should be rare.

Excessive discipline is hardly less harmful. Discipline is always excessive if it is not related to the level of development which the child has reached. It is always wrong if it is exerted not as a benefit to the child but as an outlet for the parents' offended sense of dignity. Some parents insist on obedience over a completely unimportant matter because they fear loss of face. A woman causes a scene in a bus over a trivial matter because she fears that others will be critical of her for not being able to command instant obedience from her offspring. She fails to realize that by her behaviour she merely reveals the short-comings of her own character. Some parents are far too sensitive about what people will think of their children; they think that they will frown on what any well-informed adult will know is normal behaviour for the age.

Parents who are constantly saying "No, no, don't do this, don't do that," produce the child who rebels, has temper tantrums and other manifestations of insecurity. Obedience based on repression is never permanent. Parents who apply rigid forcing methods are the parents who have most trouble with their children. As Vining[7] wrote, "Most of us are well acquainted with the food-forcing, bowel-forcing, sleep-forcing and obedience-forcing parents, to whom belong all those children who refuse to eat, to sleep, to have their bowels moved and to obey." Some children brought up in this way are unduly submissive and timid. Most react by doing the opposite of what is expected of them. They respond by dawdling, by appearing not to hear commands, or by deliberate disobedience. Some children respond by aggressiveness, negativism, and temper tantrums: some respond by excessive shyness and other signs of insecurity; others respond by rebellion and bad behaviour at school. Accident proneness commonly results from excessive discipline, just as it does from overpermissiveness.

Discipline must be accompanied by love or it fails. Excessive correction, excessive discipline which the child cannot understand, are apt to be indulged in when the parents are tired, harassed or in a hurry, so that they are irritated by trivial things. When irritated at work they take it out of their child at home. A sense of humour is essential; but unfortunately one loses one's sense of humour when tired and overworked. The mother with thyrotoxicosis or an anxiety state is apt to be excessively demanding for obedience. In Lampe's biography of Pyke,[5] educationalist, Pyke is quoted as once saying "the fundamental principle we should follow in dealing with children is to treat every child as a distinguished foreign visitor who knows little or nothing of our language and customs. If we invited a distinguished stranger to tea and he spilled his cup on the best tablecloth or consumed more than his fair share of cake we should not upbraid him and send him out of the room. We should hasten to reasure him that all was well. One rude remark from the host would drive the visitor from the room, never to be seen again. But we address children constantly in the rudest fashion and yet expect them to behave as models of politeness".

Rules should be few, but they should be obeyed. There must be a reason for them, and the child, if old enough, should know the reasons for them. All too often parents dig their heels in over something completely trivial, which does not matter—and a great deal of friction results.

The wiser the management, the less the need for punishment; and the less frequent the punishment, the less severe need it be to take effect. The most trivial scolding, the mere tone of voice, can produce a much greater effect in the wisely managed child who is rarely punished, than a severe physical punishment in a child who is used to it. The more frequent the punishment the more severe it has to be to take effect. One is commonly told that a child does not seem to care when he is beaten. The parent feels thwarted and angry if the child does not show that he has been hurt, for he fails to obtain the emotional release which he needs. With wise management, sources of friction are removed. The nursery school teacher does not teach discipline by smacking the child. She removes him from the source of danger

246

DISCIPLINE AND PUNISHMENT

instead of warning him and threatening him about what will happen if he disobeys.

Another essential principle in the teaching of discipline is consistency. It merely confuses the child if at one time he is allowed to do a thing which at another time he is forbidden to do; or if he is punished at one time for doing something which is accepted at another time. It confuses him if one parent condones what the other forbids, or if the grandparents allow him to do things which his parents will not allow. Discipline must be consistent—though parents should look the other way when there are trivial breeches. Repeated threats and occasional punishment are equally confusing; the child does not know whether his parents mean what they say or not. The same applies to alternating overstrictness and punishment with overindulgence and over permissiveness. The parents feel uncomfortable after chastising the child, and go to the other extreme of letting him have all his own way.

The parents must agree on punishment. The child does not take long to discover that what one parent disapproves the other condones. As Ogden Nash said*:

> "The wise child handles Father and Mother
> By playing one against the other.
> 'Don't,' cries this parent to the tot.
> The opposite parent cries, 'Why not?'
> Let baby listen, nothing loth,
> And work impartially on both.
> In clash of wills do not give in.
> Good parents are made by discipline.
> Even a backward child can foil them,
> If ever careful not to spoil them."

Punishment must be consistent in another way. The punishment meted out is likely to depend more on the result than on the nature of the act. No punishment, for instance, is given when the child gently rocks a small table. He is merely told not to do it. But when in the process of rocking the table a little later an expensive piece of china is caused to crash to the floor, the child gets a severe beating. It is difficult for him to understand the reason for the different attitude now adopted and he feels confused.

It is undesirable for both parents to join in an attempt to discipline the child. There is often a tendency for both parents to pounce on the child for trivial misdemeanours. I saw a disturbed child who was being constantly pounced upon and reprimanded by five adults who were living in the home.

I feel confident that the most important principle in the teaching of

* Ogden Nash (1943). "A Child's Guide to Parents," in *The Face is Familiar*. London. J. M. Dent & Sons.

discipline is this; the child should behave well because he wants to do, because he wants the approval of the parent whom he loves, and the approval of his teachers. The child who is brought up with firm loving discipline, and whose needs for love and security are met from birth onwards, is far more likely to be well behaved in later years than the child brought up without love, but with harsh strictness. The child does not learn because of scoldings, ridicule, admonitions and fear of punishment, but because of love, respect and the example set by his parents. The basis of good behaviour is praise and love, not blame and punishment. He will learn more from encouragement and judicious awards than he will from reprimands and smackings. He must never be bribed to do what he is asked to do, but an unexpected award, such as a sweet, or a word of praise for obeying an unpalatable request, is another matter. The aim should be to teach discipline without tears.

The child should always be given a chance to explain what he has done. It often happens, however, that the parent in anger says "Don't answer back." "I won't have another word." As a result the child has no chance to state that what he did was entirely unintentional or accidental.

It is essential that the child should learn that if he disobeys, there will be some unpleasant consequence. All too often one hears parents constantly remonstrating with their child, forbidding or ordering him to do something, while the child takes no notice at all, because he has learnt that it is most unlikely that anything undesirable will happen if he disobeys. Threats of punishment should never be made if it is not intended to carry them out if the child disobeys. It is most unwise to threaten punishment which the parent could not carry out if he tried. It is always wrong to threaten to put the child to bed. That implies that bed is an undesirable place, and it invites sleep problems. It is always sensible to give a child due warning that further disobedience will be punished.

Punishment, if any, must be immediate, so that the cause is related to the effect.

No attempt should be made to teach discipline until he is old enough to understand what is wanted of him. A child cannot learn discipline when he is 1 year old. He can learn when he is three. Somewhere in between is the age at which the teaching of discipline should begin. This must depend not on his real age, but on his mental age. One has seen serious trouble arising from the fact that a mentally subnormal child was being disciplined at an age at which a normal child could learn, but at an age which was far too young for him. The Newsons[6] found that two out of every three Nottingham mothers were smacking their children before they were 1 year old. I have seen many babies aged 6 to 12 months being smacked for putting their thumb into the mouth—an innocent and harmless act. They would learn nothing by this treatment.

Before punishment is decided upon it is essential to try to understand the child's motives. It is easy to punish a child for doing wrong by adult standards when, with his limited experience and undeveloped conscience, he could see nothing wrong in what he was doing. Punishment in such circumstances is wrong. An explanation and warning should suffice. A child who is old enough to understand should be reminded of the behaviour which is expected of him. It must be remembered that screaming at night may be due to a nightmare. It would be wrong to smack a child for this.

The reason for the wrongdoing may lie in boredom, jealousy or insecurity. Destructiveness and the throwing of objects about a room may be due to lack of sufficient freedom and outlet for his energies. It would be wrong merely to punish him for his wrongdoing without trying to remove the underlying cause by trying to give him space to let off some energy without doing harm, removing breakable objects, and giving him a chance to play out of doors. A child may be punished for drawing on the wall, but he should also be given paper and pencil or a black board so that his desire to scribble and draw can be satisfied.

The Method of Punishment

The method of punishment must vary with the circumstances and the child's level of development. The unpleasantness of the consequences must be greater than the pleasure of the act. In the first year at least no punishment is ever justifiable. In the second year a mere firm expression of displeasure or deprivation of privileges is usually sufficient, as soon as he is old enough to understand. He may need a tap on the hand if doing something particularly dangerous and if it is thought that he will understand its significance. The odds are, however, that he will not understand, and the punishment is therefore useless. It is easy in the latter part of the first year and first part of the second year to laugh at a child who takes no notice of "No, no," or does what he is forbidden to do with redoubled speed, laughing loudly as he does it. He will inevitably repeat the performance laughed at. This trait, together with the negativism and desire for attention so characteristic of this age, make discipline difficult.

In the third year, mild physical punishment may be needed, but only rarely. Simple deprivation and expression of displeasure is usually enough. He may be deprived of his books or taken indoors when he wants to play outside. In general the form of punishment should as far as possible be the logical outcome of what he has done, so that the child cannot fail to connect his action with the result. If, for instance, he throws cutlery or food about the table during a meal, the food can be peremptorily removed or he may be caused to eat the next meal alone. If in spite of a warning he tears paper up into small pieces and scatters them over the floor, he should be made to pick them up and perhaps be prevented from going into the garden or having his dinner until he has done so, though he may be helped in the process. He may be isolated or caused to stand in the corner on account of a temper tantrum or wilful damage. If he throws his books about or damages them, they should be confiscated. If he kicks a sibling, his shoes may be removed. If the 4-year-old fails to come in from the garden to dinner when told to do so (after being given 10 minutes' warning that dinner will shortly be ready), he is not smacked for it, and dragged in screaming: he is given one reminder, and if he fails to come in then, he just misses his dinner. He will soon learn.

No smacking should ever hurt. *It is never necessary to hurt any child.* It is not the smack which hurts: it is the parents' disapproval. In my opinion an occasional tap on the buttocks does no harm to a small child of 3 to 5, though the occasion for it should be rare; but it is never necessary to smack an older child.

I disagree with the recommendations for punishment and the principles behind them expressed by an American psychiatrist,[2] who wrote as follows:

"A properly administered spanking consists of turning the child over one's knee and holding his head down by firm pressure on the back of the neck. The parent's other leg may be used to clamp the child's wriggling legs firmly down. With his free hand, the parent administers 10 hard blows with a hair brush or similar instrument, to the bare buttocks of the child. A spanking administered with the bare hand or through several layers of the child's clothing really does not hurt. . . .

"The human buttocks are admirably designed for character building purposes.

"It is much better to spank a child on the buttocks than to slap him on the face, hands or other part of the body." Castle[2] after many years experience as a headmaster, wrote "Looking back, I am inclined to the judgement that no-one was improved by corporal punishment, that its effects were purely negative, that on rare occasions when it was brutal, the effects were bad, that it failed to make boys better behaved. It was used most by the weakest teachers. The rod is an uncivilised anachronism". Sir Alec Clegg, of the Education Department of the West Riding of Yorkshire, wrote that "attitudes of which excessive canings are symptomatic may be those which induce rebelliousness, or which do least to allay or inhibit the tendency towards delinquency which may have its roots in home conditions".

Some parents have learnt that corporal punishment is undesirable, and they use a much worse method of dealing with the child— using the weapons of ridicule, sarcasm, constant scoldings, or shaming. It is altogether wrong to try to make a child feel guilty or ashamed. It is always wrong to belittle him and make him feel incompetent. It is always wrong to make fun of him, and worse still to make him feel that he is no longer loved. Some parents "put the child into Coventry" for the whole day, refusing to speak to him. A mother tried to cure her son's fæcal incontinence by deliberately showing the boy's soiled trousers to his school friends. A headmistress of a boarding school tried to cure a child's enuresis by displaying the wet sheets to the entire morning assembly.

There is no place for retaliation. Some parents wrongly advocate the principle of "an eye for an eye, a tooth for a tooth." I heard one mother say that if her child bit her, she would bite him. This is likely to teach the child to retaliate in later years—and in married life it would be disastrous. This does not mean that the child should not be expected to stand up for himself against other children.

If the child has confessed to some heinous sin, punishment should not be severe, for if it is severe, confessions will not be likely in the future. Severe punishment is wrong for another reason. It is apt to cause repressions, insecurity and a feeling of hostility: and other behaviour problems will then arise.

The punishment should be accompanied by as little fuss as possible, for if there is a great deal of fuss and anxiety the child may repeat the performance as an attention-seeking device. After the child has been punished it is unwise to insist on repentance, for he is in no mood to give it except from fear. There must be no prolonged disapproval, as so often happens. When he has been punished he should be treated as if nothing has happened. It should not be discussed with others in his presence.

Punishment is Usually Wrong

For many reasons most punishment inflicted is wrong. George Bernard Shaw wrote that "to punish is to injure."

Most punishment is inflicted because of loss of temper. Parents lose their sense of humour and their tolerance when they are tired, hurried, worried, or feeling unwell. A mother may be bad tempered because of an unrecognized anæmia, or because of premenstrual tension. A father may have a difficult day at work and take it out of his family on return home. Furthermore, when parents become angry, they provoke, and try to find faults in the child. Parents feel thwarted by various behaviour problems in the child, because they cannot control them. They cannot make the child eat, sleep, use the pottie, or stop him blinking his eyes or fidgeting. They are exasperated, and feel that the child could easily mend his ways if he tried.

The parents' punitive tendencies commonly relate to the management which they received as a child. The father was himself punished excessively and was unable to prevent it. As he grows up he finds release from the repressions of his childhood by chastising his son. He then rationalizes his behaviour by Samuel Butler's dictum (originating from the Book of Proverbs) "spare the rod, spoil the child." He argues that "the rod did him no harm"—and fails to realize that the rod has made him the sort of father who wants to use the rod on his son. Frequent punishment commonly results from parental unhappiness and conflict.

Parents become angry when their children question parental authority. They will not allow the child to ask the reasons why.

There is a sadistic factor in punishment. The excessive beatings in public schools were sadistic in nature, the master finding sexual satisfaction in the act. At Tyburn Tree in London a charge of three shillings was made for people to witness public executions.

Punishment is usually irrational. Children are punished for acts which are in no way wrong. I have already mentioned the frequency with which one sees babies being smacked for sucking the thumb. Others are smacked for handling the genitals. Many are smacked for masturbation.

Children are punished for acts which are quite outside their control. The commonest example of this is bed wetting. It seems to me to be extraordinarily foolish to punish a child for doing something in his sleep. I knew a boy who was severely punished because his mother heard him swearing in his sleep. Children are punished for bad writing, when in fact they are clumsy children in whom abnormal neurological signs can be detected by proper examination. Children are punished for tics, for not sitting still, for overactivity—when in fact there were prenatal factors which were responsible for them. They are punished for features of the personality, such as bad temper, which they have inherited from their parents. As my colleague, Dr. Woodmansey[10] said, to punish for misbehaviour is to ignore the cause. Since a child's actions are the outcome of his feelings and unconscious urges, neither of which he can prevent, punishment is to say the least unfair, and as such will be resented. The child behaves badly because he feels insecure, and punishment merely serves to convince him that he has indeed lost his parents' love.

Woodmansey wrote about the attitude that "the child should control his feelings, but the parent need not." He added "Hostility breeds hostility. . . . The mother feels so cross if bitten by the child that she feels he should be bitten back—that in some way it will cure his aggression—despite her immediate experience that it has just had the opposite effect. . . . Adults are not only on the defensive, and ready to attack the baby when he annoys them, but they blame him for the ensuing fight."

A revealing survey of the causes of punishment in schools was made by Highfield and Pinsent.[4] Seven hundred and twenty-four teachers recorded the frequency of specified misdemeanours requiring punishment. They included the following:

Restlessness, fidgeting, lack of concentration.
Boisterous or noisy behaviour.
Forgetfulness, unpunctuality.
Deceit.
Indifference, laziness, apathy with respect to more verbal academic subjects.
Bickering, quarrelling, truancy.

Corporal punishment was thought to be justified for bullying or stealing. It should be obvious that all these conditions may well be due to factors quite outside the child's control. It is particularly irrational to cane a child for bullying; he is bullying because he is being bullied by someone else—and because of insecurity.

Most punishment reveals a lack of understanding of the developing mind of a child. Much punishment is meted out not because the child is naughty, but because he is a nuisance to adults. He may be punished because he fights his brother. He fights his brother because of the normal aggressiveness of the age. He is learning something at home which the only child misses—that he cannot have all his own way. The only child is likely to have to learn this painfully at school.

Parents tend to forget that children too are sensitive, that they become bad tempered when they are tired, bored, hungry, or bullied. To punish a child for showing bad temper when he is hypoglycæmic on coming in from school, is irrational. Much punishment is directed not at the cause, but at the symptom, and it fails.

Punishment is irrational because children, like animals, learn far better from rewards, praise and encouragement, than from punishment, blame and reprimands.

Conclusion

All children must learn discipline. It should be taught with love and tolerance and with an understanding of the mind of the child.

The child is likely to behave well because he wants the approval of his parents (and teacher), not because of fear of punishment.
Children learn better by praise and reward than by punishment.
Most punishment represents loss of temper. Most punishment is irrational.

References

1. BAKWIN, H., BAKWIN, R. M. (1951). "Discipline in Children." *J. Pediat.*, **39**, 623.
2. CASTLE, E. B. (1953). *People at School.* London. Heinemann.
3. CHAPMAN, A. H. (1965). *Management of Emotional Problems of Children and Adolescents.* Philadelphia. Lippincott.
4. HIGHFIELD, M. E., PINSENT, A. (1952). *A Survey of Rewards and Punishments in Schools.* National Foundation for Educational Research.
5. LAMPE, D. (1959). *Pyke; the Unknown Genius.* London. Evans.
6. NEWSON, J., NEWSON, E. (1963). *Infant Care in an Urban Community.* London. Allen & Unwin.
7. ROLPH, C. H. (1967). "Crime and Punishment." *J. Roy. Coll. Physcns London*, **1**, 306.
8. STOTT, D. H. (1950). *Delinquency and Human Nature.* Dunfermline. Carnegie United Kingdom Trust.
9. VINING, C. W. (1952). "Feeding Disorders in Children: Their Interpretation." *Lancet*, **2**, 99.
0. WOODMANSEY, C. (1966). "Mental Illness in the Family, its Effect on the Child." *Proc. 22nd Child Guidance International Conference.* N. Association Mental Health.

CHAPTER 21

ANOREXIA AND OTHER EATING PROBLEMS

Anorexia

Of all behaviour problems anorexia is the commonest, the mos
easily prevented, the most easily caused and the most easily cured
One pædiatrician saw so many cases in consultation that he claimed
that he built his house on anorexia. Brennemann said that the child
who will not eat represents probably 10–20 per cent. of children in
private practice between the second and fifth year inclusive. It is a
commonplace to be told in the out-patient department that the healthy
well-fed-looking child in front of one "does not eat enough to keep a
sparrow alive," "never eats a thing" or "has been losing weight ever
since the day he was born." The mother says that she has tried everything to make him eat. Therein lies the trouble, for if she had tried
nothing there would have been no difficulty at all.

In the treatment of any behaviour problem it is essential to discuss
the management of the child in detail. In order to do this one must
be conversant with the methods commonly employed by parents.

Methods commonly Employed

Brennemann's description[3] of efforts to make children eat is worth
giving verbatim: "In innumerable homes there is a daily battle.
On the one side the army advances with coaxing, teasing, urging,
cajoling, spoofing, wheedling, begging, shaming, scolding, nagging,
threatening, bribing, punishing, pointing out and demonstrating
the excellence of the food, again weeping or pretending to weep,
playing the fool, singing a song, telling a story, or showing a picture
book, turning on the radio, beating a drum just as the food enters
the mouth with the hope that it will keep going in instead of returning, even having the grandmother dance a jig—all regularly
recurrent actual procedures encountered daily. On the other side a
little tyrant resolutely holds the fort, either refusing to surrender, or
else capitulating on his own terms. Two of his most powerful weapons
of defence are vomiting and dawdling."

An excellent description of a typical food-forcing scene was given
by Benjamin.[1]

I have seen all the following methods used, many of them in scores
of children.

Coaxing Methods. The mother tries to persuade the child to eat. She watches his plate and asks him to eat just a little more to please her. She asks him to take a bite for Santa Claus, for Auntie Lizzie or for Guy Fawkes. She tells the boy that the food is good for him—but he is not interested, neither does he understand what she means (nor does the mother). She asks him to eat just a little more so that she can tell Daddy when he returns from work.

Distraction Methods. The mother turns the wireless, gramophone or television set on, or sings to him. One mother said that for a while the boy ate well when she and her husband sang to him at mealtimes, but then the boy joined in the singing and they had to try something else. The mother tells stories or recites nursery rhymes. The father neighs like a horse, or moos, and pretends to be a dive-bomber. One child would eat only if the father crept about the room on all fours, pretending to be a dog. Another child would only eat if his brother set off an alarm clock at frequent intervals near him, so distracting him and enabling his mother to slip some food into his mouth. One mother spent 4s. a week on comic papers to make him eat. Others have tried putting a mirror in front of the child so that he can race the image in getting the food down. It is a common practice to allow the child to have his meal while walking or running round the house or garden, in order, presumably, that he will forget to refuse to eat.

Bribes. Most parents faced with food refusal have offered their child bribes to make him eat. In most cases the bribes consist of sweets, ice-creams and excursions to the cinema or park. Some parents offer to let the child stay up longer in the evening if he will eat his dinner. One intelligent girl of 6 years was making between 3s. and 4s. a week in pocket-money out of the bribes. A boy of 4 would only eat if he was given a toy motor car, and he had collected a garage of between 200 and 300 motor cars in this way.

Tonics. Most parents have tried various "tonics." One mother said that the only way which she found to make her 3-year-old eat was to give her a mixture of Ribena and brandy.

Threats. The commonest threat is the warning that the child will not grow up big and strong like Uncle Bob unless he eats his dinner. The child apparently could not care less. Some mothers are unwise enough to threaten to leave the child unless he eats his meal. One mother said, "Tom, I shan't love you any more if you don't eat that." The boy replied disarmingly, "Mummy, whatever happens I shall always love you." Another told her girl that she would die if she did not eat more. The prospect did not seem to disturb her. Some mothers threaten to bring the child from next door to eat the dinner, but as this threat is never carried out the child does not take any notice. Many mothers threaten to punish the child if the food is no eaten. Others threaten to take him to a doctor, as if this is a sever punishment.

Forcing Methods. Most parents have tried and discarded food forcing methods. They hold the child's nose and push the food in wit a spoon. Any intelligent child resists violently, sends the spoon flyin with a well-aimed blow, spits the food out or vomits.

Punishment. One father regularly beat his boy with a leather stra for not eating what he was told to eat. Most mothers have trie smacking their children for not eating. As Anna Freud said, "Th meal becomes forced labour rather than wish fulfilment."

Food between Meals. The mother is so afraid that the child wi starve that she gives him food whenever he asks for it. The usual stor is that he has constant snacks of milk, sandwiches, cake, fruit or sweet When the regular mealtime is reached he refuses everything. On mother said that she always carried a packet of biscuits with he wherever she went, so that if ever the boy asked for something to ea she would be able to give it to him immediately. In another case mother was giving her well thriving little boy, aged 18 months, 25 feed a day to keep him alive!

Allowing the Child to choose the Menu. Astonishing food fads ar allowed to develop. One mother really believed that her 4-year-ol child could eat nothing but bacon and eggs. He would not touc anything else, and that was all he had. Nearly all food fads in childre arise from food forcing or over-anxiety about food.

It need hardly be added that the mother is not the only one wh employs these methods. The father joins in, tending to be firmer tha his wife and to use more physical punishment and forcing methods. I the grandmother lives in the house, she too joins in the fray. To th child's delight, the whole house revolves round what he will eat. Hi morale is good, for he always wins.

The Basic Causes of the Problem

Negativism. The Development of the Ego

Some babies suddenly between 6 and 9 months refuse the breas or bottle, and will only take food if it is given by spoon or cup. Som will refuse to eat if they are not allowed to help to hold the spoo and feed themselves. It becomes increasingly difficult to change fron breast or bottle to cup after 8 or 9 months, or to change from thickene feeds to solids. Food refusal in these babies is due to the increasin determination in the child and his developing ego.

Of all principles of infant and child feeding, probably the mos important is the avoidance of food forcing. Food forcing is by far the most important of all causes of feeding problems. Children cannot be forced to take food. There is an old saying that any man can lead a horse to water, but twenty men cannot make him drink. Children rapidly learn that they can prevent their parents from forcing them to take food. They can fight, knock the contents of the spoon on to the floor, spit food out, refuse to chew it or vomit it up when once it has been swallowed. They discover that at mealtimes there are most satisfactory opportunities for creating a fuss and for attracting attention. A child discovers that his mother is most anxious for him to take a particular foodstuff, such as milk or meat. He refuses to take it, or refuses to chew it, or else he retains the food in his mouth for an hour or two, revelling in the consternation which he causes. He particularly enjoys the scene when he spits food out or vomits it up. His parents are foolish enough to talk about his terrible appetite in front of him, and so suggest to him that he is expected not to eat. He soon has the whole house revolving about his appetite, and he certainly makes the most of the situation. It is quite an achievement for a 2-year-old to compel his parents to play games, read to him, dance jigs, creep about on all fours, pretend to be animals and dive-bombers, in order to get him to consent to eat, when in fact he is hungry, wants to eat and would on no account be prepared to do without.

Another most successful attention-seeking device is dawdling. In my opinion it is one of the commonest causes of food forcing and so of food refusal. Up to a point dawdling is normal between the ages of 9 months and $2\frac{1}{2}$ years, and all children do it. The child plays about with his food, patting it with his spoon and putting his hands into it. He drops some on the floor, puts some into his hair and anywhere but into his mouth. He has no understanding of time and therefore sees not the slightest reason to hurry. He is particularly likely to dawdle with the first course, much preferring the pudding. It is not surprising that the mother, failing to realize that all children do the same, thinks that he has no appetite and is not eating enough, and so she tries to hurry him and to persuade him to eat. This makes him all the slower, and the mother then tries to force him to take food. The mother, in addition, is in a hurry, because she wants to get the washing-up done and to clear the table, and for this reason too she hurries him, threatens him and tries to force him to eat. The dawdling, which began as a perfectly normal stage in eating behaviour, becomes exaggerated and nothing more than an attention-seeking device. This dawdling may persist for years if the parents persist in their efforts to hurry him. It passes from the conscious to the subconscious and the child cannot help it. I have seen a child who at a boarding school was compelled

to sit alone at a special table because of the time he took over hi
meals.

Early Conditioning

Infants may be conditioned to dislike food at mealtimes because o
food-forcing methods. When they are compelled to eat and are smacke(
for not eating, and the whole mealtime is a time of unpleasantness, the:
may take a genuine dislike for food, and it is hard to break. A mothe
told me that her 4-year-old child always began to cry as soon as th
meal was ready. I believe that this early conditioning against food is a•
important cause of food refusal. It is entirely due to food-forcing.

The Physical Build

A child who is small in size, either because he takes after one o
his parents, or because he was a small baby at birth (especially if h•
were dysmature), or because he has congenital heart disease or othe
physical defect, can be expected to have a smaller food intake thar
big children. He wants less to eat, and the result is commonly food
forcing—the mother feeling that he is not eating enough. In m:
experience a small build is one of the commonest causes of food
forcing and so of food refusal.

The Development of Likes and Dislikes

At 5 months a child may have firm likes and dislikes. It is amusing
to watch a 6-month-old baby sampling a food which he has not taste(
before and deciding whether he will eat more of it or not. He may
flatly refuse a dish which he does not fancy. He becomes used to :
particular dish and cup and refuses food from any other. This is harm
less within reason, but I once saw a 9-month-old baby who refused al
fluid unless it was given to him in a wine glass!

He may refuse food merely because he wants to have a drink first
After he has had a drink he will eat the rest of the dinner withou
difficulty.

He is more affected by the appearance of food than is commonl)
realized. From the age of 6 months or so he is more likely to take :
red, brightly-coloured food than a colourless nondescript mush
He likes variety and may readily become tired of a food which h•
is offered over and over again. Some mothers show little ingenuit)
in supplying variety and in making the food look attractive. Whateve•
happens, there should be no attempt to force him to take disliked foods
This would cause not only food refusal, but often a permanent dislik(
of the food in question.

The Desire for Independence and the Practice of New Skills

Failure to allow the child to practise his new manipulative skill in holding the cup or spoon may cause him to refuse food.

Children are likely to want to hold the bottle or cup when they are able to grasp objects at 5 or 6 months, and at any time from 6 months to a year they may demand to hold the spoon and help to feed themselves. The sooner this is allowed the better, for it is most desirable that they should learn to be independent and look after themselves. An independent child may be extremely annoyed if not allowed to hold the cup or spoon himself. Some babies would rather starve than be fed by their mothers in this age period. The mother is apt to refuse to let the child feed himself because she is in a hurry to get the housework done, or because she is afraid of the mess he will make. She should spread a sheet of plastic under the chair to catch the droppings and only help when it is absolutely necessary. She does nothing when the food gets into his ear or hair, but has to step in when an attempt is made to place the inverted food dish on the head as a hat. If she laughs at the mess which the child is making, he will repeat the performance and make a bigger mess. Some children of a placid disposition show no interest in this age period in feeding themselves. Others are extremely insistent. One 7-month child was referred to me on account of "acute indigestion." The story was that when the first mouthful of food was given she screamed and refused to take more. Further questioning showed that after the first mouthful the girl tried to get hold of the spoon, and the mother smacked her hand and would not let her help. The child thereupon refused to take any more.

Individual Variations in Appetite

There are big eaters and little eaters. Some children need to eat much more than others to achieve an average weight gain. The quantity of food which a child eats is in part related to his personality. The placid child tends to eat more than the highly active determined one. There is no doubt that an occasional child does have a particularly bad appetite without any parental mismanagement and without any illness or disease. These cases are rare. Thorough investigation fails to reveal any cause. In the vast majority of cases of so-called anorexia, however, the cause is simply the food-forcing methods of the parents. I have only seen two cases of severe chronic anorexia of the type mentioned above in otherwise well children.

The child's appetite varies, like that of an adult, from meal to meal and from day to day. The appetite is particularly liable to be poor at breakfast. Failure to recognize these variations causes mothers to worry about their child's appetite when they remember the appetite of a previous child or see the appetite of the child next door. Food-forcing then results.

Unhappiness

It is natural to expect that a child who is unhappy, whether because of parental rejection or insecurity or for any other reason, will have a poor appetite. When mealtimes have been allowed to become a misery for a child, it is not surprising that when he approaches the dinner table his appetite disappears.

Lack of Fresh Air and Exercise

This may be an important factor.

Association and Suggestion

Any painful experience, such as taking food when it was too hot, is likely to be remembered by a child as young as 6 months of age, and for several days he may refuse food looking like it or the dish which contained it.

Likes and dislikes are readily suggested by the parents.

The Attitude of the Parents

The Mother's Love for her Child. Realization that this is the under-lying cause of most cases of anorexia will prevent one from being critical of the mother's mistaken methods.

Undue Preoccupation with the Child's Weight. This is partly the fault of weight charts and articles in popular magazines. Mothers do not realize that there are great differences in the build of children owing to a variety of factors, such as size at birth and family history. They make the mistake of thinking that a child who is not up to the average weight is abnormal, and so they try to force him to take food. They do not know that normal children differ in the speed at which they gain weight. They do not realize that after the third month there is a rapid falling off of weight gain, and therefore of appetite. They think that at 12 months the child should be gaining about 7 oz. (200 g) a week as in the first month or two. It is my practice to explain to them that, if a child had to continue to gain weight at the rate of 7 oz. (200 g) a week, he would weigh 23 stones (146 kg) by the age of 14, which would be too much. I have seen two doctors' children who were given a test feed at every feed for 9 months.

When a child has been ill or was prematurely born, a mother is apt to consider him "delicate" and so try to force him to take more food than he wants.

A Little Knowledge of Nutrition. Many popular books teach rigidity
i feeding methods, particularly in the feeding schedule and in the
uantity of food to be given. Mothers acquire the idea that they
iust give an exact quantity of milk, and if the baby refuses it or goes
» sleep before the feed is finished they try to compel him to take more.
fter the first year parents are apt to insist on children taking foods
hich they have been told are "good" for them—vegetables, meat
nd milk. Some doctors give "diet sheets" to mothers of toddlers.
1others reading such instructions may unfortunately try to adhere
» them, and apply compulsion if the child refuses to eat what the
iet sheet recommends. They completely ignore the individual
kes and dislikes, the variations in appetite from meal to meal, day
» day and child to child. Some children show a great preference
»r the sweet course at dinner and dawdle with the first course or
ave it altogether. Mothers imbued with the vital importance of the
ieat course may try to compel their children to eat it and so meet with
od refusal.

Mothers over-estimate the quantity of food which a small child
:quires. Many fail to realize that the apparently small quantity
hich he takes is enough for an average weight gain. The inevitable
:sult is that they try to force the child to eat more.

Constant Nagging. Undue insistence on good table manners is apt to
iake mealtimes a misery. Such insistence is due to the wrong idea of
·aining and of the age at which good table manners can be expected. In
ie first 3 years all children make some mess. The amount of mess made
ipidly decreases in the second and third years and patience is necessary.

Attempts at Discipline. Many parents are obsessed with the idea
iat the child must learn from an early age that their will is law,
nd that he must be taught to do what he is told, so that he will not be
ooilt. If this is applied to mealtimes, food-forcing results, and therefore
ood-refusal.

Other Factors in the Mother. Over-anxiety and over-protection lead
» food-forcing methods. Psychologists say that the rejecting mother
:nds to concentrate on the mechanical sides of upbringing—the eating
nd elimination—and so to cause food-refusal. Impatience in the
iother as a result of pressure of work may cause the child to refuse
ood. When a mother has gone to a great deal of trouble to prepare
special dish to "tempt" the child and he refuses it, it is not surprising
iat she becomes annoyed and may smack the child or try to force him
» take it.

The majority of appetite problems commence between 6 and 18
ionths of age, at the time when the child is developing independence
f character and so resists domination.

Prevention

This lies simply in the realization that the vast majority of childre
are born in working order, with an appetite which is sufficient for thei
needs. The child's likes and dislikes should be respected within reaso
and he should be allowed to help to feed himself and, as soon as he i
ready, to feed himself completely. It should be fully understood tha
there is never any need to persuade or force a properly managed chil
to eat.

Treatment

The lines of treatment to be adopted are implicit in the remark
made above. It is futile merely to say that there is nothing wrong o
that he will grow out of it. That is untrue. There is something wrong
and it is likely that he will not grow out of it as long as the mismanage
ment persists. The worst possible advice to give is that more forc
should be used and that the child should be compelled to eat.

As with all behaviour problems, one must avoid appearing t
criticize the parents for their management. The measures which s
many of them adopt to make their children eat are so fantastic that i
is often difficult not to criticize or ridicule them. On the other hanc
they must be brought to understand that the trouble lies entirely i
them and not in the child. If the child has ever been away from hom
emphasis should be laid on the fact that he ate perfectly normall
when away from parental influence. It should be made clear that a
this is purely a matter of management, all tonics and medicines ar
totally unnecessary. All attempts at forcing the child to eat must b
stopped. When a child refuses food in the weaning period, it is a goo
plan to offer him the breast or bottle first and then to offer him the ne
food when he is in a better temper. If he still refuses it he should b
tried again a few days later. At this age, as in older children, ther
must be no persuasion, no coaxing, no bribing, no threatening and n
punishment. All tricks to make him eat must be stopped absolutel
There is no need to let him walk about the room or garden in order tha
he will eat what is set before him. He should sit up to the table an
eat the food or leave it. The mother must avoid anxious looks at th
plate. The child senses anxiety from the mother's tone of voice an
facial expression. There is no need for praise when the child eats hi
dinner. The food should be put before the child and it should b
taken as a matter of course that he will have what he wants. It is a
silly to praise a child for eating his dinner as it is to praise him fo
playing games in the garden. There must be no punitive attitude i
he does not eat and no suggestion that he is being naughty. He shoul

not be prevented from doing what he wants to do because he has not eaten his dinner. This suggests to the child that eating is a duty. If he does not want it then it is given to the cat, and no interest should be shown in the fact. There should then be absolutely nothing between meals. When a child is eating normally it does no harm to allow him to have occasional foodstuffs such as fruit, milk or sweets between mealtimes, but if he is being difficult about eating he should have nothing and be brought to realize that he will have to wait till the next regular mealtime; and mealtimes should be regular—at least after the first 6 months.

The parents inevitably ask what they should do when he will not touch a meal. The answer is that he is left without any food until the next meal. They then ask what they should do if he refuses that. It is extremely unusual for such a refusal to occur. I have never seen it happen. If it did happen the child should still be left without food. *No healthy child ever starves because he is not forced to eat.* He will soon capitulate when hunger overtakes him as long as no one makes a great deal of fuss about what he eats.

There should be no undue insistence on any particular food. It has been shown experimentally that animals show considerable wisdom in deciding what food they require. Young[22] and Richter[17] have written excellent reviews of this work. Richter showed that when rats were given complete freedom of choice between eleven pure food elements—three solid foods and eight liquid, in separate containers— they took constant daily proportions of the various food elements, all of which were necessary for life. When special circumstances were introduced, such as pregnancy, lactation or removal of a gland, the rats knew how to alter the proportion of foodstuffs taken. If, for example, the parathyroid gland was removed, the rats took additional calcium. The implication for human beings is that there need be no excessive insistence that the meat or greens be eaten before the sweet. It is no disaster if a small child eats some of the meat course, then eats the pudding and returns to the meat. It will not cause bad habits. He will grow out of it. Up to a point the child's strong likes and dislikes should be respected, but that is a different thing from allowing him to choose the menu. A child nearing his third birthday will readily, if permitted, say "I don't like this," "I don't like that," "I don't like currants," "I don't like fish." Such a child is merely asserting his ego and is displaying what is commonly termed bad manners. This should be stopped. The mother should make it plain that the food in front of him is all there is and that if he does not like it he can leave it, but there will be nothing else.

The food should be made to look attractive, bearing in mind the

10

child's fondness of bright colours. No over-facing excess is put on his plate. It is always better to put a small amount on his plate and let him ask for more than to let him habitually leave his plate half emptied. There should be reasonable variety so that he does not get tired of any one foodstuff.

As long as the child's appetite is poor it is unwise to give more than about a pint of milk per day. Excess of milk may take the appetite away and prevent him from having other more important foods. I saw a child with anorexia who was drinking 5 pints of milk a day, and the cream off a further 3 pints. As long as the child's appetite is normal there is no need to restrict the quantity of milk which he takes.

He should be encouraged to practise his new skills and to help to feed himself as soon as he is interested in so doing. At the age when domestic mimicry is a characteristic feature of the developing child—from 15 to 18 months of age onwards—he should be allowed to help to prepare the meal himself, helping with the potatoes, fruit and pastry. The child's appetite for products of his own handiwork, however horrible they look to the adult, is tremendous. Milk refusal can often be managed by allowing him to pour the milk out of the jug himself. It is a good thing for him to have his meals with his parents or with other children.

Dawdling over the food is difficult to treat. The child should certainly not be rushed. He should not be allowed to create a fuss and anxiety, or else the dawdling will continue as an attention-seeking device. He should certainly not be forced to take food more quickly. The inevitable result would be food refusal. Part of the dawdling may be due to over-insistence on the meat course. The child is much less likely to dawdle with the pudding or sweet course. One has to decide exactly how long the meal will be allowed to take. If the child is still playing with his food when the rest of the table has been cleared, and certainly when the washing-up has been done, the food should be removed. There may be a wail of dismay. The only way to deal with the problem is to make no fuss, but simply to allow a reasonable time for the child to eat, and then, without further ado and without any threats or argument, remove the food.

The child should get as much outdoor exercise as possible, and over-fatigue should be avoided.

It is not always easy to persuade the parents to carry out this treatment. In my experience most parents do, and the response is extremely satisfactory. As soon as the child realizes that he cannot cause any more fuss and attract any more attention in this way the food refusal abruptly stops.

Other Eating Problems

Obesity

The word "obesity" is derived from the word "*obesus*," which is translated in Lewis and Short's Latin Dictionary as meaning "Fat, stout, plump, stupid, that has eaten itself fat." Obesity is becoming a common problem in the first five years, and can be a serious problem as soon as the latter part of the first year. Obesity at this period often rights itself, in that there is usually a notable loss of fat in the second year, but this excessive deposition of fat should act as a warning that the child is liable to respond in future to a positive food balance by laying down fat. Eid[6] showed that excessive weight gain even as early as six weeks of age is strongly correlated with obesity at the age of six to eight years. It is now known[9,19] that the number of fat cells is decided in the early weeks of life, undernutrition reducing the number and overnutrition increasing it. It may be that excessive food intake in early life may program excessive secretion of insulin and growth hormone, with a permanent effect on cell size, number and metabolism.[4]

It is difficult to define obesity because it is not possible to draw a line between normal weight and the abnormal. It is not entirely a behaviour problem, but it is in part, and for that reason it is discussed here. Those interested should read the extensive review by Börjeson,[2] who described data concerning 718 overweight girls and 687 overweight boys.

Jean Mayer[13] suggested that measurement of skin fold thickness is the simplest and most practical available method of determining the extent of obesity. Suitably standardized calipers measure this at the midpoint of the back of the front arm flexed at 90°.[18]

Ætiology. The ætiology of obesity is obscure. Few will disagree with Newburgh's[15] statement that "obesity is invariably caused by an inflow of energy that exceeds the outflow."

The factors related to obesity may conveniently be discussed under the following headings:

(1) Increased Intake. This is the main factor in obesity. It is then important to consider why overeating occurs. It may begin because the mother regards the child as delicate, because he was prematurely born, or had frequent illnesses, or one serious illness, and she then gives him particularly rich food. Psychiatrists consider that overfeeding and over-protection may be manifestations of rejection by the mother. She uses these as symbols of motherly care and as substitutes for real affection.

Overeating is commonly the direct result of habit formation. Sibling rivalry may play a part. When one child has a second helping of pudding, the sibling feels that he must have the same. Sweet eating is very largely a habit, and is a potent cause of obesity.

Overeating results from insecurity. An unhappy child may find solace in overeating.

Imitation is a factor in some children. The child sees his parents and adolescent sibling eat large quantities and he feels that he should do likewise.

Unwise selection of foodstuffs for the young child is an important factor. The common practice of introducing cereals and soups in the first few weeks of life may lead to an excessive weight gain because of the high carbohydrate intake. (Chapter 3.)

An important cause of obesity is the eating of constant snacks between meals. It is easy to see that most really fat children are constantly eating. They become fat because they overeat. The mother thinks that her child needs a lot of food because he is such a big fellow and she gives him more.

Mothers commonly consider that the bigger a child is, the better he is. They refer to their ugly obese child as being "Bonny." They commonly like him to be fat and are proud of it.

(2) Reduced Output of Energy. Fat children tend to be less active than thin ones. It is difficult to say which of these is the cause and which is the effect. When a child is rendered inactive by a condition such as amyotonia congenita, obesity is particularly liable to occur.

Mayer[13] regarded abnormal inactivity as a much more frequent finding than compulsive eating.

(3) Hormonal Factors. There are still many doctors who consider every fat child they see to be a case of Fröhlich's syndrome of adiposo-skeletogenitodystrophy. I have never seen a case. It is associated with glycosuria, polydipsia and polyuria. Wilkins[20] wrote that in 18 years experience in endocrinology, he had only seen one or two cases of this syndrome.

Others make the mistake of diagnosing thyroid deficiency. Wilkins found only two obese children in over 200 cases of hypothyroidism.

Many are confused by the way in which the penis of a fat boy is buried in fat and looks unduly small.

It is incorrect, however, to say that there are no hormonal factors in obesity. There are. It is known that there are two centres in the hypothalamus which are responsible for the regulation of appetite. In experimental animals the destruction of one of these causes polyphagia and polydipsia, while the destruction of the other causes aphagia and adipsia. These centres are affected by many influences, such as stimuli from the nose (smell), mouth (taste), stomach, and the blood sugar level. It was shown that damage to the appropriate centre in the hypothalamus caused overeating and therefore obesity, but that after a time the appetite returned to normal. The animals, however, remained fat. One should remember this when faced with a fat child, whose mother insists that he eats very little. In the great majority of fat children, however, investigation does in fact prove that intake is excessive.

Almost all fat children are tall for their age. X-ray studies show that they have advanced skeletal maturation. It is thought that this is related to secondary adreno-cortical overactivity. They excrete large quantities of 17-ketogenic steroids in the urine. The output falls when their weight is reduced[5]

(4) Hereditary Factors. When a child is obese, one almost invariably finds that one or both of his parents is overweight. It is difficult in this matter to distinguish the hereditary factor from the familial liking of good food and plenty of it. There have been many studies, however, of strains of animals, such as mice, rats and sheep dogs, in which obesity was proved to be a hereditary feature.

In one study[2] it was shown that 10 per cent. of children were overweight when their parents were of normal weight; 40 per cent. were overweight when one parent was overweight; and 80 per cent. of children were overweight when both parents were similarly affected.

(5) Social Factors. Obesity is more common in the lower social classes than in the upper classes.

(6) Unknown Factors. It would be incorrect to say that the whole problem of obesity is now fully understood. Some have an enormous appetite but do not grow fat. Some have a small appetite and readily become fat.

Treatment. Prevention is better than cure. It is far easier to prevent obesity developing, when a child is beginning to show an excessive weight gain, than to treat it when obesity is fully developed. Although preoccupation with weight is undesirable, there is much to be said for a weight chart on which a child's weight is plotted at intervals. I would only advise this in a child who showed any sign of excessive weight gain, especially if there was a family history of obesity. An excess weight gain of 1 kg a year may easily pass unnoticed; but it adds up to a considerable excess as the years go by. The earlier excessive weight gain is checked the better, and the easier is it achieved by a simple modification of food habits.

Many doctors make the mistake of telling the mother that "it is only puppy fat. He will grow out of it." An occasional baby or toddler has an enormous appetite, and is extremely cross if his food intake is restricted. It is not always easy, therefore, to cut down the food intake. Such children, however, are rare.

Early weaning is advisable in breast-fed babies who show a tendency to obesity. In bottle-fed babies a gradual change from an all-milk diet to mixed feeding should be made. In general it is wise to commence mixed feeds when a child reaches 12 lb (5·5 kg) if he has not already started them on account of his age. He may otherwise take an excess of milk and continue to put on weight excessively. Care should then be taken to avoid giving excess of starchy food, such as cereals. The quantity of milk taken should be limited to 20–30 oz. (570–850 ml) per day. Puréed vegetables are to be preferred to tinned puréed fruits, which have a high carbohydrate content. Jelly is useful for the second course at dinner, because it is liked by most babies and has little food value. Vitamin D may be given in concentrated form instead of cod-liver oil, because of its low caloric value.

In the case of the older child aged one to three, care to avoid excess of starchy and fatty foods may be enough to correct the tendency to excessive weight. Fried foods should be avoided. Milk should be limited to 1 pint per day. Sweets should be eliminated and no food should be given between meals. Potato crisps and ice creams should be avoided. Fruit drinks should be discouraged because of their carbohydrate content.

Drugs are used only in the most extreme cases because of the danger of addiction. Thyroid extract should not be used, as there is no thyroid deficiency, and there are possible undesirable side actions. Amphetamine should not be used, because it is a drug of addiction. Fenfluramine is a much safer drug to use, with fewer side effects, but its exact value is uncertain. Methyl cellulose wafers ("Melozets"), which swell in the stomach in contact with fluid, may be of some use in older children, but are unnecessary in younger ones.

Attempts to make the child lose a great deal of weight are dangerous. Rigid dieting is apt to stop linear growth, and therefore to render him unduly small in height. The growth needs must be remembered, particularly when he is tall for his age, as most obese children are. Fasting causes weight loss due to loss of water and protein, but not fat. Most dietary regimens accelerate weight loss, but not loss of fat.[10] It is safer to aim at keeping the weight fairly stationary while he is growing in height, at the same time giving him an adequate supply of vitamins (e.g. a mixed vitamin preparation). Every effort, instead, should be made to increase the exercise which he takes.

It is much more important to discuss details of management with the parents, and to deal with their attitudes and habits. Care must be taken not to talk to the older pre-school child so much about his diet that anxiety is conveyed to him, with resulting insecurity. The parents should themselves set a good example, particularly in the avoidance of sweets.

Prognosis. Fully developed obesity is difficult to treat. There is usually an initial satisfactory response to treatment, but relapse is common. The prognosis is worse if one parent is fat, and worse still if both parents are fat. Heald and Hollander[8] showed that 75 to 80 per cent. of juvenile obesity persists into adult life. Woolf[21] showed that the outlook is worse for girls than it is for boys.

Vomiting of Psychological Origin

Vomiting may occur from a variety of psychological causes. Excessive crying at almost any time in the first 3 years may make a child vomit. In the infant it is probably largely due to air swallowing which results from prolonged crying. The cause of the vomiting associated with crying in the 2–3-year-old child is not clear. The difficult problem of the child with sleep refusal, who when left to cry makes himself vomit, is discussed elsewhere. Food forcing is a common cause of vomiting in a child after the age of 5 or 6 months of age. It is commoner after the first birthday. It may occur when he is given food which he does not like, as an attention-seeking device. It inevitably causes considerable disturbance if it takes place at the tea-table, and other children may imitate it.

Any sort of excitement may make a child vomit. The excitement of an impending party may be enough to make him sick. In travel sickness there is a psychological element, the excitement of the prospect of a long trip in the car to the seaside or other desirable place being at least a contributory factor in causing the vomiting. If the vomiting is the subject of unwise conversation in front of the child, and if he realizes that there is a great deal of anxiety about it, it is likely to recur, partly as an attention-seeking device and partly as a result of suggestion.

Pica

Pica (dirt eating) is an annoying habit in some small children. I have known children eat live black snails or roundworms from the garden. One small boy regularly caused consternation in his anxious mother by appearing in the kitchen with his mouth full of pebbles. Some children bite painted objects and acquire lead poisoning as a result. Among the substances eaten by children described by Kanner[8] were dirt, rags, splinters, wallpaper, ashes, plaster, match heads, shoestrings, sand, hair, rubber, coal, stones, toys, buttons, clothes, soap, thread, paper, sticks, worms, bugs, fæces, polish, oilcloth and filth from the dustbin. Other objects eaten include crayons, wood, string, cigarette ashes and butts, laundry starch, celluloid and the soles of shoes. The problem merges into that of poisons, of which the number taken by children is legion. Lourie[12] found that sixty-seven per cent. of children admitted on account of poisoning were dirt eaters.

A question on paper-eating was asked in the Question and Answer Section of the *British Medical Journal*.* The reply ran as follows: "The eating of paper, which symbolizes cleanliness through its toilet use, is likely in the logic of infancy to represent inner cleanliness. Practical measures would include the avoidance in the diet of food which may arouse disgust, such as sausages or anything brown, or of messy consistency"! Pica is more common in the lower social classes, in mentally subnormal or emotionally deprived children,[11,12] especially when there is inadequate mothering, economic deprivation, and prolonged absence of the father. In one study of children with pica, 65 per cent. of the children had a mother who also had the condition. Some mothers gave their children clay to eat, and most of the mothers gave them a dummy to suck. Pica may be associated with various body manipulations, such as head banging, thumb sucking or rocking. Neumann[14] questioned whether it is a behaviour problem at all. He wrote that it is almost universal in West Africa, and represents an instinctive desire to chew on something. I think that Neumann was confusing dirt-eating and chewing—the desire to chew something hard.

It has been suggested that pica is related to iron deficiency. A controlled study of 30 negro children and of 28 controls from the same socio-economic background did not confirm this.[7] Like others, Laurie found that pica was not related to malnutrition or iron deficiency anæmia. On the other hand Ohara and Shibata in a study of 63 dirt eaters found that all had hypochromic anæmia, and that 55 of 59 were cured of their dirt eating by injections of iron. They had no controls, however, and they did not make it clear why they gave iron by injection instead of by mouth. When dirt eating is so much more common in the lower social classes, in which malnutrition is prevalent, it is difficult to prove that iron deficiency is causally related to pica.

Polydipsia

Infants do not usually show polydipsia, and babies with nephrogenic diabetes insipidus have to be strongly persuaded to drink sufficient fluid.

Thirst in normal older children is likely to be due to excessive perspiration, due to a high external temperature, overclothing or fever. It is commonly due to a habit and is then termed compulsive drinking. It has to be distinguished from organic causes of polydipsia, which include all conditions causing polyuria, such as diabetes insipidus.

* *Brit. med. J.*, 1948, 2, 768.

References

1. BENJAMIN, E. (1942). "The Period of Resistance in Eearly Childhood." *Am. J. Dis. Child.*, **63**, 1019.
2. BÖRJESON, M. (1962). "Overweight Children." *Acta Pædiat. Uppsala*, **51**, Suppl. 132.
3. BRENNEMANN, J. (1932). "Psychological Aspects of Nutrition in Childhood." *J. Pediat.*, **1**, 145.
4. CHEEK, D. B., GRAYSTONE, J. E., READ, M. S. (1970). Cellular Growth, Nutrition and Development." *Pediatrics*, **45**, 315.
5. COHEN, H. (1958). "17-Ketogenic Steroid Excretion in Obese Children before and after Weight Reduction." *Brit. med. J.*, **1**, 686.
6. EID E. E. (1970). "Follow up Study of Physical Growth of Children who had Excessive Weight Gain in the First Six Months of Life." *Brit. Med. J.*, **2**, 74.
7. GUTELIUS, M. F., LAYMAN, E. M., MILLICAN, F. K., COHEN, G. J., DUBLIN, C. C. (1962). "Nutritional Studies of Children with Pica." *Pediatrics*, **29**, 1012.
8. HEALD, F. P., HOLLANDER, R. J. (1965). "The Relationship between Obesity in Adolescence and Early Growth." *Pediatrics*, **67**, 35.
9. HIRSCH, J., KNITTLE, J. E., SALANS, L. B. (1967). "Cell Lipid Content and Cell Number in Obese and Non-obese Human Adipose Tissue." *J. Clin. Invest.* **46**, 1112.
10. *Journal of the American Medical Association* (1970). "Obesity, a Continuing Enigma." **211**, 492.
10a. KANNER, L. (1957). *Child Psychiatry*. Springfield. Charles Thomas.
11. LOURIE, R. S. (1965). "Pica." *Clin. Proc., Children's Hospital, Columbia*, **21**, 175.
12. LOURIE. R. S., MILLICAN, F. K. (1969). "Pica." In Howells J. G., *Modern Perspectives in International Child Psychology*. Edinburgh. Oliver and Boyd. p. 455.
13. MAYER, J. (1966). "Some Aspects of the Problem of Regulation of Food Intake and Obesity." *New Engl. J. Med.*, **274**, 610, 662, 772.
14. NEUMANN, H. H. (1970). "Pica—Symptom or Vestigial Instinct?" *Pediatrics*, **46**, 441.
15. NEWBURGH, L. H. (1942). "Obesity." *Arch. Inter. Med.*, **70**, 1033.
16. OHARA, T., SHIBATA, F., "Personal Communication."
17. RICHTER, C. P. (1942). "Self Selection of Diets." *J. Pediat.*, **20**, 230.
18. TANNER, J. M., WHITEHOUSE, R. H. (1962). "Standards for Subcutaneous Fat in British Children, Percentiles for Thickness of Skin Folds over the Scapula or Below the Scapula." *Brit. med. J.*, **1**, 446.
19. WIDDOWSON, E. (1970). "Harmony of Growth." *Lancet*, **1**, 901.
20. WILKINS, L. (1957). *The Diagnosis and Treatment of Endocrine Disorders in Childhood and Adolescence*. Oxford. Blackwell.
21. WOLFF, O. (1963). *Final Report on the Symposium on Obesity*. London. Royal College of Physicians.
22. YOUNG, P. T. (1941). "The Experimental Analysis of Appetite." *Psychol. Bull.*. **38**, 129.

CHAPTER 22

SLEEP PROBLEMS

The majority of children, either sooner or later in their first 4 years, develop sleep problems. These include crying when put to bed, refusal to go to bed for one parent and not for the other, refusal to lie down, awaking with or without crying in the night, prolonged failure to go to sleep, sleep rituals and early morning awakening. Often the "crying" begins as soon as the mother's back is turned. It starts as a mere shout without tears, the so-called "testing cry," but sometimes if she does not return promptly tears are shed and true crying begins.

The fussing and crying when the toddler is awakened from a nap are of no importance.

Sleep problems in children can be divided into two main groups— those dependent on normal or natural processes of development, and those dependent on the interaction of environmental and developmental factors. In the former group are variations in sleep requirements, early morning awakening in the toddler, thumbsucking, rocking and other rhythmical movements on going to sleep, and fussing on awakening (between the age of 2 and 3). In the latter group is refusal to go to sleep for one or for both parents, refusal to lie down, the testing cry on being put to bed, and repeated awakening and crying in the night.

Methods commonly Employed

The usual story is that the parents coax the child and tell him to be a good boy and go to sleep. They play games with him, sit and read to him or tell him stories. They smack him for staying awake, lie at his side till he falls asleep, leave his light on or even bribe him to go to sleep. It is a common practice for parents to take the child into their own bed. One 3-year-old child seen by me kept both parents occupied for 4 hours every night in trying to get him to sleep. Another bounced about the bed so much that the parents, aided by the grandparents, tried to get him to go to sleep by holding his four limbs down on the bed. Some doctors, and others, drug their child every night for months.

Relevant Developmental Trends

(i) THE DURATION OF SLEEP. The duration of sleep depends on a child's age, personality and intelligence and on the duration of his afternoon nap. The new-born baby sleeps most of the day. At 3 months the average baby has three or four sleep periods, at 1 year two or three, and at about 3 years of age he discards the afternoon nap. The more placid child sleeps a great deal more and may still sleep for most of the day at 4 or 5 months. He may continue to have an afternoon nap until he is 4 or 5 years old. The active child sleeps a great deal less. At 5 months he is awake for the greater part of the day and may refuse to have an afternoon nap by the age of two. Various workers found that the more intelligent child tends to sleep less than the less intelligent.

The duration of the child's sleep at night is related to the duration of the nap during the day. Many parents make the mistake of allowing the 2- or 3-year-old to have a three-hour nap from 2–5 p.m. and then expecting him to be ready for the night's sleep at 6 p.m. It is convenient to have a rest from the child in the afternoon and to get on with one's work, which is impossible when the child is around, but it does very often mean that the child will be wide awake and active for the rest of the evening. Over-fatigue may delay sleep and shorten the duration of the night's sleep. Sometimes parents awaken their child from the mid-day nap too soon, and he is then tired in the later afternoon and sleeps badly. Over-fatigue can shorten sleep in some children as much as the absence of fatigue does in others.

It is normal for any child from 18 months onwards to lie awake for a long time in the evening talking or playing, or to waken up in the early hours of the morning and sing. It is normal for a child to finish his sleep by 5 or 6 a.m. Some children are not tired at the time when one would expect them to be ready for bed. Gesell remarked that the bedtime of the 2½-year-old is often 8–10 p.m. It is remarkable how a small child may go to bed tired out and awaken half an hour later, having apparently lost all fatigue, sleepiness and complete desire to sleep. He is then liable to cry for company. If taken downstairs he is then socially at his best.

It is wrong to lay down rigid times for the amount of sleep required. The best guide to the adequacy of sleep is the absence of fatigue in the daytime: but even if the child is unduly tired during the day it may be difficult to increase the duration of his sleep. He is particularly liable to be tired in the afternoon when he is first doing without his afternoon nap. If he refuses this there is nothing that one can do about it. It rights itself in a few weeks.

(ii) GOING OFF TO SLEEP AND FUSSING ON AWAKENING. Whereas the new-born baby cannot help going to sleep, after about 9 months it becomes a voluntary process which can be inhibited at will. A child can resist sleep for hours on end if he wishes, even though tired. Between 9 and 21 months going to sleep may be associated with rocking on the hands and knees, bed shaking, head banging, head rolling and finger sucking.

The child between 2 and 3 years often shows difficulty in awakening, crying and fussing for a while. Such difficulty is more likely to occur if there is also resistance to going to sleep. It is better not to hurry the awakening process.

(iii) THE SOUNDNESS OF SLEEP AND THE CAUSES OF AWAKENING. The older the child the less sound the sleep. Practically nothing will awaken a young baby who is sleeping after a good feed, but from 4 months or so noises may readily awaken him. There is no doubt that some babies sleep much more soundly than others. Boys tend to be more restless in their sleep than girls. It is said that the more intelligent child tends to be more restless in sleep than the less intelligent. A late evening meal is associated with restlessness in sleep. Children, like adults, may sleep badly in unduly hot weather.

In the first 4 weeks most babies awaken twice for feeds in the night. Most of them drop the night feed by about 10 weeks. After that age babies only waken up for a feed under special circumstances, such as thirst on a very hot night or as a result of the compensatory increase of appetite after an illness such as gastro-enteritis. Discomfort of any sort may awaken a baby—colic, flatulence, excessive heat or cold, a rash, a wet napkin, teething or tight clothes around the limbs. I saw a child brought downstairs on a cold winter's night on account of crying. The overclothing was so excessive that clouds of steam were rising from the child. When the cause is merely a wet napkin the child goes to sleep when he has been changed. Contrary to popular belief, teething does not cause sleep disturbance. Most sleep disturbances, which are ascribed to teething, are in fact due to bad habit formation and therefore to mismanagement.

A common cause of sleep disturbance is the presence of parents in the same room. The child is disturbed by their coughing, snoring, arguing or by the squeaks of the springs. When a child awakens in his own room he is likely to go to sleep again without difficulty. When he awakens in his parents' room he soon realizes that his parents are there and he may cry for them. His mother, furthermore, would not know that her child had awakened if he were in another room, provided that he did not cry or talk, while if he is in her own room she is apt to get out of bed and look to see if he is safe. The child is then further disturbed.

It is an undesirable practice for the parents to have to creep about the house in the evenings for fear of awakening the child. Every effort should be made to get the child used to sleeping in spite of the ordinary household noises.

After the age of about 6 months children are apt to awaken with a sudden scream. It is not due to a wet napkin or other discoverable cause. It is probably a form of nightmare, and the child rapidly settles when the parent goes in to see him and gives him the desired security.

Often there is no discoverable cause for the child's awakening.

Between the age of 2 or 3 years children usually acquire sphincter control at night, and the full bladder may awaken the child and cause him to cry for help.

(iv) HABIT FORMATION AND ASSOCIATIONS. The child rapidly forms associations with sleep. The association of sleep release with head banging, head rolling and finger sucking has already been mentioned. It was also mentioned that a child with "three-months' colic" who was rightly picked up frequently in the evenings may continue to cry for the parents long after the colic has disappeared, until it is realized that the colic has been replaced by a habit. When a toddler is picked up at every whimper a bad habit is rapidly created, and the child then cries until picked up. If he can postpone bedtime by arguing or throwing temper tantrums, it becomes a habit and he causes trouble every night when bedtime comes.

The child becomes used to his surroundings, and even at 16 weeks a move from a bassinet to a crib may cause trouble. At 28 weeks a baby may refuse to sleep in a strange room. The whole rhythm of sleep may be upset as a result of taking the baby away on holiday. If he is allowed to sleep with his mother on account of an illness he may refuse to sleep alone for a time after recovery.

A child who is frequently rocked or sung to sleep soon becomes unable to sleep without it. Most children above the age of 18 months come to associate a particular rag, teddy or other object with sleep and will not go to sleep if deprived of it. Sometimes a double association can be seen. As soon as the child is given the special teddy he puts his fingers into the mouth and goes to sleep. After about 21 months the majority of children develop some sort of sleep ritual, demanding this, that and the other before going to sleep. The child demands a drink, asks to be placed on the pottie and then asks for a doll. He commonly asks for the door to be left open for a specific width. If the parent is not careful he will keep adding to the ritual and successfully delay the departure of the mother from the bedroom. Most children discard these rituals shortly after the third birthday.

(v) THE EGO AND NEGATIVISM. These are major factors in sleep disorders. If the child discovers that he can cause a great deal of fuss and anxiety and can attract attention, causing the whole house to revolve round his sleeping, he will certainly continue to be difficult. Many parents are unwise enough to discuss the child's sleeping problem in front of him. Attempts to force him to lie down or go to sleep will inevitably cause sleep resistance. In a fight the child almost always wins.

(vi) DESIRE FOR LOVE AND SECURITY. Most of the crying in bed is due to the desire for the parents' company. The phase of increased dependence on the parents between 18 months and 2½ years makes the child's separation from the mother a matter of difficulty. This separation is all the more difficult if he has been deprived of her company all day because she has been at work or for other reasons. If the mother works all day in industry or leaves the child for long periods during the day so that she can "get away from him," playing Bridge and so forth, he may cling to her in the evening and be particularly reluctant to leave her. It is always wrong to go out in the evening and leave the child without telling him, as soon as he is old enough to understand. He must never feel that he is being put to bed so that he can be out of the parent's way; he will feel resentment at being excluded from the family circle.

The happier the child is during the day, the greater his feeling of security, and the fewer the scoldings which he receives, the more likely it is that there will be little trouble at night. The more tense he is during the day, the more tired and impatient the mother, the greater is the likelihood of difficulty at night. As a result of his bad behaviour at night the mother has insufficient sleep and so is impatient and irritable with him during the day, and a troublesome vicious circle is set up.

A child's sense of security may be broken by admission to a hospital, particularly if he undergoes a painful experience there, such as an operation.

(vii) FEARS AND NIGHT TERRORS. Fear of the dark is extremely common in children, especially after the age of 2. Not only is there fear of the dark but there may be fear of strange shadows or moving curtains. The fears may be suggested by alarming stories about ghosts and giants before bedtime.

Sleep walking is not usually a problem in the pre-school child. There are no known causes of the condition. It has been suggested that it is related to insecurity, but I doubt this. It may follow a late meal just before going to bed, and this can readily be avoided. Otherwise no specific treatment can be recommended, nor is it necessary.

(viii) THE USE OF BED FOR THREATS AND PUNISHMENT. It is common to threaten to put a child to bed if he is naughty. This is always wrong, for it inevitably causes the child to associate bed with punishment.

(ix) OTHER PSYCHOLOGICAL CAUSES. Psycho-analysts offer various theories about the causation of sleep disturbances. Sperling[3] wrote: "According to psycho-analytic theory and practice, repressed infantile sexuality, particularly the œdipal conflict, is the principal cause of neurotic sleep disturbances in children. Sibling rivalry, with the repressed hostility and resentment towards the mother and death wishes directed toward the sibling, I would place second highest in the ætiology of such disturbance." She thought that sleep rituals were aimed at counteracting such repressed feelings. Night terrors she regarded as "the repression of intense sexual and aggressive impulses stemming from the œdipal complex."

(x) UNEXPLAINED PHASES. When children misbehave, parents can always take refuge in the excuse that they are teething, or that they are merely "going through a difficult phase." There are often good grounds for such excuses. There is no doubt that children do go through such phases, for which no adequate reason can be found. Properly managed they rapidly pass; badly managed they become perpetuated and fixed.

Parental Attitudes to Sleep

(i) A WRONG IDEA OF THE AMOUNT OF SLEEP NEEDED. Parents are often ignorant of the normal variations in sleep requirements and are seriously disturbed when the child lies awake, happily playing or talking with her dolls, or awakens at 1 a.m. and sings a few songs. Instead of leaving her alone they go in and try to persuade her to go to sleep. Rigid ideas of sleep requirements are liable to lead to sleep-forcing methods and so inevitably to sleep refusal.

Those parents who are most concerned about the importance of adequate sleep, are the parents whose children are most likely to have resulting sleep problems.

(ii) FAILURE TO SATISFY THE CHILD'S BASIC NEEDS IN INFANCY. Moore and Ucko[2] in an excellent study of night awakening, found a strong correlation between night disturbances and fear of spoiling and failure to nurse the child in earlier months and pick him up when he wanted it.

(iii) OVER-ANXIETY AND EXCESSIVE DOMINATION. Over-anxiety, over-protection and excessive domination are important factors in the genesis of sleep problems. Many mothers frequently visit their children in the evening to see if they are safe and are apt to disturb them. Children often stay awake expecting such visits. The mother's anxiety is soon sensed by the child. Others go in to see the child and pick him up when there is the smallest whimper. Impatience of the parents to go out for the evening often causes trouble. A child is apt to be put to bed before he is ready for it or deliberate efforts are made to force him to go to sleep, with the opposite of the effect desired. The child may sense the fact that the parents want to get rid of him, as in fact they do. They want to eat their meal in peace and be on their own, but the child reacts accordingly and cries. Attempts to discipline the child and to make him obey, cause sleep refusal just as much as food refusal.

(iv) RIGID METHODS OF MANAGEMENT. *It is thoroughly desirable to create good habits in the child, and as far as possible a fixed bedtime is eminently desirable.* The child becomes used to a regular routine and accepts bedtime as a matter of course. One cannot, however, agree with Blatz[1] who wrote: "The most common error of training is to permit the child to put off the sleeping time even for 5 minutes." Such rigidity of management, though working well in many children, leads to a great deal of trouble in others, for it completely fails to take into account the different sleep requirements of children. It is not reasonable to expect small determined children to go to sleep smoothly when they are in no way fatigued.

(v) SOCIAL FACTORS. A major cause of trouble after 4 or 5 months of age is allowing the baby to share the room with the parents. It is almost inevitable that he will be awakened. Overcrowding frequently makes the provision of a separate room impossible, but it can often be arranged in a flat that the baby's cot is carried out of the bedroom and put into the kitchen or bathroom when the parents go to bed.

Of equal importance is the proximity of neighbours or the presence in the same house of complaining relatives. The mother who has a small child in part of the house, particularly in part of one floor of a house, is in a difficult position. If the child cries, immediate complaints come from the neighbours. As a result she is almost compelled to keep picking the child up and trying to force him to go to sleep. The inevitable result is the opposite of the effect desired.

Prevention of Sleep Problems

There should be some elasticity with regard to bedtime, for reasons stated. If the toddler is not ready to go to bed at the usual time in the evening, one should try the effect of cutting down the afternoon nap.

Open-air exercise is a good source of healthy fatigue. Fatigue must not be excessive, for an over-tired child is apt to be difficult about going to sleep.

A wise pre-bed routine is essential. It is a good practice to read a story before the child goes to bed. There must be no argument about whether it is time to go to bed or not. Once the child sees that the mother is undecided, or changes her mind when pressed by him, he will certainly take advantage of it and try it again another night. Tears at this or any subsequent stage should be avoided. It is easy to become impatient when the child dawdles in putting his toys away or in putting his toys down to come up to bed. He should be allowed to help to prepare the bath—to turn the tap on, to throw the sponge in and to undress himself, even though it takes a lot longer than doing it all oneself. Children from earliest infancy enjoy the bath, and this should be encouraged. Much as one would like to complete the job as quickly as possible, the child should be allowed some time to have fun in the bath and help to wash himself. He should then be allowed to help to dry himself if he is old enough (2½–3 years) and put his nightie on. The bed in winter should be warmed by a bottle, which is taken out when he gets in. From the age of about 5 months, when he learns to grasp objects, he should be allowed to have toys in bed with him. It is no use expecting the toddler's bed to be tidy. The wise mother does not mind if he lies asleep in strange positions in bed, with his feet on the pillow (as long as he can be covered up), with a mass of toys all around him—his bits of rag, bobbins, bricks, old tins and toy dogs—for she knows that he is much more likely to be quiet in the morning after early awakening if he has some toys than if he has none. He should not be tucked in excessively if he does not wish. The room should be well ventilated. The effect of a dark blind may be tried if there is difficulty in the summer. It is exasperating after fitting a dark blind, however, to be compelled to supply a nightlight because of the development of fear of the dark. Overclothing must be avoided. The child should be put to bed with an air of certainty, for the child recognizes uncertainty and anxiety with astonishing rapidity. It is wise for the parents to take turns, because if no one else but the mother puts him to bed, difficulty might arise in the event of the mother's illness. It is wrong to tell him to be a good boy and go to sleep. This is asking for trouble in the shape of negativism. No one can go to sleep on request.

The rapidity with which children form habits must be remembered. There is no need to fear that bad habits will be started if a child is given night feeds in the first in the first 10 weeks if he demands them. It is wrong to refuse to pick up a child with colic, pain from teething or other discomfort because of the fear of habit formation and of spoiling him. A child should be given all the love and security which he needs when he is suffering discomfort. Habit formation may arise as a result, but once diagnosed it can readily be treated. It is not always easy, however, to draw a distinction between crying from discomfort and crying from habit. When one is readily satisfied that the child is no longer having colic or other discomfort and that a habit has developed, the habit must be broken.

It is harmless to rock a child or sing him to sleep occasionally, but it readily leads to habit formation, so that he cannot go to sleep with out such rocking or singing. He must get used to going to sleep with out such devices. They may be used on odd occasions, as when for instance, a child who normally sleeps without trouble awakens without apparent reason and seems to be unable to go to sleep again In the same way it is harmless on occasion to take the crying chilc downstairs, but such a procedure readily becomes a habit and it mus not therefore be frequently repeated.

No hard and fast rules can be laid down about the advisability o: lifting a child out in the late evening to pass urine. It is futile before about 18 months of age, because he has not sufficient retention span to make it profitable. It should only be practised after that age, wher the retention span is such that if lifted out he is likely to be dry in the morning, and if not lifted out he is liable to be wet. The practice should in any event be dropped as soon as possible in order to allow him to take responsibility for being dry in the night. Such lifting ou does not usually disturb him. In my opinion there is no need tc awaken him when lifting him out. He should otherwise only be visited when necessary, in order to see if he is adequately covered up. Children are likely to learn soon after the second birthday to cover themselves up if cold. Before that much anxiety can be avoided by the use ot a sleeping bag in winter, and by clips which hold the blanket in place. Care must be taken, however, when a sleeping bag is used, or when bedclothes are tightly tucked in or held in place by clips, to see that there is no chance that the baby can wriggle down and suffocate himself. Many children kick all the bedclothes off in the process ot finding a comfortable position in which to go to sleep, and the bed is in such a state of confusion that they can hardly be covered up without being disturbed. The mother should in these circumstances keep a blanket on a chair at the side of the bed so that this can be put over the child after he has gone to sleep. She may keep his hands warm by sewing mittens to his bed jacket so that they cannot be pulled off.

The Treatment of Sleep Problems

The treatment can be difficult, and it is wrong merely to tell the mother to leave the child to cry out, to smack him or to put him to sleep every night with drugs. The treatment is not nearly so simple. It has already been explained that the whole daytime management ot the child has to be reviewed. It is necessary to explain the relevant features of normal child psychology in order that she can understand the reason for the approach suggested and the reason for the necessity of avoiding forcing methods, loss of temper and anxiety. The mother needs to lose any sense of guilt she may feel for failing to manage the child better. She needs to understand that the child's behaviour is in no sense naughtiness, a sign of nervousness or other abnormality. She needs to understand habit formation and the importance of being consistent. It is wrong, if a child cries when put to bed, on one day to take him downstairs, on the next to sit and play games with him and on the third to leave him to cry. He can never learn that way. She must realize the importance of breaking a bad habit which has already formed. The mother herself may have to be given a sedative drug so that she is calmer in her management of the child in the day-time as well as at night. Psychiatrists tend to think that it is wrong to break the habit by leaving the child to cry. I am convinced that it is a kindness in the long run to do this. It is better for the child to have a proper night's sleep. It is essential for the parents that they should have a good night. A mother who is tired and worn out by bad nights with her baby is not able to cope with her child adequately by day. The child benefits in the long run by having a rested mother to look after him instead of a bad-tempered, tired, overwrought one.

It is important to see that the child does not go to bed hungry. If there is inadequate breast milk, a bottle feed last thing at night may make all the difference. When a baby is fed on the bottle, a feed with cereal last thing at night may prolong the night's sleep.

The treatment of specific problems can be summarized as follows:

Crying. It is normal for the 6–12-month infant to cry for a minute or two when put to bed (the "testing cry"). No treatment is necessary. The child is put to bed and the mother leaves the room.

It is another matter if there is prolonged crying every night when he is put to bed. This is a habit, and it has to be broken. In the first place, he should be left to cry. If there is a danger that he will fall out of his cot he should graduate to a bed. If there is a danger that he can open the bedroom door (as many children can at about 2 years of age) and fall downstairs, then a catch may have to be put on the door. It must be emphasized that it is thoroughly undesirable to lock a child in the bedroom, and it must only be done as a very temporary expedient.

It is difficult to say how long a child should be left to cry. A good mother finds it difficult to leave him crying at all, but it must be done to break the habit, which otherwise may continue for years. Some children show an astonishing capacity for crying for hours on end even though extremely tired. It is incorrect to say that if a child is left to cry it out for 3 or 4 days the habit will be broken. It is broken in most children but not in all. Most cry for less than half an hour on the first night, 15 minutes on the second, and not at all after that, but some cry longer. In any case it is essential for the mother to glance into the room at intervals to see if he is safe. A mother would never forgive herself or the doctor if, acting on his advice, she left a child to cry and he met with a serious accident as a result. The greatest difficulty of all is the fact that many children make themselves vomit by crying. In infants the vomiting is probably due to air swallowing. The increasing distension of the abdomen of a screaming baby is easy to observe. When a child can make himself sick by crying he cannot be left to cry for long. As has already been said, social factors, particularly the proximity of complaining neighbours, make it impossible to leave a child crying for long. In such cases there is only one way of breaking the habit, and that is the use of a drug.

Drugs should be used as a preventive rather than as a therapeutic measure. They should be used not after the child has begun to cry, but rather to prevent him crying. The drug is used not merely to break a bad habit, but to start a good one. It should be given before the child goes to bed, so that when he gets to bed he is sleepy. It may have to be used to break a habit such as taking the child into the parents' bed. One of the safest drugs to use is chloral. The dose has to be adequate and can only be determined by trial and error. In a child of 1 year of age one could begin with 180 mg, and increase each day if necessary by 120 mg, till the desired effect is achieved. As much as 0·6 g may be required even at that age. It should only be necessary to use the drug for 5 or 6 days. The prolonged daily use of the drug is quite unnecessary and merely a sign of defeat. Drugs are no substitute for careful history taking and a frank detailed discussion of the child's needs and management.

It is impossible to say with certainty in an individual child whether shortening or lengthening the afternoon nap will help. It is a matter for trial and error. It is certainly unreasonable on the one hand to expect a child to go to sleep when he is not in the least fatigued. On the other hand, excessive fatigue often postpones sleep. However tired a child is, he possesses the power of screaming and resisting for prolonged periods if he so wishes.

When a child of any age wakens up in the night and cries, the line of action depends on the nature of the cry and on the frequency with which it occurs. When there is a sudden half-hearted cry, gradually decreasing in intensity, it is usually better not to go in to see the child. It is another matter if he emits a full-throated shriek. It is then essential to go in to see him immediately. He does not make such a noise without reason. The causes of night awakening have already been mentioned. He may have vomited, had a nightmare or be strangling himself. He may want to empty the bladder. Whatever the cause, his needs should be attended to without delay. The longer he is left to cry the longer it takes to pacify him. Crying, if allowed to continue, becomes hysterical, the child becomes greatly distressed and continues to show the sudden jerky respirations known as sobbing long after he has been picked up. A stay of a minute or two is usually enough to give the 2-year-old awakened by some fear the security which he needs. When the younger child has been awakened by a wet napkin, the napkin is changed and the room is then immediately left. As has already been said, if he is occasionally rocked or sung to sleep no harm is done.

It is another matter when the child wakens up every night and screams. One mother complained that her child awakened twelve or fifteen times every night and screamed, and she went in to see her every time. Such crying is a habit, and the habit must be broken. It is always wrong for the parents to take the child into their own bed. This inevitably creates a habit rapidly, and sooner or later the habit has to be stopped. It is always wrong for the same reason to sit and play games with him or to make a practice of taking a hot drink to him whenever he awakens and cries. The necessity of avoiding a scene, of not having a fight with the child or smacking him has already been described. It is stupid to smack a child for wanting the company of the mother whom he loves, for that is the cause of the crying. Only occasionally is smacking justified in the older child, when there is deliberate screaming in the night unrelated to night terrors.

Refusal to go to bed for one parent and not the other. As has already been said, this may be due to the child's greater dependence on the mother, especially between 2 and 3 years. The father should, if possible, put the child to bed every day for a week or so, and then the mother should take over, being careful to avoid any show of anxiety or doubt about what the child will do. The habit may have to be broken with the aid of a drug.

Refusal to lie down when put to bed. He should be left sitting or standing up. The child of 2 is usually able to cover himself up in bed. The use of a sleeping bag in the winter is a help to keep the child warm. The mother may have to look in on him as soon as he has gone to sleep in order to cover him up.

Sleep rituals. These have to be broken, especially when the child is adding to them.

Failure to sleep or awakening without crying. It is normal for children, especially after 1 year, to lie awake in the evening and talk and play. It is normal for a child of $2\frac{1}{2}$ to waken up at 1 a.m. and sing. On no account should the mother go in to see him or do anything about it. He will go to sleep when he is ready to do so.

Early-morning awakening. I do not know any answer to this problem,

The child has no sense of time. He cannot be blamed for thinking it is time to get up at 5 a.m. The problem is almost confined to the child of 18 months onwards. There is not likely to be much difficulty if there are two children who are old enough to play with each other. If he merely awakens and plays with his toys and sings, there is no need to do anything about it. When he cries or insists on going into his parents' room, it is not so easy. It is futile to leave him to cry out, hoping to break the habit that way. Not being tired, he will continue to cry incessantly until the parents are worn out. He should be given a plentiful supply of toys to have in his room. One can try the effect of changing the napkin or giving him a drink or placing him on the pottie, but it usually does not help. He is wide awake and full of energy, and he sees no reason why his exhausted parents are not as pleased to see him as he is to see them. One may try changing the child's napkin or lifting him out at 10 or 11 p.m. in the hope that he will at least not be awakened early by a wet napkin or a full bladder. One might think that if the child were put to bed later that he would awaken later, but the reverse may occur. One can only console oneself with the thought that this is usually a temporary phase. When the child is old enough to sit on the pottie without help (from $2\frac{1}{2}$ onwards) and when the bladder capacity increases, as it does with age, there is likely to be less early-morning disturbance. The greater the child's intelligence at this age the greater the likelihood that one can persuade him the previous evening not to cry for his parents when he awakens in the morning. An average 3-year-old child is certainly old enough to understand that he should not disturb his parents when he awakens. Often no measures succeed, but he grows out of it.

Conclusions

Enough has been said to indicate the difficulties which may arise with sleeping problems. Every sympathy should be shown with the mother, who feels at her wit's end. She feels powerless with the child. She has discovered that smacking is useless. She cannot reason with him, because he does not understand. She cannot explain to him that she is tired out and longing for sleep. She cannot leave him to cry, because the neighbours complain or he makes himself sick. A full, careful history is essential in order that the mother can be helped to deal with the problem. It is wrong to think that the problems are easy to solve. They can be difficult and there is no answer to early-morning awakening. One cannot agree with Blatz[1] when he said: "There are no problems of training so easily dealt with and which espond so readily to adequate treatment as those connected with sleeping. A reasonable routine rigidly but patiently enforced is always successful." Would that it were always so easy.

References

1. BLATZ, W. E. (1933). In Murchison, C., *A Handbook of Child Psychology*. Worcester. Clark Univ. Press.
2. MOORE, T., UCKO, L. E. (1957). "Nightwaking in Early Infancy." *Arch. Dis. Childhood*, **32**, 333.
3. SPERLING, M. (1949). "Neurotic Sleep Disturbances in Children." *The Nervous Child*, **8**, 28.

CHAPTER 23

PROBLEMS OF SPHINCTER CONTROL

Most children develop minor problems of sphincter control. Most of them have phases of refusing to sit on the pottie. Other problems include delay in the acquisition of control of bowel or bladder, or loss of control when once it has been acquired; deliberate withholding of urine or stools, either at all times or merely when placed on the pottie; constipation, sometimes causing diarrhœa and incontinence; frequency of micturition and stool smearing.

The Normal Development of Sphincter Control

The frequency of urination in babies varies from child to child. There is often a temporary phase of increased frequency at the age of about 21 months. At 2½ years there is often a retention span of about 5 hours. The retention span then rapidly increases with age.

Babies commonly empty the bowel and bladder immediately after a meal, especially in the first 8 months, and they can often be "conditioned" to use the pottie any time after 2 or 3 months of age. This conditioning frequently breaks down as a result of teething or some disturbance of routine, particularly between 12 and 18 months. It is important to realize that there is no voluntary control at this time, for voluntary control does not begin till about 15–18 months of age.

The first indication of voluntary control is awareness at about 15 months of having passed urine, the child pointing it out to the mother. By about 16–18 months the child is able to say "No" with reasonable correctness when asked if he wants to urinate. He now begins to tell the mother just before he passes urine, but he does not give her time to "catch" him. The urgency decreases as he grows older, and by 18–24 months he tells the mother in sufficient time for her to place him on the pottie. By 2–2½ years he is able to pull his pants down and go to the lavatory and may climb on to the lavatory seat unaided. He takes pride in so doing and may refuse to pass a stool if his mother tries to attend to him. Bowel control is usually acquired before bladder control. Children at a similar age also take responsibility for not wetting their pants, and as a result the napkin is discarded during the day. The child is still wet at night. By 2½ the retention span is longer, and between 2½ and 3, if he is lifted out at 10 or 11 p.m. he is dry in the morning and the night-time napkin is discarded. The pottie is placed at his bedside and he gets out of bed and attends to his own needs. At about 3–3½ he is dry by night, though occasional accidents may occur till he is 4 or older. He rarely soils his pants after the age of 2 years, though an accident may occur if the stools are temporarily loose. Girls tend to acquire sphincter control earlier than boys. In the Newcastle 1,000 Family Survey 8·9 per cent. wet the bed regularly or frequently at the age of 5 years. Newson[18] found that at the age of four 46 per cent. still had some trouble with wetting.

Temporary relapses of control occur as a result of teething, an infection, a change of surroundings or some other change in routine. Short phases of refusal to sit on the pottie occur form time to time without apparent reason. In some instances such refusal occurs with the eruption of each new tooth, the child's behaviour returning to normal in 2–3 days.

The extreme urgency in the early days of voluntary control is worthy of emphasis. Once the child feels the urge to pass urine or a stool he cannot wait a minute without doing it. He soon develops a genuine desire to be clean and the desire to pass urine is often shown by a shriek, as if some dreadful accident has occurred. The urgency rapidly disappears. There is a gradual transition from the entirely unconscious voiding of the baby through the stage when the child is fully conscious of the act (15 months), past the stage when he becomes conscious of the desire immediately before emptying occurs, to the stage when he can wait as long as circumstances make it necessary.

Shortly after control has been acquired children commonly go through a phase of deliberately withholding the urine or stool. The child knows that he wants to empty the bowel or bladder but does not want to drop his toys or stop his game. He "holds" himself below, characteristically jerking himself up and down, and has to sit down as if he dare not stand up. Accidents commonly do happen at this stage. He emits a shriek and is unable to move from the spot. Even though the child is old enough to look after himself, the wise mother sees that accidents are avoided when he is concentrating on some exciting game, and reminds him to go to the lavatory. Some children find it difficult to pass urine after a long span and have to be placed in a warm bath before they can empty the bladder.

Muellner[17] wrote a valuable paper on the development of bladder control. He described how every child has to pass from the stage of the automatic emptying of the bladder in infancy to the stage of awareness of the full bladder (normally 12 to 18 months, when he first tells his mother), to the stage of learning to inhibit the contraction of the detrusor muscle and to hold the urine through the use of the levator

ani and the pubococcygeus, to the stage when he can control intra-
abdominal pressure through the use of the diaphragm and abdominal
muscles, to the final stage when he can start and stop the flow of urine
at any degree of bladder filling. He wrote that bladder capacity should
double between the age of 2 and $4\frac{1}{2}$.

Children often pass through a stage of stool smearing between the
age of 1 and $2\frac{1}{2}$, especially at 18 months. They have a tremendous
interest in the elimination at this age.

There are considerable variations in the age at which sphincter
control is acquired. In some, conditioning is acquired early and there is
no breakdown. Voluntary control is acquired without difficulty and the
child is completely dry by day from 9 months or so. This is exceptional
but not rare. In others there is little sign of voluntary control until
after the second birthday.

Historical Methods of Treating Enuresis

There have been several interesting articles on the historical
methods of treating enuresis.[9] They include placing burning leaves
between the legs (Okinawa), eating the crop of a cock, chrysanthe-
mums, the testicle of a hare cooked in wine, or hedgehog flesh, sprink-
ling dried sow's bladder over the bed; applying blistering agents to the
sacrum; cauterizing the urinary meatus in order to make micturition
painful; applying stinging nettles to the penis; inflating a bag in the
vagina; pouring collodion into the prepuce in order to seal it; and
applying bandages or clamps to the penis. In 1544 Thomas Phaer in
his "Boke of Children" wrote a section "Of Pyssying in the Bedde"—
recommending the trachea of the cock or the claws of the goat for treatment. For generations roast mouse or mouse pie was advocated.

In 1830 Nye[19] suggested that one should "attach one pole of an
electric battery to a moist sponge fastened between the shoulders of
the patient and the other to a dry sponge placed over the urinary
meatus. The sound of the battery will soon lull the patient to sleep
While the sponge is dry, no electricity passes through the body of the
patient, and his slumber is not disturbed. The moment the sponge is
moistened by urination, it becomes a conductor of electricity. The
circuit is completed through the body by the patient and he is aroused
and caught in the very act. A repetition of a like experience for a
sufficient number of times ought, I am inclined to think, to cure the
patient."

Methods commonly Employed

I have frequently seen all the methods described below.
Mothers try to insist on the child passing an "adequate" and

regular stool, and compel him to sit on the pottie for long periods
(e.g. 20 minutes three times a day) in order to "train" him. They
coax him, offer bribes (trips to the town, sweets), threaten punishment
if a stool is not passed and smack him for "failure." He screams and
kicks to get off the pottie, but he is held down by force. He learns
to withhold the urine or stool until he is off the pottie and then passes
it in his pants or under the carpet. I have seen several cases in which
paper was regularly spread out on the floor for the child to pass a
stool on, as he would never pass it into the pottie. Such children
usually pass the stool away from the paper. One child who was
accustomed to receiving bribes for passing a stool would daily say,
"What will you give me if I use the pottie?" Trouble begins even
before the child is placed on the pottie. I was impressed by the screaming and kicking of a boy who was being undressed so that he could
be examined. The mother said: "He is always like that. He thinks
that he is going to be put on the pot." Mothers sit with their children
when they are on the pottie and play games with them. They may
sit on the lavatory themselves in order to set the example. They
place hot water in the pottie, thinking that the steam will enable
the child to pass a stool. Even when the child is 8 or 9 years old the
mother insists on staying with him and inspecting the product to see
if it is adequate. Some go to the trouble of building a special seat
for the child, as he refuses the ordinary seat. One child of 9, with fæcal
incontinence as a result of constipation, was every morning placed
in the charge of his elder sister, whose duty it was to see that he passed a
stool.

Mothers say that they have "tried everything" to get the bowels
moving. They have "really persevered." They have tried numerous
patent medicines, inserted soap sticks into the rectum and given
enemas, and still the child is no better. The mother says that his
bowels are the despair of her life. One despairing father said that his
daughter regarded "all time spent on the pot as so much time wasted."
A mother told me that she had inserted several different sizes of cork
into the child in order to stop soiling.

Some Causes of Toilet Training Problems

These include:

The wrong idea that children need to be trained to be clean. They are
not trained. They can only be helped when they are developmentally
ready to learn. Numerous books advocate strict "training" methods.
As Halliday[12] put it, "When the clock strikes certain hours little
pots are punctually applied to little botts." Such methods frequently

cause the mother to keep the child on the pottie against his will, and rebellion then results.

Ignorance of the normal variations. Variations which occur in the age of acquisition of control are great. If the first child acquires control early the mother is apt to expect the second one to acquire control at the same age, and she punishes the child for his "failure."

Ignorance of the normal bowel action. Mothers have a greatly exaggerated idea of the importance of a daily action. When a child misses a day they try to force him to have a motion or give purgatives. Many cases of chronic constipation have started with the mother's anxiety about the infrequent motions of a breast-fed baby. The child who normally has motions at irregular times is the one who is apt to be forced to sit on the chamber for long periods against his will. Parental over-anxiety is a major factor in the genesis of the problem. The mother who carefully inspects every stool which the child passes in order to decide whether it is adequate or not is the sort of mother who owns the child who refuses to empty his bowels.

Ignorance about the development of sphincter control. Mothers think that the "conditioning" of a child to pass a stool or urine is synonymous with voluntary control. When conditioning breaks down, as it does in the majority of babies, they interpret it as a refusal by the child or naughtiness and punish him. The child then rebels.

Mothers fail to understand the normal sequence of events in the development of control and think that a child is naughty for telling them about his need too late. The boy is then smacked. Later, when accidents occur, he is punished and a display of fuss and anxiety is shown. He then deliberately does the opposite of what is wanted.

Development of the ego and negativism. Nothing pleases the child more than to have the whole house revolving round his bowels. He discovers that not only can he refuse to take food in without his parents being able to do anything about it, but he can refuse to let anything out. Both achievements cause untold anxiety, fuss and attention, and he delights in it. As with food refusal, his morale in fights is good, for he always wins. He delights in the fuss which occurs when there is an accident or when he deliberately passes the stool into his pants as soon as he has been allowed off the pottie. He finds that there is no more successful way of annoying his parents. He likes to have his mother sitting with him in the bathroom, playing games with him, coaxing and trying to persuade him to have a motion, and he delights in refusing to oblige. He uses the pottie for anything but what it is intended for. He roams the room on it, plays games when sitting on it or wears it as a hat.

A baby may withhold stools deliberately because he has passed a hard one which hurt him or because he has a painful fissure *in ano*. More often he withholds it because he finds that by so doing he can draw attention to himself and cause a great deal of fuss and anxiety. It should be understood, however, that when this voluntary inhibition of defæcation continues for some weeks stools become hard, considerable dilatation of the colon (megacolon) occurs and dyschezia develops, so that the rectum becomes insensitive to distension. The final result is that the child cannot have a motion if he tries. The hard scybala irritate the mucosa and cause diarrhœa, and there is frequently associated fæcal incontinence. The picture is then a strange one of diarrhœa with masses of hard fæces to be felt in the rectum, and often in the abdomen. The abdomen may become severely distended and the diagnosis of tuberculous peritonitis or even of malignant disease is not uncommonly made. Hirschsprung's disease is closely simulated, but fæcal incontinence and a full rectum make it unlikely. The hard scybala may themselves cause anal fissures, so that further retention occurs as a result of painful defæcation.

A child can satisfy his ego, his craving for attention, by means other than the mere retention of stools or of urine. He enjoys the fuss which is made when he has an accident and is apt deliberately to repeat the performance. It is unfortunate that the period of the early acquisition of sphincter control coincides exactly with the phase of resistance or negativism. The majority of functional disturbances of sphincter control are due to efforts to force the child and the child's refusal to be forced.

Another attention-seeking device is frequency of micturition. The child discovers that when he asks to use the pottie the mother immediately drops everything, and probably carries him upstairs. He is then apt to demand this attention every few minutes. It is difficult for the mother to refuse to answer his call, because she assumes that the request is genuine and that he will not learn to be dry unless he is given immediate attention. It is true that there is genuine urgency at this age and that children genuinely desire to be clean and dry if properly managed. It is not easy to decide just how much is natural urgency and how much is a deliberate attention-seeking device. If it is decided that it is the latter, it has to be treated in the usual way by ignoring the call except at what are considered suitable intervals. The urine should always be examined in these cases so that a urinary tract infection or polyuria can be eliminated.

Laziness. On a cold night, particularly if the lavatory is at the other side of a yard, a child may prefer to wet himself rather than to go to the lavatory.

Unhappiness and other psychological causes. Unhappiness or insecurity for any cause may lead to a reversion to infantile habits, including the loss of sphincter control. The insecurity may be the result of jealousy, a spell in hospital, domestic friction and over-strictness on the part of the mother.

Freud[8] explained the deliberate withholding of stools as follows: "Children utilizing the erogenous sensitiveness of the anal zone can be recognized by their holding back of fæcal masses until through accumulation there result violent muscular contractions. . . . One of the surest premonitions of later eccentricity or nervousness is when an infant obstinately refuses to empty his bowel when placed on the chamber. . . . The retention of fæcal masses, which is at first intentional in order to utilize them as it were for masturbatic excitation of the anal zone, is at least one of the roots of constipation so frequent in neuropaths." I personally feel that the problems mentioned are due simply to the developmental trends and parental attitudes described above.

Neglect and failure to help the child. The acquisition of sphincter control is later in children brought up in an institution than in children at home. Unhappiness together with a failure to help them in the learning stage is primarily the cause of this.

Mothers who have themselves had enuresis may regard it as an act of God and fail to help their children to acquire control. They regard them as having "weak kidneys" or "a weak bladder" and do nothing to help them when they show a desire to pass urine. One mother told me that she had never placed her 4-year-old daughter on the pottie because "she did not mind washing nappies."

There is often a strong history of nervous instability in the parents of enuretic children.

Conditioning. If the child is compelled to sit on the pottie when he wants to get off, in spite of his crying and lamentations, and if he is smacked and scolded for not using it, he naturally revolts and tends to regard the whole matter as thoroughly unpleasant. He becomes conditioned against normal bladder and bowel action.

Delay in helping the child to learn. Though some child psychiatrists advocate that no effort should be made to train the child at all until he shows the desire to use the pottie (normally at about 18 months), various workers[6,7,18] have shown that there is less likely to be trouble when mothers begin "potting" their children early rather than late.

Primary and Secondary Enuresis

By the term primary enuresis, one refers to bed-wetting continuing without intermission after the end of the third year. By the term secondary enuresis one refers to the development of bed-wetting in a child who has been dry at night for a long (though undefined) period. I believe, as do many others, that primary enuresis is due mainly to delayed maturation of the complex mechanism required for control of the bladder. Just as some children are later than others of comparable intelligence in learning to sit, walk, talk, or read, others are later in learning to acquire control of the bladder. In primary enuresis there is usually a family history of the same complaint. In a study of 20 consecutive children with this type of enuresis, I found that there was a family history of the same complaint in nineteen. Hallgren[11] found that another person was affected in 70 per cent. of families of 203 sufferers. He reported that there was a higher incidence of enures is in both of uniovular twins than in both of binovular twins—evidence which supports the theory that there is a genetic factor. As in other fields of development, the basis of the variation in age of control is probably myelination of the relevant part of the nervous system, and this commonly has a familial pattern. Bakwin in his invaluable book on behaviour problems,[1] wrote that enuresis is looked on as a hereditary abnormal bladder function, the principle characteristic of which is an urgent need to empty the bladder. Cerebral control is normal, but the call to micturition is so intense that voluntary inhibition may be overcome and wetting takes place. Muellner[17] regarded primary enuresis as due to improper development of bladder capacity as a result of delay in the development of the bladder mechanism. It is certain that the primitive urgency of micturition, present in all normal children at about 18 months, persists in many primary enuretics. When at school, for instance, they cannot wait long when once they feel the urge to void. In some cases this urgency persists into adult life.

Miller,[15,16] writing about the findings in the Newcastle 1,000 family survey, wrote that "the social correlations were such that it is reasonable to think that most enuresis occurs in a child with a slow pattern of maturation when that child is in a family where he does not receive sufficient care to acquire proper conditioning. We doubt if the continuous type of enuresis is caused by major psychological difficulties at the outset, though we acknowledge that psychological difficulties can occur as an overlay." He went on to say that most enuretics over the age of 10 come from a low social class and a low level of intelligence.

Werry[22] examined the causes of enuresis. He wrote that "in a majority of enuretics, no psychopathology will be discernible". In a study of 58 children with secondary enuresis, he found that "the overwhelmingly commonest cause was environmental variables likely to provoke a high level of anxiety in the child, such as hospitalisation, separation from the mother, or other emotionally traumatic incidents."

The shorter the period over which the child has been dry, the more likely is he to develop enuresis when subjected to psychological trauma "The most reasonable position to assume seems to be that enuresis i not an etiologically homogeneous condition, and facile overgeneralisa tions are to be deplored". MacKeith[14] suggested that anxiety in th third year of life, at the time when bladder control is being learnt or ha just been acquired, is an important factor.

It would be idle to suggest that there is no psychological factor ii primary enuresis. It is obvious that coercive measures and parenta anxiety will superimpose a psychological problem on to the delay ii maturation. Such management may prolong the enuresis in a chilc whose bladder mechanism has matured sufficiently to provide control.

There is no evidence that there is polyuria in enuretic children a night. Studies have shown that the urinary output is no different ii enuretics from that in other children.

There is no evidence that the depth of sleep is any greater ii enuretic children than in others.

The organic causes of enuresis were reviewed by Smith.[21] The causes include an ectopic ureter opening into the urethra, or betweer the urethral and vaginal orifice, or near the hymen; obstruction of the urethra in the boy; diverticulum of the anterior urethra; spina bifida with meningomyelocele; sacral agenesis; diastematomyelia; sacra lipoma; ectopia vesicæ; epispadias; absent abdominal muscles with gross expansion of the posterior urethra; and a complication of cir cumcision. He pointed out that infection is a factor in enuresis if there is cystitis, because then a lesser degree of distension causes the desire to micturate; but that pyelonephritis is not related to enuresis unles there is associated cystitis. Spina bifida occulta is never related to enuresis. Constant dribbling in the male suggests urethral obstruction while in the female it suggests an ectopic ureter.

When an epileptic child has enuresis, one should always remembei the possibility that he is wetting the bed in fits during sleep.

Secondary enuresis results mainly from insecurity and tension anc other psychological factors. It may also result from anything whicl causes polyuria or frequency of micturition such as diabetes mellitus diabetes insipidus, renal insufficiency, or cystitis. I believe tha urinary symptoms, such as polyuria, or emotional upsets, are o especial importance in causing enuresis when they develop shortly after the aquisition of sphincter control. It is essential to examine the urine for the specific gravity, albumin, sugar, excess of white cells in the deposit and for organisms, in order to try to eliminate an organic lesion.

Primary and Secondary Constipation. Soiling

The infrequent bowel action in many breast-fed babies has been described elsewhere. Fully breast-fed babies do not have hard stools unless they have Hirschsprung's disease.

Constipation in artificially fed babies in the first few weeks has also been discussed. It can usually be corrected by adjustment of the diet.

Constipation after the first few weeks may arise as the result of the passage of a hard stool which has caused pain. In the same way an anal fissure may lead to deliberate withholding of stools. The rectum may become so loaded that the child cannot empty it if he tries.

Constipation may result from anorectal stenosis. As in Hirschsprung's disease, attacks of enterocolitis may occur, with diarrhœa. The stenosis is readily found by rectal examination. Hirschsprung's disease is an important cause of constipation. As the rectum is not loaded, soiling does not occur.

There remain many children with severe constipation, some of them with soiling and spurious diarrhœa—the constant leakage of semi-liquid material around the hard fæcal masses in the rectum. Psychiatrists tend to ascribe all these to psychological causes. Recent studies of the motility of the lower colon have indicated that many of these are due to increased muscular tone in the terminal colon, associated with excessive drying of the stool and unco-ordinated muscular activity.[4] One certainly sees many severely constipated children whose toilet "training" has apparently been managed in an exemplary manner, and in whom there does not appear to be insecurity or other emotional factors.

Secondary constipation is readily caused by over-enthusiastic toilet training. A child who is compelled to sit on the pottie against his will, or one who is punished for not using it, is liable to react by constipation.

Bellman[2] in his 151 page monograph on encopresis, found that at the age of 7 to 8 years, 1·5 per cent. of Stockholm children soiled their pants. The symptom was more than three times more common in boys than in girls. The incidence declined after the age of 7, and none persisted after the sixteenth birthday. Half the children had never acquired bowel control, but half had developed control and then started to soil. Two-thirds of the children who acquired the encopresis started soiling when they started school, or when separated from their mother, or when a new sibling was born. In several cases, a sibling or parent had had the same complaint. Other behaviour problems, such as enuresis and food refusal, were more common in affected children than in controls. They tended to have more difficulty in handling their aggressive feelings than did controls, and they were less successful in making and keeping friends. Their average level of intelligence

11

was the same as that of controls. The children tended to be anxious, tense, and immature in their behaviour. Their mothers were more tense, anxious, overprotective and indulgent than mothers of control children and had tended to use coercive methods in toilet training: their fathers had tended to exert excessive discipline.

Prevention

The management of the child must be adapted to the level of his development. He will not learn voluntary sphincter control until he is developmentally ready for it, and all attempts to "train" him before he has shown himself ready are likely to lead to the opposite of the result desired.

There is a difference of opinion as to when "conditioning" should be attempted. I do not think that it matters as long as the difference between conditioning and voluntary control is fully understood, so that there is no anxiety when breakdown occurs. Provided that there is never a fight to keep the child on the pottie and the child does not resist, "potting" is a harmless procedure, and it does undoubtedly save dirty napkins. When there is a phase of resistance to the pottie there must on no account be anxiety and attempts to compel the child to sit on it. Most children sooner or later develop such phases. The motto should always be "Placid painless potting." The child is placed on the pottie when he awakens from a nap, immediately after a meal and when he comes in from outside. If he does not void in a minute or two he should be taken off it. Enemas and suppositories should never be given unless absolutely necessary.

Muellner[17] found that there was no relation between the age at which "training" was started and the acquisition of control. Dimson[5] studied 165 families containing 225 enuretics and 174 dry siblings. The age at which toilet training was initiated was the same in each group. He thought that there was more resistance to "potting" when toilet training was postponed until after the age of 3 months. Douglas and Blomfield[6] found that those who were "trained" early were less likely to relapse than those "trained" later. Younger mothers and mothers in lower social classes tend to "train" their children later than others, and there is a higher incidence of enuresis in those two groups.

The mother should know the normal development of control and realize the great individual variation in the age at which it is achieved. She should get out of the idea that she is training the child. All she can do is to help him when he is ready by enabling him to reach the pottie in time. She can also help him by allowing him to take responsibility for looking after himslef as soon as he is ready—thus satisfying his ego, his pride in new skills.

It is futile to allow him to do without a napkin too soon, before he has shown himself able to tell the mother when he wants to void. When he is able to manage without a napkin during the day, he should be tried without one in his daytime nap. At night it is wrong to let him do without a napkin until, having been picked up at 10 p.m., he is usually dry in the morning, unless he can persuaded to get out of bed and use the pottie unaided. This is not likely to happen till after the age of 2½. If the napkin is discarded too soon, frequent accidents are inevitable, and they upset both mother and child. If the child is allowed to wear a napkin after the time that he is ready to do without, the mother merely retains all responsibility for his dryness and the child is late in learning control.

The age at which a child should be picked up at 10 p.m. is a matter of trial and error. It is a mistake to think that one is "training" a child by picking him up. Usually the child is not even awakened. I cannot agree with those who feel that it is essential that the child so picked up should be thoroughly wakened so that he knows what he is doing. Parents are rightly reluctant to waken children at this time. They may be slow to go to sleep again and be fatigued next day as a result. If a child is disturbed by being picked up it should as a rule be avoided. It is useless to pick a child up if he is found to be wet at that time. This would mean that his retention span is not long enough. On the other hand, it is sometimes found that picking a child up delays his early-morning awakening. Sooner or later it will be found that if a child is not picked up he is wet in the morning, while if he is picked up he is dry. Picking him up will now enable him to do without a napkin and so take responsibility himself.

Some children are not dry at night unless they are given a chance (without a napkin) to get out of bed to use the pottie when they want. This is impossible if the child is in a cot, but most children after the second birthday are ready for a bed. Naturally, he cannot get out of bed in winter if he is in a sleeping bag.

Every effort should be made to prevent the stools being hard and so causing painful defæcation. Any tendency to this should be treated by attention to the diet (giving more fruit) and if necessary by giving a mild aperient such as milk of magnesia.

The child should become accustomed to using a toilet outside home; otherwise he may refuse to void when visiting friends.

The most important single point in the normal establishment of sphincter control is the absolute necessity of avoiding a fight with the child, of trying to force him to sit on the pottie or to void when he does not wish to do. At all costs there must be no fuss when a lapse occurs, when he refuses to sit on his pottie or when accidents happen.

The placid understanding mother who takes everything in her
stride has little trouble with her child in the difficult days when
sphincter control is being acquired. A few extra weeks of napkin
washing when the child is 1 or 2 may save months of pants and sheet
washing when he is 3 or 4.

Treatment

The treatment is implicit in the remarks made above. A careful
detailed history of the whole management of the child has to be taken
before the treatment can be discussed with the mother. It is essential
to know how the mother tried to "train" the child and how she dealt
with "accidents." One has to understand her attitude to the problem
and that of her husband and relatives in the house. The mother must
know a little about the normal development of sphincter control and
the relevant features of the psychological development of children, in
particular the negativism and desire for fuss and attention in the age
group in question. She must learn that no harm will befall the child
who fails to have a motion every day as long as the stool is not hard.
Every effort, in other words, has to be made to remove her anxiety,
which is usually the basic cause of the whole trouble. All forcing
methods must stop. She must stop showing anxiety or making a
fuss when accidents occur or when the child refuses to sit on the
pottie. She must on no account punish the child for an accident,
scold him try to shame or ridicule him or show anger. She must
not discuss the problem with anyone in front of him or do anything
else which encourages him to use the difficulties as an attention-seeking
device. She should, in fact, show no interest in accidents apart from
clearing up the mess. There is no place for bribes or rewards in
treatment. She must be told about the wide normal variations in the
age at which control is acquired, and she must be brought to understand
that forcing methods and anxiety will do nothing more than postpone
the age at which control is established.

Even without any mismanagement most children have temporary
phases of refusal to sit on the pottie. The refusal should be respected
and no attempt should be made to persuade the child to change his
mind. An effort may, of course, be made to distract him by giving
him a toy, but if he still refuses, nothing further should be done about it.
Provided that no forcing methods are applied, the phase will be a temporary one only.

When serious harm has already been done the problem is indeed
a difficult one. When a child has for some weeks displayed complete
rebellion against the pottie, there are only two alternatives which
are likely to work. One is for the mother to stop "potting" him at

all for a sufficiently long period for him to forget all about it—and this depends on the child's memory. The period may be one of, say, 3 months. The mother then starts again after the doctor has given the necessary advice about management. The other alternative—in many ways undesirable but sometimes necessary—is to take the child into hospital, where a tactful nurse will soon cope successfully with the problem. The disadvantage of this method is that the child is likely to relapse as soon as he returns home. It is better for the mother herself to correct the mischief that has been done.

When a child, aged about 18 months, who is in the process of acquiring voluntary control of the bladder, demands the pottie every few minutes, one has to decide whether this is purely an attention-seeking mechanism or a genuine fear of an accident. It is usually the former. It is difficult for the mother to decide on the correct course. She will have to try to ignore the frequent demands and only place the child on the pottie at reasonably frequent intervals—say, after a meal and halfway between mealtimes. If the diagnosis of an attention-seeking mechanism is correct the problem will then resolve. It is important that frequency of this nature should be distinguished from the constant dribbling of urine which is sometimes found in boys in association with urethral obstruction, or in girls with an ectopic ureter.

When a serious relapse occurs in a child who has acquired full control of the sphincters, there is usually an underlying emotional disturbance, which must be sought and treated. An organic cause should be eliminated by examination of the urine for an infection or for polyuria, but it is unlikely that an abnormality will be found. Much the most likely causes are rigid training methods, with an excessive display of anxiety when accidents occur, or some cause of insecurity, such as jealousy. As with the other problems mentioned, the less anxiety which is shown about it and the less scolding which the child receives, the more rapidly is it likely to clear, particularly when the underlying emotional disturbance is properly managed.

When the child is nearing his third birthday and is not showing any sign of acquiring control of the bladder, in spite of reasonable management on the part of the parents, the problem is a difficult one. One often sees children like this, who show no resistance to the pottie, who have been given every chance to urinate into one or in the lavatory without any undue fuss or anxiety having been shown, and yet they constantly wet their pants. In the majority of these there is a family history of similar lateness in the acquisition of control, and the age at which control was established in other members of the family may provide a useful indication of when control can be expected in the child in question. It is worth while performing a routine examination of the urine to exclude a renal lesion, such as a chronic pyelonephritis or chronic renal insufficiency, but the chance of finding an abnormality is a remote one.

In my experience medicines are of little value. Some have found the tranquillizing drugs imipramine or amitryptiline useful. I have tried them with some success, but it must be remembered that a wide variety of side effects have been ascribed to them. Ephedrine and belladonna are useless. Amphetamine acts only by reducing the depth of sleep, or keeping the child awake.

Nothing will be achieved by fluid restriction in the evening. In fact Hägglund[10] found that fluid restriction might even have the opposite of the effect desired.

In older children with primary enuresis, the electric buzzer is an effective treatment. It is not normally used, however, in the child under five. The use of the buzzer was reviewed by Lovibond[13] and Young[2]. The child sleeps on a special pad, and as soon as any wetting occurs the circuit is completed, an alarm sounds, the child awakens, gets out of bed and turns the alarm off, and passes urine. Young wrote that "The theory of conditioning treatment is derived from the strengthening of incompatible reactions. If to one response, another incompatible response, initiated by the same stimulus, is added and repeatedly presented, it is probable that the evocation of the first response will progressively decrease until it is extinguished." The enuretic responds to the stimulus of a full bladder by urination. Treatment consists of associating the same stimulus with an awakening stimulus—namely the bell. The response to urination is inhibited by awakening and this inhibition of micturition, by a conditioning process, ultimately occurs spontaneously without the necessity for the operation of the bell.

The buzzer cures some 75 per cent. of children. Relapse is commonly due to discontinuing the use of the alarm too soon. It should be continued for at least a month after the last wet bed. Failure may be due to the child not being awakened by the buzzer. This can be remedied by obtaining a louder buzzer, or giving amphetamine to reduce the depth of sleep. Failure may result from the child being able to switch off the alarm without getting out of bed.

In the case of gross constipation, especially if there is diarrhœa and incontinence, it is often advisable to admit the child to hospital in order to ensure that the bowel is completely cleared out. This is achieved by olive oil enemas and colonic washouts. Manual removal of hard scybala is sometimes necessary, an anæsthetic being used for the purpose. Tremendous dilatation of the colon occurs, and the rectum is apparently quite insensitive to the loading and distension. The bowel, therefore, has to be re-educated. After it has been cleared out, normal bowel actions are maintained with the aid of non-irritating aperients. A combination of syrup of figs and magnesium sulphate is satisfactory, the dose given being adjusted to give the desired action without causing diarrhœa. Preparations which act entirely by increasing the bulk of the motions, such as agaragar, are ineffective.

If the problem can be dealt with without enemas, it is better to do so. Berg and Jones[3] secured an 80 per cent. remission rate in 59 affected children at the Great Ormond Street Hospital by combined psychiatric and therapeutic measures.

A wetting agent, dioctyl sodium sulphosuccinate, has been recommended, the idea being that it would promote penetration of water or mineral oil into the hard fæces. A controlled study at Sheffield[20] indicated that the drug was not of value. In my experience prostigmine does not help. It is doubtful whether rectal suppositories are useful. The objection to them is that they involve further interference with the anal region. Every effort should be made for psychological reasons to discard the use of enemas and suppositories as soon as possible. It is obvious however, that unless sufficient doses of the drugs (syrup of figs, salts) are given by mouth, the motions become hard and are either not passed for a long time or cause pain when they are passed.

An essential part of the cure consists of encouraging the child to pass a stool in the usual way without forcing or fussing. As soon as he is passing a normal daily stool without the help of enemas or suppositories he is returned home, the necessary advice being given to the mother. For a time a mild aperient is needed every day, but this is reduced and stopped as soon as possible. It should not be thought that cure of this condition is easy. It is very difficult.

With the exception of the treatment of gross constipation there is no place for drugs in the treatment of the problems of sphincter control.

The problem of stool smearing is discussed in the section on Attention-seeking Devices.

References

1. BAKWIN, H., BAKWIN, R. M. (1960). *Clinical Management of Behavior Disorders in Children*. Philadelphia. Saunders.
2. BELLMAN, M. (1966). "Studies on Encopresis." *Acta Pædiat. Scand. Suppl.*, 170.
3. BERG, I., JONES, K. V. (1964). "Functional Faeceal Incontinence in Children." *Arch. Dis. Childh.*, **39**, 465.
4. DAVIDSON, M., KUGLER, M. M., BAUER, C. H. (1963). "Diagnosis and Management in Children with Severe and Protracted Constipation and Obstipation." *J. Pediat.*, **62**, 261.
5. DIMSON, S. B. (1959). "Toilet Training and Enuresis." *Brit. med. J.*, **2**, 666.

6. DOUGLAS, J. W. B., BLOMFIELD, J. M. (1958). *Children Under Five.* London. Allen and Unwin.
7. DRILLIEN, C. M. (1959). "A Longitudinal Study of the Growth and Development of Prematurely and Maturely Born Children." *Arch. Dis. Childh.*, **34**, 487.
8. FREUD, S. (1938). *Three Contributions to the Theory of Sex.* New York. The Modern Library.
9. GLICKLICH, L. B. (1951). "An Historical Account of Enuresis." *Pediatrics*, **8**, 859.
10. HÄGGLUND, T.-B. (1965). "Enuretic Children Treated with Fluid Restriction or Forced Drinking." *Ann. Pæd. Fenn.*, **11**, 84.
11. HALLGREN, B. (1959). "Nocturnal Enuresis—Ætiological Aspects." *Acta pæd. Uppsala*, Suppl. **118**, 66.
12. HALLIDAY, J. L. (1946). "Epidemiology and the Psychosomatic Affections." *Lancet*, **2**, 185.
13. LOVIBOND, S. H. (1964). *Conditioning and Enuresis.* Oxford. Pergamon.
14. MacKEITH, R. C. (1968). "A Frequent Factor in the Origins of Primary Enuresis; Anxiety in the Third Year of Life." *Develop. Med. Child Neurol.*, **10**, 465.
15. MILLER, F. J. W., COURT, S. D. M., WALTON, W. S., KNOX, E. G. (1960). *Growing up in Newcastle-upon-Tyne.* London. Oxford University Press.
16. MILLER, F. J. W. (1966). "Childhood Morbidity and Mortality in Newcastle-upon-Tyne." *New Engl. J. Med.*, **275**, 683.
17. MUELLNER, S. R. (1961). "Obstacles to the Successful Treatment of Primary Enuresis." *J. Amer. med. Ass.*, **178**, 843.
18. NEWSON, J. E., (1968). "Four years old in a Urban Community." London. Allen and Unwin.
19. NYE, S. (1830). "Incontinence of Urine." *Med. and Surg. Rep.*, **45**, 389.
20. RENDLE-SHORT, J. (1956). "Dioctylsodium Sulphosuccinate in the Treatment of Constipation in Children." *Lancet*, **2**, 1189.
21. SMITH, E. D. (1967). "Diagnosis and Management of the Child with Wetting." *Australian Paed. J.*, **3**, 193.
22. WERRY, J. C. (1967). "Enuresis—a Psychosomatic Entity?" *Can. Med. Ass. J.*, **97**, 319.
23. YOUNG, G. C. (1965). "Conditioning Treatment of Enuresis." *Develop. Med. Child Neurol.*, **7**, 557.

CHAPTER 24

CRYING—TEMPER TANTRUMS—
BREATH-HOLDING ATTACKS

Crying

Crying may begin *in utero*. It is termed *vagitus uterinus*. King and Bourgeois[10] collected 127 cases from the literature after 1800. St. Bartholomew and Mahomet are said to have cried *in utero*. Mclane[14] described a case in an operating theatre. The cry was heard by all present, and a superstitious nurse spent the rest of the time on her knees in prayer. It can only occur when the membranes are ruptured and air has entered the uterine cavity.[1] It is of no significance.

According to Adler the first cry represents an "overwhelming sense of inferiority at thus suddenly being confronted by reality without ever having had to deal with its problems." This feeling of inferiority at least serves a useful function in ventilating the lungs. Another psychologist[16] wrote that birth represents "a loss of paradise," but it is not clear how he knew this. After birth crying is largely a signal for need. Babies can demonstrate their displeasure long before they can show pleasure, yet there are not many stimuli for displeasure in the new-born period. I have reviewed the subject fully elsewhere.[6]

As a result of repeated statements by mothers in six bedded wards in the Jessop Obstetric Hospital, Sheffield, that they were awakened only by the cry of their own baby and not that of other babies, we decided to put the matter to the test.[2] In the first place, tape recordings of the cries of 31 newborn babies were played to mothers: 12 of 23 mothers recognized the cry of their own child in the first 48 hours, and thereafter all successfully recognized the cry of their own baby. Secondly, with the mother's permission, we recorded the mothers' awakening in response to babies' cries; in the first three nights 15 of the 23 awoke only in response to the crying of their own baby, but after the third night 22 of the 23 mothers responded only to their own baby.

Any pædiatrician knows that there are certain characteristic cries—the shrill high pitched cry of the child with cerebral irritability, the hoarse cry of the cretin, the whimper of the severely ill baby, the grunt of the infant with a respiratory infection, the cry of the mongol, the child with laryngitis or with the cri-du-chat syndrome, or with amyotonia congenita. Analysis of cries by the method of sound spectography[10,20] has confirmed the clinical impression that the cries of cerebral irritability, hunger and pain are different in quality. Karelitz and Fisichelli[7] traced the normal development of the cry by the same method. They showed that the cry of the mentally defective infant corresponds with that of the younger normal infant. Defective children require a more painful stimulus to cry and take longer to cry after the stimulus. They found that there was a high correlation between the nature of the cry and the Apgar score.

It is unusual for a baby to shed tears when crying in the first 4 weeks or so. After the age of about 6 months many infants cry at night for their mothers without shedding tears. (Animals do not shed tears, though it is said that marine turtles shed tears when laying eggs.)

By far the commonest causes of crying in the new-born period are discomfort and loneliness. The chief cause of discomfort is hunger. On a self-demand schedule crying is quickly checked by a feed, provided that the quantity of food is adequate. Even in the new-born period personality differences manifest themselves. Some cry more readily than others. Some will not brook a moment's delay when they are hungry and scream so vigorously that the mother is compelled to take action. Others are more tolerant of hunger. Some babies are well suited by a rigid feeding schedule because the times laid down for their feeds happen to coincide with their needs. Others find themselves hungry long before the clock says that they ought to feel hungry, and cry a great deal as a result. There are still many who say that a child should never be fed in the night in the first few weeks because it may leads to bad habits. Instructions to this effect inevitably cause unnecessary crying at night.

Crying from hunger may also be due to fixed ideas of the duration of feeds or of the quantity which a child should take. Babies are individuals and some suck better and more quickly than others. The milk flows from some breasts more slowly than others. The crying may be due to nothing more than not allowing the baby sufficient time on the breast. Some babies require more than the average amount of milk for an average weight gain and for satiation of their hunger and thirst. Wallgren investigated the amount of milk taken by normal healthy breast-fed babies and found that the variations were considerable. If "heavy eaters" were compelled to take a quantity of milk which was an average one and sufficient for most babies, a great deal of crying resulted. Rigid rules for the duration and quantity of feeds should not be laid down. They are apt to cause unnecessary crying.

Some babies are of the irritable type and scream when they approach the breast, or suck for a minute and then withdraw and scream.

Some scream vigorously when taken off the first breast prior to being given the second. Others do not fuss in this way.

Another cause of discomfort in the new-born period is flatulence, the causes of which are discussed elsewhere. Colic is a common cause of crying in the first 3 months. It occurs mostly, but not entirely, in the evenings. Colic may also be due to substances in the milk if the mother is taking senna, excess of fruit or pickles.

Other causes of crying are overclothing, excessive heat or cold, a wet or soiled napkin, an itching rash or an unpleasant smell or taste, such as that of vomit. A baby cries when there is a sudden noise or when a light shines in his face. Sometimes the new-born baby cries when the light is put out and he finds himself in the dark.

Another common cause of crying in the new-born period and onwards is loneliness. It is surprising how many mothers fail to realize that even the very young baby cries for company. The crying stops as soon as he is picked up, whereas the crying of hunger does not stop, or else there is a minute's quiet and then he cries again even though he is in his mother's arms. I saw a mother who was completely worn out as a result of following the instructions given to her by a nursing home. She had been told never to pick her baby up when he cried, never to feed him at night and always to feed him strictly by the clock. The baby did not approve of this. He settled immediately when managed with common sense. The usual cause of excessive crying due to loneliness is the fear of spoiling. It does not spoil a baby to pick him up when he wants it.

Failure to realize that loneliness causes crying leads many mothers who are using the self-demand method to give unnecessary feeds.

Crying commonly occurs when the position of the baby is suddenly changed, particularly if he is allowed suddenly to fall back from the sitting position. He is likely to cry when his clothes are being changed or when his cot is being made, but this may be partly a cry to be picked up and loved. Some babies cry when placed in the bath, but most enjoy this. An almost certain way of making a baby cry is to hold his limbs or head so that movement is impossible. For the same reason clothing which prevents movement should be avoided.

As the baby grows older crying decreases, though the number of different stimuli which cause crying increases. At 6 months a child endures hunger, thirst or a wet napkin longer than a month-old baby does. Any sort of discomfort still causes crying, though some cry more readily than others. The commonest causes of discomfort are a wet or soiled napkin, hunger, fatigue or teething. A baby may emit a scream when he passes urine, as if it causes discomfort. He cries if he feels tired or poorly. He objects to having his nose or ears cleaned.

The breast-fed baby may cry at the time of the mother's menstrual period.

After 5 or 6 months fears may cause crying. The baby may cry when he sees a strange face, particularly when a stranger speaks to him. He cries when he gets into difficulties in his cot. Any time after 5 months he may cry when put to bed in a room to which he is not accustomed. He may awaken with a sudden shriek which is not due to a wet napkin or to other discoverable cause. It may well be a nightmare. From 9 months onwards the baby may show signs of jealousy and cry when he sees his mother pick up another baby. A 6-month-old baby may cry when he sees his brother fall and hurt himself or when he sees him smacked.

Loneliness comes into greater prominence as a cause of crying after the new-born period. The importance of loneliness as a cause of crying depends on the child's personality. Some babies are quite content to be left out in the pram all day. Others at 3 or 4 months cry incessantly if left outside. They are perfectly content when lying in the pram in the kitchen where they can see what the mother is doing. At 4 months the baby may cry when approaching the cot. He is reluctant to see his mother leave the room.

Any thwarting of the baby's developing powers is apt to cause crying. Reluctance to be left outside in the pram is partly due to the child's developing interest in the activities of the kitchen. Many mothers fail to realize this and think that the child is crying to be picked up. Fearing that they will spoil him, they leave him to cry. It is surprising how many mothers are apparently deaf to the crying of their babies, leaving them to cry for hours on end. When a child is ready to be propped up in the pram he is reluctant to be left lying down. When he can sit, he may well cry if not given the opportunity to do so. When he can grasp objects, he may cry if not given a chance to play. It is common to see a baby over the age of 5 or 6 months left for hours without any toys; he cries from sheer boredom. A baby cries when a pleasurable experience is stopped, as when he is removed from his bath or when the mother stops playing with him, or when, having held him in her arms, she puts him into the cot. He cries when he is unable to reach for an object which he wants or when a wanted object is removed from him.

The development of the ego and personality leads to crying from 6 months or so onwards. Even at 5 months the baby may show striking likes and dislikes and cry when given food which he does not like, or when fed from a cup or dish which is not the usual one. A determined independent child at 6 or 7 months may refuse to take food unless he is allowed to help to hold the spoon. Efforts to make the child take food which he does not want or to sit on the pottie against his will, lead to crying. *Excessive crying in this period is almost always due to failure to answer the child's basic needs for comfort, love and security, and for opportunities to practise his new-found skills.*

After the first birthday there is a further reduction in the frequency of crying. Crying is liable to be the result of conflict with the developing ego and with his newly-found interests. Many tears are the result of wounding of the child's pride. When he has learnt to do things for himself— to help to set the table, to dress himself, to attend to his eliminations— he is likely, if of an independent character, to respond to interference by tears. He becomes more and more determined to have his own way. He wants to play without interference. Adults often interfere unnecessarily in children's play and thereby cause tears. The father, for instance, steps in when he sees his boy pushing his engine about on the floor instead of winding it up and letting it run on its own. The child does not want to stop doing what he is so much enjoying, and has no sense of time. He wants to do something which for reasons of safety his parents forbid. He wants a toy which another child has. Crying as a result of the most trivial knocks or falls is often purely an attention-seeking device.

He may find wailing during play an effective way of getting an older sibling into trouble. It is stopped by ignoring it or by punishment.

His great need is for love and security, and any apparent deprivation of this causes tears. His fears of the dark may be largely fear of separation from his mother. He cries when he feels lonely or when he is left behind because he walks so slowly. If given a chance he will cry every night for company. After the age of $1\frac{1}{2}$ he develops a variety of fears and cries for the security of his mother's company. He may cry outside because of the discomfort of wind and rain. He cries because of the pain of teething, because he is tired or because he feels unwell.

As in the case of the younger child, the frequency of crying depends in part on his personality. Excessive crying is almost always due to mismanagement, in the form of failure to give the child the love and security which he needs and failure to allow him to learn independence and practise his newly-found skills. It is greatly increased by constant interference—by perfectionism, domination and attempts to "train" him before he is developmentally ready. It is increased by insecurity, whatever the cause. It is greatly increased by irritability and fatigue in the parents. It is similarly increased in the child as a result of insufficient sleep.

Psychoanalysis have other explanations for the cry of babies. According to Melanie Klein[17] "a hungry infant, screaming and kicking, fantasies that he is actually attacking the breast, tearing and destroying it, and experiences his own screams which tear him and hurt him as the torn breast attacking him in his own inside. Therefore not only does he experience a want, but his hunger pain and his own screams may be felt as a persecutory attack on his inside.

A hungry raging infant, on being offered the breast, instead of accepting it, turns away from it and will not feed. Here the fantasy may be of having attacked and destroyed the breast, which is then felt to have turned bad and to be attacking in turn. The breast is distorted by these fantasies into a terrifying persecutor."

There are many who feel that a child is spoilt by picking him up when he cries. I do not agree. No child is spoilt by being picked up when he cries for love and security, or when he has fallen and hurt himself or has pain or discomfort. It is never right to leave a child to cry for prolonged periods. The less he is allowed to cry in the first 2 or 3 years the happier he is likely to be in later childhood. This does not mean that he should always have his own way. It does mean that the wiser the parental management, the greater the parents' tact, patience, common sense and sense of humour, the fewer tears will be shed by their children. There is no place for drugs in treatment, except only in certain sleep problems.

It is interesting to note that Lipton, Steinschneider and Richmond[11] in their fascinating monograph, confirmed by scientific methods the clinical impression that swaddling reduces the amount of crying. Wolff,[21] in an interesting analysis of crying, showed that crying is stopped not only by swaddling, a pacifier, talking to the child, or picking him up, but by rhythmical tapping of the spinal column at the rate of 80 to 140 per minute.

Temper Tantrums

The usual age for temper tantrums is 15 months to 3 years or more. A determined child may give displays of temper long before that age, from 6 months onwards, but typical tantrums hardly occur before the first birthday. Their appearance corresponds with the period of resistance, of the development of the ego and negativism, and of the normal aggressiveness in the transition stage from infancy to the independence of the mature child. The frequency and character of temper tantrums are familiar to all. In the worst forms the child may do considerable damage by throwing china on to the floor, valued objects into the fire and by kicking the furniture. Breath-holding attacks are intimately related to temper tantrums, but owing to their distinctive nature they are discussed in a separate section.

The methods used to deal with tantrums are also well known. The child is likely to be soundly smacked and he often succeeds in getting his own way after them.

The Basic Causes

(i) *The personality of the child.* Tantrums are not a problem in the placid, easy-going child. They occur in the active, determined child with abundant energy.

(ii) *The period of resistance and the development of the ego.* In essence tantrums represent the clash of the child's developing personality with the will of his parents. His increasing desire to show his powers, to gain attention and to have his own way gets him into trouble, particularly when his parents are perfectionists and of the domineering type. If he finds that by screaming and a display of temper he can attract attention, secure bribes or sweets to pacify him, or get his own way and do something which he wanted to do or avoid doing something which he did not want to do, he will certainly repeat the performance. His tantrums give him control over his environment. He finds a tantrum a successful device for avoiding punishment. When parents have been foolish enough to talk to friends in his presence about his dreadful tantrums, he realizes immediately the anxiety and interest which they have aroused and repeats the performance. A single tantrum badly managed is liable to develop into a habit. The child soon realizes that he has discovered a most satisfactory way of annoying his parents. This reaction is not one of naughtiness. It is merely a normal sign of the development of the ego.

It is an obvious fact that the child's negativism is increased by fatigue and boredom, and to a certain extent by hunger.

(iii) *The desire to practise new skills.* Bound up with the above is the child's desire to practise new skills and to take responsibility for doing things which he has recently learnt. There is little doubt that many tears are due to the thwarting of this pride because the parents, perhaps in order to save time or to prevent possible accidents (e.g. with china), have not allowed him to help or do things for himself which he is able to do.

(iv) *Imitativeness.* The child who sees his parents display bad temper, throwing things on to the floor and banging the doors in rage, is likely to copy them. He is also likely to imitate tantrums thrown by his friends.

(v) *Insecurity.* Insecurity for any reason is a potent cause of temper tantrums.

(vi) *The level of intelligence.* Though temper tantrums are common in children of any level of intelligence, including those of mental superiority, they are especially liable to occur in children with some degree of mental retardation. Such children are apt to be thwarted because too much is expected of them or because they are unable to understand the limits of their freedom.

(vii) *Ignorance of the normal personality differences in children*. An attempt to bring children up by rigid rules instead of by elastic methods adjusted to the needs of the individual is apt to lead to various difficulties, including tantrums. When a first child has been of a placid easy-going disposition and the second one has an active determined character, methods applied to the first often cause considerable trouble in the second.

(viii) *Over-indulgence, over-protection and domination*. One of these is almost always present. The temper tantrum is one of the commonest manifestations in the child who has suffered from over-indulgence or over-protection. The child who has never been taught discipline, when eventually he goes too far even for his over-indulgent mother and is rebuked, throws a tantrum in order that he can still have his own way. If ever he has difficulty in getting his own way he knows that he will get what he wants if he has a tantrum.

Excessive strictness with the child is equally liable to cause temper tantrums. Insistence on unreasonable demands which are unsuitable for his level of development and on immediate obedience inevitably causes trouble. Excessive interference with the child's normal pursuits by the mother or grandmother because of perfectionism, an excessive desire for tidiness or a determination to make the boy "good," is apt to be met by rebellion. The mother who is saying "No, no" to the child all through the day, when in reality his pursuits are harmless, must expect to meet resistance if the child has any character at all. The temper tantrum is the child's best defence reaction against such repression. A vicious circle is apt to be set up, the resistance being met with more repression, and the repression by more resistance.

Sometimes the excessive repression is due to a social problem, the mother being compelled to prevent the child making a noise because of unpleasant critical neighbours or relatives in the house.

(ix) *Parental inconsistency*. If the parents vacillate, sometimes insisting on a particular line of behaviour and sometimes not taking any notice, or if they constantly threaten and never carry out the threats, the child becomes confused or reacts by a tantrum when eventually the parents take action. More often the parents disagree with each other. If one parent forbids a child to do a particular thing and the other permits it, the child is apt to throw temper tantrums in order to get what he wants.

(x) *Parental fatigue, impatience or unhappiness*. The irritating characteristics of the small child have been mentioned elsewhere. They are particularly relevant here. The mother has to put up with her very exasperating offspring morning, noon and night. One can hardly blame the mother who complains that the child is getting on her nerves and is driving her to distraction. The more tired she gets, the more irritable she becomes, and the more her fatigue and irritability is reflected in the child's behaviour. He is worse when she snaps at him or tries to hurry him. Domestic unhappiness has a similar effect. When the mother is badly treated by her husband and is not happy in her relationship with him, the child suffers from her irritability, over-protection or fatigue.

Prevention and Treatment

It is essential to look behind the temper tantrums for the underlying cause. In the first place, organic disease must be eliminated. A chronic infection such as tuberculosis may cause undue fatigue in the child and so lead to bad temper. Bad behaviour with screaming attacks may be due to deafness, the child being unable to make his wants known. When in addition to the bad temper there are personality changes, one must not forget the possibility of a cerebral tumour or of a degenerative disease of the nervous system. Some children thought to have simple behaviour problems may have abnormal electroencephalograms.

In the majority of cases, no sign of organic disease will be found. One then has to review the whole management of the child in order that the parental attitudes can be understood and corrected. Any underlying insecurity in the child, over-protection, over-indulgence and over-strictness in the parents, has to be remedied. No excessive demands must be made on him. The opportunities for resistance must be cut down to a minimum, for the essence of treatment lies in prevention. He should be kept occupied. He should have playmates of his own age. He should frequently have them in his own house and go out to visit them in their homes. He should be encouraged to practise skills, and to take pride in what he can do. As far as possible sources of danger must be removed, and he should be removed bodily when he is approaching them or when it is seen that a storm is brewing. Most children at this age are distractable, and this trait should be utilized. It is far better to remove him and distract him than to sit and say "No, no," thus inviting defiance. The mother must be reasonable in her requests and not rush him, but she must be consistent and there must be no disagreement between the parents. Once she has given the child an instruction she must see that it is carried out.

If the request involves tidying up after games, she should help him rather than risk meeting with resistance. She may reduce opportunities for resistance by deciding on a course of action for the child rather than asking him if he would like to do it. For example, when she wants to take the child out for a walk, instead of saying "Shall we go out for a walk now?" her attitude will be "We are going to go out for a walk now." She must on no account try to break the child's will. He will need his determination and force of character in later years. Excessive inhibition of a child's normal aggressiveness is apt to lead to timidity, morose withdrawn behaviour, an inferiority complex, or, later to rebellion and excessive aggressiveness.

When a temper tantrum occurs there must on no account be a fight, a fuss, anger, anxiety or argument. There must be no reasonings and no attempt to force him to stop his behaviour. Reasonings and repression are useless. Scolding a rebellious child is as much use as pouring petrol on a fire to extinguish it. It is essential that the mother should herself not lose her temper. Smacking is likely to be merely the result of loss of temper and should be avoided. The best way to treat a tantrum is to ignore it. A display of indifference is a much more severe and effective punishment than any disciplinary method. On no account must the child be given the centre of the stage for his effort. He should certainly not be given what he wanted after the tantrum. As soon as he finds that he is achieving nothing by tantrums he will stop having them. He can be picked up and given a feeling of love and security after one, but he should not be given sweets or other awards.

After the tantrum the mother should ask herself exactly why the tantrum occurred. Was it really necessary to stop him doing what he wanted to do or to try to force him to do what he did not want to do? Was she too hasty in scolding him? Could she have achieved her ends by a loving request rather than by a hasty rebuke? Was it because he was tired? Did she insist on obedience or on a particular line of action to satisfy her own pride? Was her request reasonable for a child of his age who was engaged in a fascinating game which he did not want to stop? Many tantrums arise as a result of unreasonable insistence on something which does not matter. Discipline and obedience are essential, but they must be reasonable. There is no doubt that the greater the parental wisdom, patience, common sense, tact and sense of humour, the rarer will be the temper tantrums.

Finally, when a vicious circle has developed as a result of maternal fatigue and loss of patience, the best immediate solution to the problem may be a short holiday for the mother away from the child, if that can be arranged. She will come back rejuvenated and rested and better able to deal with her exuberant children. Far too many mothers never have a chance to get away from their offspring and a stage comes when each gets on the nerves of the other.

The Dummy

I have been unable to obtain information about the history of the Dummy—termed by some the "Pacifier," "Comforter" or "Titty." A variant of the dummy is the Dormel, a glass or plastic bottle, containing rose hip syrup, golden syrup, glycerine, blackcurrant juice or sweetened water, with a teat which the child is left to suck on in his cot or pram.

The dummy is introduced in the first few weeks of life. The Newcastle team found that only 9 per cent. of babies had been weaned from it by the time of the first birthday. I have seen a child sucking a dummy while learning to swim in the public swimming baths. Newson and Newson, in their Nottingham survey, found that mothers, instead of merely throwing the dummy away, an act which they considered cruel, would scold, ridicule or smack older toddlers for using a dummy.

The dummy is a feature of lower social class mothering. Newson and Newson[15] found that 65 per cent. of 709 Nottingham mothers provided their babies with a dummy; and that 74 per cent. of mothers in social class 5, but only 39 per cent. of those in social classes 1 and 2, provided a dummy. The Newcastle Thousand Families survey's figures[19] were comparable—81 per cent. for social class 5, as compared with 23 per cent. of social classes 1 and 2, the overall figure being 62 per cent. of 967 families. Newson and Newson found that middle-class mothers tended to be ashamed of using the dummy, and to be embarrassed by it, concealing it or aggressively defending it. Spence et al., in the Newcastle survey, wrote "In our frequent visits to the homes we have seen it (the dummy) in the infant's mouth, resting on the shelf, trailing over the side of the pram, hiding beneath the sofa or the kitchen table, and, often with a preliminary suck by the mother, returned to the baby's mouth."

Theoretically, one would anticipate that the dummy would be responsible for introducing infections into the mouth and alimentary tract, though it is difficult to see why it should be responsible for more infection than the child's own fingers, which he sucks. I know of no study which relates the incidence of stomatitis to the use of the dummy. The Newcastle survey found that babies with dummies suffered no more gastroenteritis than did those without. They did find that the dummy was used more by mothers who were unable to cope effectively with their infants.

The dummy does great harm to the teeth if it is soaked in a sweet substance, or if it is used as a dormel, leading to gross caries of the incisor teeth. It does not cause permanent malplacement of the teeth.

A dummy may cause a palatal ulcer if the dummy collapses, the hard plastic central core damaging the palate.

There is no evidence other than the above that the dummy is harmful. There is no need to take active steps to persuade a mother to discard the dummy. The toddler or older child looks absurd when running about the street sucking a dummy. Sucking a dummy does seem to provide some comfort to the baby, but it should never be regarded as a good substitute for picking the baby up and loving him. There is little to be said for the use of a dummy, and little against it (except when it is used in conjunction with a sweet substance). Its use is firmly established in the lower class.

Breath-holding Attacks

Breath-holding attacks are closely related to temper tantrums. They occur any time from 1 year to 5 years of age, but the great majority begin in the first 18 months. They are rare before 6 months and after 5 years. In a minor form they are fairly common; in the severest form, which is associated with major convulsions, they are rare. Affected children are almost exclusively of normal intelligence.[12] There is commonly a family history of the same complaint.

Hippocrates described an attack as follows: "The onset may be from some mysterious terror or a fright from somebody shouting, or in the midst of crying the child is not able quickly to recover his breath, as often happens to children; but when any of these things happens to him, at once the body is chilled, he becomes speechless, does not draw his breath, the breathing fails, the brain stiffens, the blood is at a standstill."

The attack is caused by pain, anger, thwarting or punishment. It may be due to a toy being snatched from him by another child or to an unsuccessful attempt to get a toy from him. It may be due to insistence of the parents that he should put his toys away, or to their refusal to allow him to do something which he has set his heart on.

Some children have the attacks only when they experience pain, as from a fall or knock, or fear. It is certainly not true to say that they are purely and simply a behaviour problem, though some may be. Pet monkeys have been said to have breath-holding attacks when infuriated by being kept in a cage.

There are two types of attack—the cyanotic or the pallid types.[9,13] The cyanotic type is more likely to be due to thwarting, the pallid type to pain. In the cyanotic type the child utters two or three loud cries and then holds the breath in expiration. In trivial cases the apnœa lasts 5 or 10 seconds, he becomes blue and then promptly recovers. In slightly more severe cases the breath is held for an additional 5–10 seconds, he becomes severely cyanosed and loses consciousness, becoming pale and limp. He may fall. There is then a feeble cry followed by more vigorous crying, and after a few moments of confusion he is his normal self again, though an occasional child may sleep after an attack. If the apnœa is prolonged for more than 30 seconds or so the child develops generalized rigidity and has a major convulsion indistinguishable from epilepsy. There is a marked bradycardia in the attacks. There may be only one attack in his life or they may frequently recur. I have seen children have several attacks in a day. If no treatment is given they tend to occur at less and less frequent intervals and disappear by about the fourth birthday. If they are due to pain they are less likely to be repeated than if they are due to a behaviour problem, unless undue fuss is made of them, when they will continue as an attention-seeking device. Livingston[12] studied 242 cases; eighty-seven had one or more a day, thirty-three had less than one a month. In all but three the attacks disappeared by 5, and in the remaining three at 6. Electro-encephalograms are normal. In the pallid variety, the child, immediately after experiencing some discomfort, becomes pale and limp and falls or becomes unconscious, without a preceding cyanotic phase, and usually without a preceding cry. The attack closely resembles a faint.

The mechanism of the attacks was discussed by Gauk[3,4] and Sharpey Schafer and his co-workers.[18] The latter workers, describing similar attacks in schoolboys and adults brought about voluntarily as a trick, concluded that the unconsciousness is due to the drop of blood pressure caused by the increased intrathoracic pressure due to breath-holding in expiration. Sharpey Schafer pointed out that, amongst other actions, over-ventilation increases muscle blood flow and increases cerebral vascular resistance. Breath-holding in expiration then causes a greater than normal drop in effective cerebral blood pressure and, since the cerebral vascular resistance is simultaneously increased, a considerable drop in cerebral blood flow results. The cerebral anoxæmia then causes unconsciousness and possibly convulsions. That the kink cannot be due to spasm of the glottis was well shown by Gauk et al.[3,4] who described a case of breath-holding attacks in a child with a tracheotomy. A study by Holowach and Thurston[5] indicated that there is a strong association between breath-holding attacks and anæmia. The reason for the association is unknown. The finding does indicate that one should have a hæmoglobin estimation carried out on all children with breath-holding attacks. If anæmia is found, it should be treated.

The differential diagnosis is important. As the attacks are rarely seen by the doctor, the diagnosis rests essentially on a careful history. The orderly and rather slow sequence of events in the breath-holding

attack, a few cries after a known precipitating factor, followed b
breath-holding in expiration, the rapid onset of cyanosis, followed b
limpness and convulsion in that order, differ from epilepsy, in whic
fits rarely follow a precipitating factor, except occasionally over
ventilation. In epilepsy, the so-called epileptic cry before a convulsio
is unusual in children, and when it does occur it is usually differen
in nature from the child's ordinary cry. In epilepsy the clonic phas
is preceded not by limpness but a tonic phase, and cyanosis, instea
of preceding the onset of the fit, follows the beginning of the toni
spasm. The whole sequence of events in an epileptic fit is mucl
quicker. After an epileptic fit the child, instead of being just momen
tarily confused, is likely to fall asleep. Though many epileptic fits ar
short lasting, some may last for many minutes or even for hours
while breath-holding attacks never last longer than 2 or 3 minutes
It is by no means always easy to distinguish the two conditions.

If the attacks are due to pain, nothing can be done to prevent them
Otherwise the methods of prevention and treatment are the same a
those for temper tantrums. Drugs are of no value. When an attacl
occurs every effort must be made to prevent injury. There must be ;
minimum of fuss and interest in the event. A colleague found tha
attacks in his own child were effectively stopped by holding him upsid
down. A parent stopped attacks by blowing strongly into the face, o
pouring cold water over it. On no account must the child have hi
own way as a result of the attack. Some adopt the method of giving
the child a sound slap as soon as breath-holding is observed, and there
is much to be said for this. It must be admitted that whatever the line
of treatment, the attacks may persist for a time, gradually becoming
less frequent and finally ceasing. They are not easy to stop.

References

1. BLAIR, R. G. (1965). "Vagitus Uterinus." *Lancet*, **2**, 1164.
2. FORMBY, D. (1967). "Maternal Recognition of Infant's Cry." *Develop. Med*
   Child Neurol., **9**, 293.
3. GAUK, E. W., KIDD, L., PRICHARD, J. S. (1963). "Mechanism of Seizure
   Associated with Breath-holding Spells." *New Engl. J. Med.*, **268**, 1436.
4. GAUK, E. W., KIDD, L., PRICHARD, J. S. (1966). "Aglottic Breath-holding
   Spells." *New Engl. J. Med.*, **275**, 1361.
5. HOLOWACH, J., THURSTON, D. L. (1963). "Breath-holding Spells and Anemia."
   New Engl. J. Med., **268**, 21.
6. ILLINGWORTH, R. S. (1955). "Crying in Infants and Children." *Brit. med. J.*
   1, 75.
7. KARELITZ, S., FISICHELLI, V. R. (1969). "Infants' Vocalisations and their
   Significance." *Clin. Proc. Children's Hospital of District of Columbia*, **25**, 345.
8. KING, H. L., BOURGEOIS, G. A. (1947). "Vagitus Uterinus." *Bull. U.S. Army*
   med. Dep., **7**, 147.
9. LAXDAL, T., GOMEZ, M. R., REIHER, J. (1969). "Cyanotic and Pallid Syncopa
   Attacks in Children (breath holding spells)." *J. Pediat.*, **75**, 755.

10. LIND, J., WASZ-HOCKERT, O., VUORENKOSKI, V., VALENNE, E. (1965). "The Vocalization of a Newborn Brain-damaged Child." *Ann. Pædiat. Fenn.*, 11, 32.
11. LIPTON, E. L., STEINSCHNEIDER, A., RICHMOND, J. B. (1965). "Swaddling, A Child Care Practice. Historical, Cultural and Experimental Observations." *Pediat. Suppl.*, 35, 521.
12. LIVINGSTON, S. (1970). "Breath-holding Spells in Children." *J. Am. Med. Ass.*, 212, 2231.
13. LOMBROSO, L. T., LERMAN, P. (1967). "Breath-holding Spells. Cyanotic and Pallid Infantile Syncope." *Pediatrics*, 39, 563.
14. McCLANE, M., quoted by Clouston, E. C. T. (1933). *Brit. med. J.*, 1, 200.
15. NEWSON, J., NEWSON, E. (1963). *Infant Care in an Urban Community.* London. Allen & Unwin.
16. RANK, quoted by Ruja, H. (1948). *J. Genet. Psychol.*, 73, 53.
17. SEGAL, H. (1964). *Introduction to the Work of Melanie Klein.* London. Heinemann.
18. SHARPEY-SCHAFER, E. P., HOWARD, P., LEATHART, G. L., DORNHURST, A. C. (1951). "The Mess Trick or Fainting Lark." *Brit. med. J.*, 2, 382.
19. SPENCE, J. C., WALTON, W. S., MILLER, F. J. W., COURT, S. D. M. (1954). *A Thousand Families in Newcastle-upon-Tyne.* London. Oxford University Press.
20. WASZ-HOCKERT, O., VALANNE, E., VOURENKOSKI, V., MICHELSSON, K., SOVIJARVI, A. (1963). "Analysis of Some Types of Vocalisation in the Newborn." *Annales Paed. Fenniae.*, 2, 1.
21. WOLFF, P. H. (1969). "The Natural History of Crying and Other Vocalisations in Early Infancy" in Foss, B. M., *Determinants of Infant Behaviour.* Vol. 4. London. Methuen.

CHAPTER 25

BODY MANIPULATIONS

Finger and Thumb Sucking

All children suck their fingers or thumbs at one time or another. A few suck their toes. Some suck part of the wrist or forearm. The sucking may be so frequent that soreness or callus formation occurs. It is said that bullae have been seen on the wrist or fingers in new-born babies as a result of intrauterine sucking.[25] The act is often associated with ear pulling, hair pulling or twisting, handling of the genitals, or with rubbing the nose or chin on some soft fabric or doll, or with sucking the blanket. Finger sucking occurs in baby monkeys.

There is a surprisingly extensive literature on the subject. Views expressed as to its ætiology differ considerably. Gesell[9,10] considered that it is a developmental phenomenon. Most babies suck their fingers in the new-born period. There is then a lull in the activity until the child can voluntarily take his fingers to his mouth at about 3 months of age. When he can grasp objects voluntarily, at about 5 months of age, he takes everything to his mouth, for the mouth becomes the exploratory organ and it is natural that his fingers should go to it.

Finger sucking is apt to be associated with hunger, shyness, teething, fatigue and sleep. It may disappear at 5 months, only to reappear when each new tooth comes. The child is then seen to rub the affected part of the gum with his fingers and then to suck them. About half of all babies suck their fingers at 1 year of age—some much more than others. Finger sucking is apt to reach its peak between 18 and 21 months. It is apt to become associated with sleep, and the insertion of fingers into the mouth may actually induce sleep. The child who is wearing gloves out of doors may, when tired, remove his gloves so that he can suck his fingers and then fall asleep. The association with sleep becomes less marked by about 3. Whereas previously he had sucked his fingers throughout the night, by 3 or so he may merely suck his fingers when about to go to sleep.

Freud[9] wrote: "Thumb sucking is a model of the infantile sexual manifestations. ... No investigator has yet doubted the sexual nature of this action. ... The child does not make use of a strange object for sucking, but prefers its own skin, because it is more convenient, because it thus makes itself independent of the outer world which it cannot yet control, and because in this way it creates for itself, as it were, a second even if an inferior erogenous zone. The inferiority of this second region urges it later to seek the same parts, the lips of another woman. ('It is a pity that I cannot kiss myself' might be attributed to it.)" Melanie Klein[14] explained thumb sucking in a 6-year-old child who was being psycho-analysed as being due to "phantasies of sucking, biting and devouring her father's penis and her mother's breasts. The penis represented the whole father, and the breasts the whole mother." According to English and Pearson[6] the cause of much of the unnecessary alarm in parents is that they unconsciously realize the connection with masturbation, and their own early conflict with masturbation is brought to the surface.

Levy[20] thought that the most important ætiological factor is insufficiency of sucking experience in feeding. He found that there was more often a history of spontaneous withdrawal from a too rapidly flowing breast or bottle, or forced withdrawal from sucking at the end of a set period of time, in thumb suckers than in controls. They had a longer interval between feeds and a shorter feeding time than controls. In the controls there were more unscheduled untimed feeds, more frequent feeds and more frequent night feeds, and there was a greater use of dummies. He could find no relation between the type of feeding—breast or bottle. He showed[18,19] that when the feeding of animals was interfered with before satiety was reached, corresponding sucking habits developed. Dogs would lick the paw or body of another dog and suck various inanimate objects. Calves licked the ears of other calves, painted boards, clothes or other objects. Chicks pecked excessively. Puppies fed from nipples with large holes, so that the sucking time was short, acquired vicarious sucking habits to a greater extent than puppies fed from nipples with small holes. Margaret Mead[24] wrote: "In most primitive societies of which we have any knowledge children are suckled whenever they cry; as a result infants seldom cry for more than a few minutes, unless they are sick. This suckling at any time seems to have one important result—no primitive child whom I have ever seen or heard of sucks its thumb or fingers." Freeden,[8] on the other hand, after 10 years' experience of feeding babies by cup from the new-born period onwards, found that there was no greater incidence of thumb sucking than in those fed on the breast or bottle.

Spock,[29] probably rightly, thought that no one explanation is sufficient for all cases, and suggests that the ætiology may vary with the age. In the younger age group the satisfaction of the sucking instinct may be of importance, whereas after the first birthday insecurity and boredom may be important factors, though he agreed with Gesell that the finger sucking in connection with sleep is probably related to neither, but is merely a developmental phenomenon. It seems to me that not all finger sucking is related to insufficient sucking experience. Two children in a family fed in precisely the same way on the breast may differ considerably in the extent of their finger sucking. There are probably constitutional factors which govern the amount of finger sucking in which children indulge. It might be supposed that Nature made sucking a pleasant occupation so that babies would suck to keep themselves alive. It would then be expected that babies would enjoy sucking the nipple, bottle or thumb, and that they would suck the thumb or other object when tired, bored or unhappy.

Prognosis

Bragman[4] and Mazzini[23] found thumb sucking in various paintings and sculptures of Italian masters of the early Renaissance. As Kanner[1] wrote, the notion that it is bad and harmful did not arise till the end of the nineteenth century. Alarmists then stated that thumb sucking causes scoliosis, enlargement of the tonsils and adenoids, flatulence and colic, dental caries, digestive disorders in adult life and changes in facial expression. It was commonly believed that the habit was the cause of severe malocclusion.

Sillman[24] took serial casts from impressions of upper and lower jaws from birth to 14 years in 60 children, 20 of whom were thumb suckers. The habit did cause some deformity of the jaws, but by the age of 4 it had corrected itself. He thought that hereditary factors were more important in governing the development of oral structures. Gardiner[10] at Sheffield showed that in a survey of 1,000 unselected school children, only 14 per cent. did in fact have a deformity of the teeth as a result of thumb sucking after the age of 5. Lewis[21] in a study of 170 children over a 5-year period, found that in 24 or 30 thumb suckers there was some malocclusion of the deciduous teeth, but that if the habit was stopped before the age of 6 the deformity corrected itself spontaneously. Freud[9] claimed that "children in whom this (thumb sucking) is retained are habitual kissers as adults and show a tendency to perverse kissing, or as men they have a marked desire for drinking and sucking."

Treatment

In the past a wide variety of ingenious mechanical devices was used to stop thumb sucking. It is unanimously agreed now that no devices should be used, at least until the age of 5 or 6. They cause considerable psychological disturbance in the child and do nothing but harm.

In the new-born baby no treatment should be given, because it is normal. Nothing should be done in the first year to check the habit. In view of Levy's work some recommend that the duration of breast feeds should be lengthened, or that the hole in the teat should be made smaller so that sucking is prolonged. This would seem unwise, as such a measure might well cause flatulence and colic. After the age of a year thumb sucking associated with sleep or indulged in occasionally during the day is a harmless procedure, and the child will almost certainly grow out of it. No treatment should be given. Dental or other appliances should not be used. Bitter substances should not be painted on the fingers. A direct attack on the problem is useless.

When in a 2- or 3-year-old child the thumb sucking is excessive and occurs in the daytime as well as at night, or when thumb sucking starts after a long period without it, every effort should be made to determine the cause. If it is boredom the child should be kept occupied. If it is insecurity, repression or jealousy, the cause should be treated. On no account should threats or punishment be used. If a lot of fuss is made, the child may deliberately continue to suck the thumb as an attention-seeking device. By about 3 years of age a direct appeal can be made to him to stop it on the grounds that it is an infantile habit and that he is too old for it.

Over-enthusiastic efforts to stop thumb sucking do a great deal of harm. There is apt to be constant nagging and reprimands, which cause unhappiness, resentfulness and insecurity. Ridicule is always undesirable as a means of dealing with such problems. All ridicule, teasing, shaming and threats should be avoided. The danger of thumb sucking lies not in the thumb sucking but in what the parents do about it. It can cause some soreness of the thumb, but that is all.

The vast majority of thumb suckers grow out of the habit by the age of 5 or 6.

Nail Biting

According to Massler and Malone[22] nail biting does not occur before the age of 3. This is not true, but it is not a common habit in the first 3 years. I have seen it in a 15-month-old child. Billig,[2] in a 90-page review, wrote that it usually begins between the ages of 8 and 10. Of 346 boys in Chicago aged 8 to 11,[22] two out of three were nail biters. In another study 44 per cent. of boys and girls aged 12 to 14 were biting their nails at the time of examination. Similar figures were given by Birch.[3] He found that 51 per cent. of 4,000 school children in South Yorkshire were biting their nails at the time of examination.

Although these figures apply to the older child, they are quoted here because they suggest that the popular idea that nail biting is always a manifestation of insecurity seems hardly tenable. It is true that children (and adults) often begin to bite their nails when nervous, tense, or in deep thought. It may be learned from another child. According to Billig[2] nail biters are nonconformists. "The nail biting is a form of revolt at having to comply." Wechsler[30] wrote that "it is nothing but a particular form of unconscious masturbating activity, a symptom of an incompletely resolved œdipus situation."

An American expert wrote[12] that it is "a means of oral gratification, and or a form of unconscious masturbating activity that carried with it the punishment (cutting off) which this tabooed act called for. ... By biting the claws oral sadistic impulses are released. ... Guilt is expiated by the infliction of pain upon the self." I know of no evidence which supports these psycho-analytical theories.

It is commonly said that nail biting starts as condemned thumb sucking. I very much doubt this. The sort of mother who vigorously condemns thumb sucking might well be likely to have the sort of child who later bites his nails.

Nail biting itself does no harm, but the attitude towards it certainly may.

Punishment and restraining devices will do nothing but harm. It must be treated by distracting the child when he is biting the nails, attending to any cause of insecurity, and seeing that the child is fully occupied. In the older pre-school child, an appeal to his pride may help. Ridicule and teasing never works.

Nail picking This is a habit similar to nail biting, and on inspection of the finger or toe nails it is probably impossible to distinguish the two. It is of no importance.

Lip Biting

Kravitz[15] found that 94·3 per cent. of 177 normal infants bit their lip. The average age of onset was 4·8 months, and it usually ceased by 10 months. It usually ceased with the appearance of the mandibular central or lateral incisors. Kravitz suggested that lip biting may be a specific sign of teething.

Rocking

Rocking in the bed begins especially between the age of 5 and 10 months. It usually stops after one or two months, but may last for many months. Some children cause their cots to disintegrate by the constant rocking. It pleases them to find that they can rock the cot from one side of the room to the other. It is a difficult habit to stop. If a soft rug is placed under the cot, it may help by reducing the pleasing vibrations. It is useful to move an older child with this complaint from a cot into a bed. In an intractable case the child may be put into a hammock. Body rocking is sometimes a feature of the mentally defective child, especially if there has been previous restriction of movement.[7]

Head Rolling

Head rolling is practically confined to the first 3 years. It may cause the hair of the back of the head to be worn off. It is of no importance and no particular treatment helps.

Spasmus Nutans

This condition occurs in normal children and is not associated with any known disease or with malnutrition. It has been reviewed by Norton and Cogan.[26] It is characterized by head nodding, anomalous head positions and nystagmus. The head nodding is usually an irregular horizontal movement, but the movement may consist of turning or tilting. The frequency is about 1 to 2 per second. The movements decrease with efforts to fix the eyes on an object, and disappear in sleep, or if the eyes are bandaged.

The nystagmus is always asymmetrical in the two eyes, and varies with different positions of gaze. It is lateral, vertical or rotary in type. It is a fine rapid nystagmus, and it is increased by forced fixation of the head. It may be associated with a convergent strabismus. There is a tendency to look at objects out of the corner of the eyes, with the head partly flexed. The nystagmus is more constant than the head nodding, and is usually the last sign to subside.

The onset is usually between the fourth and twelfth month. It is rarely seen after the second year, but may last up to 8 years. There is no particular sex or familial incidence, and there is no relationship to mental deficiency or rickets. It is usually said that it is due to poor lighting conditions, but this is thought now to be untrue. The cause of the condition is unknown. No treatment is of value.

Head Banging

This occurs particularly in the child aged 7–12 months when put to bed. The head is banged against the mattress, top of the bed or other hard object. It occurs in perfectly normal children as well as in mentally retarded ones. Head banging sometimes occurs during sleep. A mother of a head banger told me that her child seemed to find some strange solace in head banging, and that he banged his head instead of sucking a dummy. It may be a manifestation of insecurity or an attention-seeking mechanism, particularly if the parents show great anxiety about it and try forcible means of stopping it. It is a relatively harmless pursuit which usually stops spontaneously between the age

of 2 and 3 years, and no treatment is either advisable or necessary.
In severe cases head banging in bed can be cured by putting the child
into a hammock, but head banging involving furniture can be difficult
to stop.

A rhesus monkey developed head banging after liberation from
early social and visual deprivation.[17] Various workers[5] found that head
banging was sometimes related to discomfort from a wet nappy, otitis
media, teething, or thwarting, as from removal of a favourite toy.

According to De Lissovoy,[5] 27 out of 33 children bang their heads
primarily at bedtime. Fourteen out of the 19 stopped at or before
the fourth year, but in the remainder it continued into school age. All
the children had shown other rhythmical activities, such as head or
body rolling, prior to head banging. "Sessions" lasted $\frac{1}{2}$ to 4 hours.
The number of "head bangings" ranged from 19 to 121 per minute.

There have been several papers on a late sequela of prolonged head-
banging, namely cataracts.[28] It is said that many head bangers develop
cataracts in adolescence or adult life, years after cessation of the symptom. Ophthalmological inspection of a group of head bangers in an
instititution showed that the majority had cataracts. It is suggested that
periodical ophthalmological examination is desirable for chronic head
bangers.

Hair Plucking

This is sometimes called trichotillomania. It is apt to occur when
the child feels frustrated or angry. It may be associated with finger
sucking. When the cause has been removed and the act is ignored the
habit stops.

Hair plucking is sometimes a feature of Pink disease (erythrœdema).

Ear Pulling and Tongue Sucking

These are similar habits. The tongue sucker twists the tongue
round the mouth with a loud sucking noise. The practices are harmless
and disappear spontaneously.

Tooth Grinding

Though more frequent in mentally defective children or in children
seriously ill with a disease such as tuberculous meningitis, it may occur
in normal children. In such a case it is likely to be an attention-seeking
device, perpetuated by the anxiety which parents show about it. It
also occurs in sleep. No treatment can or should be given. If it is
ignored it will stop.

Masturbation

Levine and Bell[16] quoted Vogel (1890) as writing that "Boys who masturbate become visibly emanciated and anæmic, remain backward in their bodily and mental development, the integument of the lower eyelid turns to a brownish or bluish colour; they develop an apathetic expression of the countenance and flaccid muscles. They become indifferent to amusements which they once enjoyed and withdraw from all society, preferring to be alone, in order to indulge their passion. The gait becomes unsteady and lumbersome and the knees fall inward. The emaciation is most strikingly seen in the lower extremities and lumbar region, while the penis increases disproportionately in length and thickness. Tabes dorsalis and paralysis of the lower extremities are occasional though rare effects of this practice."

They described drastic methods of treatment advocated 50 years ago. They include cauterization of the clitoris, blistering of the vulva or prepuce, and sending the child away from home.

Masturbation is practised at all ages, but it is rare before the age of 5 months. It must be distinguished from simple non-rhythmic manipulation of the genitals which is not accompanied by any excitement or evidence of particular satisfaction. It is natural that when a child learns to grasp objects, at about 5 months, he should grasp the penis. This is often thought by mothers to be wrong and efforts are made to try to stop it. They think that it is dreadful for the child to touch his genitals, although they themselves try to retract his foreskin in bathing him, and in the girl they clean the vulva. The less attention which is paid to such manipulations the sooner they will stop.

True masturbation is another matter. In the infant it is usually practised by rubbing the thighs together. This is often achieved by a variety of rocking movements—rhythmic elevation of the pelvis in the supine position, or rocking back and forth on hands and knees in the prone. This begins any time after the age of 5 or 6 months. It may be associated with head banging and is often particularly noticed at bedtime. A little later the child may learn to rub the genital area against the arm of a chair or against part of the play pen. Rhythmic manipulation of the genitals by the hand rarely occurs before the age of $2\frac{1}{2}$.

In all these rhythmic activities the child's face may become flushed while doing it, and the sweating of the face, fixed eyes, and sometimes pallor, with the bodily contortion, may well lead to a diagnosis of epilepsy. It frequently arises as a result of some local irritation, such as vulvovaginitis, pruritus from threadworm infection, balanitis, napkin rash or eczema. It could arise from excessive handling of the genitals by the mother when washing the child. It is also learnt by imitation of others. Bergman[1] offered various other explanations. He wrote "He may masturbate because he wants to call another person's attention to the excellent little organ he owns. He may do it because he wants to shock or irritate or shame the other person. Or he may want to convince himself that he can still produce pleasure in himself in spite of some frightening experience he may have undergone. He may wish to reassure himself that his organ is all right in spite of the fact that it is different from the organ he has noticed in the other sex. He may try to transform his organ into that of the other sex. He may have nothing else to do and resort to masturbation because of boredom. He may feel unhappy in his interpersonal relationship and console himself with masturbation. Masturbation may give a child the feeling of strength he needs to be stubborn and hostile towards his parents."

The practice is carried out quite openly unless the mother has scolded the child for it, when it is practised in secret. Mothers are apt to be shocked by seeing their child masturbate and smack him hard, threaten that his penis will fall off or that something dreadful will happen to him. On no account should he be scolded, frightened or threatened. It is a mistake to "catch him" in the act and then try to shame him. He should simply be distracted as soon as it is seen and nothing should be said to him about it, the actual act being ignored. Any local cause of itching must be removed. There should on no account be any fuss about it. If there is it will be prolonged as an attention-seeking device.

In severe cases it is important to try to find the cause of the problem. It is likely to be due to worry or insecurity, and it has almost certainly been exaggerated and perpetuated by parental efforts to stop it.

It is essential to treat parental attitudes, for it is those attitudes and the resultant actions which do the harm, rather than the actual masturbation. The parents must be made to understand that all children do it at one time or another and that their child is not therefore a sexual pervert. They must have their fears allayed that he will develop insanity, epilepsy or other disease.

References

1. BERGMAN, P. (1946). "Neurotic Anxieties in Children and their Prevention." *The Nervous Child*, **5**, 37.
2. BILLIG, A. L. (1954). "Finger Nail Biting—Its Incipiency, Incidence and Amelioration." *Genet. Psychol. Monogr.*, **24**, 125.
3. BIRCH, L. B. (1955). "The Incidence of Nailbiting among Schoolchildren." *Brit. J. Educ. Psychol.*, **25**, 123.
4. BRAGMAN, L. L., quoted by Kanner, L. (1948). *Child Psychiatry*. Springfield. Charles Thomas.
5. DE LISSOVOY, V. (1962). "Head Banging in Early Childhood." *Child Development*, **33**, 43.

6. ENGLISH, O. S., PEARSON, G. H. (1937). *Common Neuroses of Children and Adults.* New York. Norton.
7. FOREHAND, R., BAUMEISTER, A. A. (1970). "Body Rocking and Activity Level as a Function of Prior Movement Restraint." *Am. J. Ment. Def.*, **74**, 608.
8. FREEDEN, R. C. (1948). "Cup Feeding of Newborn Infants." *Pediatrics*, **2**, 544.
9. FREUD, S. (1938). *Three Contributions to the Theory of Sex.* New York. The Modern Library.
10. GARDINER, J. H. (1961). "The Care of Children's Teeth." *Practitioner*, **187**, 196.
11. GESELL, A., ILG, F. L. (1943). *Infant and Child in the Culture of Today.* New York. Harper.
12. *Journal of Am. Med. Ass.* (1962). "Nailbiting." **162**, 1066.
13. KANNER, L. (1938). "Thumbsucking." *J. Pediat.*, **13**, 422.
14. KLEIN, M. (1937). *The Psychoanalysis of Children.* London. Hogarth.
15. KRAVITZ, H. (1964). "Lip Biting in Infancy." *J. Pediat.*, **65**, 136.
16. LEVINE, M. I., BELL, A. I. (1956). "The Psychological Aspects of Medical Practice." *Pediatrics*, **18**, 803.
17. LEVINSON, C. A. (1970). "The Development of Head Banging in a Young Rhesus Monkey." *Am. J. Ment. Def.*, **75**, 323.
18. LEVY, D. M. (1928). "Finger Sucking and Accessory Movements in Early Infancy." *Amer. J. Psychiat.*, **84**, 881.
19. LEVY, D. M. (1934). "Experiments on the Sucking Reflex and Social Behavior of Dogs." *Amer. J. Orthopsychiat.*, **4**, 203.
20. LEVY, D. M. (1935). "A Note on Pecking in Chickens." *Psychoanal. Quart.*, **4**, 612.
21. LEWIS, S. J. (1930). "Thumbsucking—A Cause of Malocclusion in the Deciduous Teeth." *J. Amer. Dent. Ass.*, **17**, 1060.
22. MASSLER, M., MALONE, A. J. (1950). "Nailbiting, a Review." *J. Pediat.*, **36**, 523.
23. MAZZINI, quoted by Kanner, L. (1948). *Child Psychiatry.* Springfield. Charles Thomas.
24. MEAD, M. (1933). In Murchison, C., *A Handbook of Child Psychology.* Worcester. Clark University Press.
25. MURPHY, W. F., LANGLEY, A. L. (1963). "Bullae Due to Intrauterine Sucking." *Pediat.*, **32**, 1095.
26. NORTON, E. W. D., COGAN, D. G. (1954). "Spasmus Nutans." *Amer. med. Ass. Arch. Ophthal.*, **52**, 442.
27. SILMAN, J. H. (1957). "Thumbsucking and the Oral Structures." *J. Pediat.*, **39**, 424.
28. SPALTER, H. F., BEMPORAD, J. R., SOURS, J. A. (1970). "Cataracts Following Head Banging in Autistic Children." *Arch. Ophthalm.*, **83**, 182.
29. SPOCK, B. (1946). *Baby and Child Care.* New York. Pocket Books Inc.
30. WECHSLER, D. (1931). "The Incidence and Significance of Finger Nail Biting in Children." *Psychoanal. Rev.*, **18**, 201.

CHAPTER 26

JEALOUSY, FEARS, SHYNESS AND MISCELLANEOUS PROBLEMS

Jealousy

Jealousy is a normal reaction which most normal children feel at one time or another. As Ziman[31] wrote in his excellent book on the subject, "Children are jealous as a matter of course. It is normal and proper and to be expected." Some of the manifestations of jealousy are obscure, and parents, not realizing this, are apt wrongly to think that their children have never shown jealousy. Jealousy is not a problem unless it is mismanaged.

Ætiology

The child fears that he is losing something which he had before—love, a feeling that he is important and that he is wanted. It is greatly exaggerated by anything which causes a feeling of insecurity—a feeling that he might lose his mother's love, that he might be deserted. Such feelings arise from any of the causes of insecurity—over-protection, excessive domination, parental impatience and irritability, domestic friction or indiscipline. They are especially liable to occur if the mother has ever been foolish enough to threaten to leave the child if he will not do what she wants him to do, or if she has been in the habit of leaving him a great deal. In a child rendered insecure in this way problems of jealousy are precipitated by the arrival of a new baby, and more still by what he rightly or wrongly interprets as loss of love and interest in him. He has already had a foretaste of what is to come when he was moved out of the bedroom which he loved so much to make way for the baby, and when later he was sent away from home to some people he did not know while his mother was in hospital. The mother on arrival home has little time for her first-born. She is tired and therefore irritable, when the latter, feeling the first pangs of jealousy, is more than usually demanding of her love. Tactless friends come and admire the baby and bring him presents, not saying a word to the 2- or 3-year-old, who till then has held the centre of the stage. The more stupid ones make jokes to the older child about his feeling put out by the new baby. It so happens that the second baby is apt to come just at the time that the first one is passing through a phase of increased dependence on the mother. According to Levy, the larger the age difference between one child and the next the less likely is jealousy to occur.

When the child is a little older, there are new ways in which the older child is made to feel that he has lost his parents' love. The father, when he comes home from work, may make the mistake of always picking up the younger one. The child is apt to be constantly warned not to touch the baby or to be careful not to hurt him. The baby snatches toys from the first-born's hands, and when the latter protests there is a chorus of reprimands from the parents. It is difficult for the parents to do anything else but come to the defence of the little one and to punish the older child for acts which are ignored in his young brother, for the simple reason that the brother is not old enough to understand that they are wrong. It is difficult for the older child to understand this difference in treatment, and he is apt to feel hurt and upset as a result. There is no doubt that the first-born's discovery that he is not the only one is painful and does cause a considerable emotional disturbance. The disturbance is all the greater if he has not been accustomed to mixing with other children and if he has been given all his own way.

Comparisons with siblings are a potent cause of ill-feeling in the home. The mother says, "John does not cry when he falls"; "John would never do a thing like that"; "Watch John and see how he eats." Not only does this sort of remark produce enmity between the children, but it leads to a feeling of insecurity, inferiority or rebellion. The little girl who is compelled to wear the clothes of her elder sister is apt to feel jealous when her sister has new clothes in place of the discarded ones. When the 3-year-old is taken with his baby brother into a restaurant or other public place, people admire and talk to the baby and never speak a word to him. The child may be jealous of his parents if they constantly caress each other in his presence and leave him out. The boy is apt to rush up and demand to be cuddled too.

The younger child may feel jealous when his older sibling first goes to school (and the older child may feel jealous when his younger sibling starts at school—the older one realizing that he is no longer quite so important as he was).

The importance of favouritism has already been discussed. If one child is more advanced than another in the family, jealousy is apt to occur. Jealousy in twins may be troublesome.

Manifestations

The manifestations of jealousy may be obvious, but there are frequently occult signs and symptoms of emotional disturbance which only the most discerning can ascribe with confidence to underlying jealousy. When a child hits the new baby on the head or fusses when the baby or another child is picked up, it is not difficult to see that he is jealous. But when, shortly after the baby's arrival, he reverts to infantile behaviour, sucking his thumb again, wetting the bed, demanding to be fed, talking baby talk and constantly asks to be carried, or when he becomes quarrelsome and aggressive with his friends, becoming destructive and negative again, the cause of the behaviour may not be obvious. Observation of a girl's play with her dolls and of her conversation with them may give the mother a clue to the real nature of the disorders. The child cannot express his feelings in words, but his feelings are there and various behaviour disorders result. He may react, in fact, by any of the manifestations of insecurity.

When jealousy becomes a serious problem and is allowed to continue, it may well have a permanent effect on the child's character, leading to aggressiveness, selfishness or an inferiority complex, which he will carry with him for the rest of his life and which will in time affect the character of his children.

Prevention

The most important preventive for jealousy is love, understanding and security with judicious discipline. When a new baby is expected, plans calculated to prevent undue jealousy should be made early in the pregnancy. The child should not start at a nursery school at the time of the baby's arrival, move from one bedroom to another to make way for the baby, or move from the cot to a bed. These changes should be made long before the birth of the baby. He should be allowed to help in shopping for the baby and be given money with which to buy necessary objects for it. When the mother goes to hospital it is better in general for the child to stay at home as long as there is someone whom he likes to look after him. Otherwise he should go to a relative whom he loves. It would certainly be a mistake to leave him in the hands of strangers, if this could be avoided. When the baby is brought home the importance of the child's first impressions should be remembered. The whole house is apt to revolve around the new arrival. Though inevitable, it should be minimized, and on no account should the older child feel that no one has any time for him. He should be encouraged to help in bathing the baby and changing the napkin and in fetching things for him. It is easy to overdo this, however, and so let the "helping" become an unpleasant duty. When he wants to play with the baby, the playing has to be supervised until he can be trusted not to hurt the baby, but parents are apt to issue so many admonitions and reprimands that he is reduced to tears or plays on his own. It is most desirable that the child should play with and get to love the baby. Jealousy then is much less likely to be a problem. When the mother picks the baby up, the father or other person should go out of his way to pick the older child up. Every possible effort should be made to ensure that the elder child is just as sure as he ever was that he is loved and wanted. Some parents go too far in their effort to prevent jealousy, and if giving a present to one child also give one to his sibling. This is undesirable. The children should feel so secure that if one child receives a present, the others know that in the course of time their turn will come.

Treatment

Half the battle is won when the parents understand the nature of the problem. They must on no account have a feeling of guilt that they have let the child down. They should realize that jealousy is not a crime, but that it is normal, and as long as it is managed with common sense and understanding it will not be a problem which will last. The whole management of the child has to be reviewed in order that the various manifestations of jealousy can be properly treated. All possible causes of jealousy have to be avoided. When an overt act of jealousy occurs it has to be treated wisely, or great harm can be done. When the child hits the baby he should not be unduly scolded or smacked, for punishment will merely make him worse and increase his feeling that he has lost his parents' love. The cause of the incident should be treated, not the symptom, and the cause is the child's fear that his mother no longer loves him. This fear must be attended to so that he is given that love and security which he needs. Smacking for bed wetting or other manifestations of jealousy would be equally harmful, for it would lead to greater insecurity. It is far better to try to prevent a child injuring the baby than to warn him or smack him after the act. He should be prevented from the act by distraction— by lifting him bodily away from temptation and giving him something interesting to do. Anything which contributes to the insecurity— anger, irritability, constant warnings and reprimands—must be avoided. Above all, there must be no favouritism and no comparisons with other children.

Fears

Probably all normal children have fears. Up to a point they are desirable, for a completely fearless child is particularly liable to become involved in accidents. Severely mentally defective children have practically no fear. Fears constitute a natural normal defence mechanism. It is only when they are exaggerated and anxiety develops that they are harmful.

It is always difficult to draw a line between normal and excessive fears. The infant in his first year is likely to show fear when there is a sudden noise, a sudden falling movement or when there is some sudden unexpected event which he cannot understand. At about 6 months he may show fear of strangers. Children between the ages of 2 and 3 characteristically develop fears of everyday objects—dogs, motor cars, the hole in the bath, the water-closet, noisy machines and darkness. During the phase of increased dependence on the parents, at about the same age, they may fear being deserted by their mother.

Ordinarily fears are not a problem in the first 3 years. They may become a problem if they are exaggerated by an underlying insecurity or by mismanagement by their parents.

The number and extent of fear reactions shown by children is governed in part by the sex and the personality of the child. Girls tend to show fear more than boys. Some show fear a great deal more than others. One factor is the child's imagination, the imaginative child being more apt to develop fear.

Ætiology

According to some workers, all fears are the result of suggestion. There is no doubt that many fears are suggested by adults. Caution has to be taught and used by parents and it is almost inevitable that some fear is engendered in a susceptible child as a result. This particularly applies to fear of motor cars, animals, fires and other hot objects. The parents may themselves show fear of thunder or of the dark, and the child by suggestion and imitation shows the same fear. Dislike of certain foodstuffs can readily be suggested by the parents if they express their own dislikes in front of a child. Fears may be caused by foolish threats made in an attempt to force him to eat, sleep or have the bowels moved. Fear of desertion is commonly suggested by stupid threats by the mother that if he does not do what she wants him to do she will go and leave him or send him away. Fears may be suggested by fairy stories which are unsuitable for his age or by other gruesome tales or pictures, particularly if he has a vivid imagination. Excessive shyness may almost amount to fear. It may result from his having been prevented from mixing with people outside his own home. He may show fear of objects and of noises when he is alone but not when he is in the presence of his mother. He feels unable to cope with the situation on his own. Fear may develop as a result of transference. Arlitt[4] described how in a party a paper napkin caught fire as a boy blew out the candles on his birthday cake. Thereafter the boy cried with fear whenever birthdays were mentioned. Fear may arise in the same way as a result of a fall from a tricycle. The child after such a fall may be afraid of all tricycles.

Gesell[10] thought that the role of suggestion is overdone. He emphasized the developmental aspect of fear, pointing out that the nature of fear stimuli is related to the child's developmental level and to the level of his experience. The child is afraid of those objects which his experience has not equipped him to cope with, so that objects, for instance, of which some immature 3-year-olds are afraid, have stopped frightening the more mature 2½-year-old, who has learned to cope with the situation in question.

There is no evidence that fears are inherited, but the personality which renders a child particularly likely to show fear because of his timidity or imaginativeness is largely a hereditary characteristic.

Prevention and Treatment

Fears cannot be entirely prevented, and in any case they may serve a useful purpose. Some excessive or undesirable fears can be prevented by care to avoid suggesting them. Still more important is the prevention of a feeling of insecurity by over-protection, domination and the other faults of management discussed elsewhere.

Fears cannot be stopped by teasing, ridicule, force or distraction. They are not stopped by reassuring the child (that a dog, for instance, will not hurt him), or by ignoring his fear. Children are not likely to forget their fears or to lose them by getting used to the feared objects. It is wrong to be impatient or unsympathetic with a child who is afraid. Such an attitude increases rather than decreases his fear, because he feels that he cannot rely on his parents for protection as much as he had hoped. It is wrong when a child is afraid of the dark to deprive him of a light in the hopes that he will get out of the fear. He should be given security, protection and reassurance. His fear is a real one to him and it should be respected. It is a good thing to try to let him become more familiar with the feared object. If he is afraid of the vacuum cleaner, he may be willing to play with some of the components and then with the machine as a whole. If he is afraid of water he should be encouraged to play with water with a bucket and ladle. If he is afraid of the dark he may play at putting the lights on and off. His natural imitativeness should be remembered. He should be enabled to see other children playing with the feared objects, such as a dog.

In every case the whole child must be treated. Children with excessive fears are often insecure, and as a result they show other behaviour problems. It is essential to review the whole of the management and to correct unwise parental attitudes. Most fears will be outgrown.

Shyness

Though all will agree that shyness is a common and important problem, there is a remarkable dearth of literature on the subject. It is not mentioned in the index of any of the books by Arnold Gesell referred to in the reference lists in this book.

Perhaps the first sign of shyness is at about 4 months of age, when the baby shows some coyness when spoken to by strangers. After his first birthday he tends to cover his eyes up with his forearm when spoken to, he becomes notably quiet, pulls faces and hides behind his mother. The child of 2 or 3 cries if his mother leaves him with other children. He fails to play either alongside or with other children, merely standing immobile, quiet and unhappy. He will not say a word when he is spoken to.

Shyness is partly an inherited characteristic, but it is also partly developmental and partly environmental in origin. Any parent of two or more children knows how one child is more shy than his brother, although there has been no known difference in the management of the two children. This difference is probably due to inherited character traits. It is also developmental in origin, for almost all children go through stages of shyness. Environment is obviously a factor. The child who is never given a chance to mix with others, adults and children, is likely to be shy.

Shyness can be partly prevented by allowing the child from earliest infancy constantly to mix with others. It can partly be prevented by wise upbringing in other directions—by giving him love, security and self-confidence and giving him a sense of pride in the skills which he has learnt.

Treatment is not easy. The causes must be treated. He must certainly not be ridiculed or scolded for his shyness. It is wrong to say anything at all about his shyness in front of him. It is stupid to tell him not to be shy. He cannot help it and ridicule can do nothing but harm. He should be allowed to have friends into his home at frequent intervals and he should go out to visit friends, at first with his mother. He should be encouraged to play alongside friends in the first place and not be pushed into playing with them. Above all, his shyness must be respected.

Stuttering

Johnson[14] made the remark that stuttering develops after the diagnosis has been made rather than before it. He considered it a consequence of the diagnosis. Some lay person—the parent, grandparent or neighbour—suggests that the child is beginning to stutter.

The parents become seriously concerned and do their utmost to check
it. They tell the child to take a deep breath before he speaks, to repeat
himself and to speak more slowly and distinctly. He becomes self-
conscious about his speech and it becomes forced and artificial instead
of natural. One is reminded of the story of the centipede:

> "The centipede was contented quite,
> Until the toad one day in spite
> Said, 'Say! which foot comes after which?'
> This so wrought upon her mind,
> She lay distracted in the ditch,
> Considering which came after which."

Johnson, at the Iowa Child Welfare Research Station,[14,15] became
interested in the normal repetitions made by children in learning
speech. He found in a large group of normal children that 15–25 per
cent. of their words figure in some sort of repetition. The initial sound
or syllable of the word is repeated, or the whole word is repeated, or the
word is part of a repeated phrase. Johnson considered that much
stuttering is caused by the diagnosis being made as a result of failure
to realize that such repetitions are normal. Children from $2\frac{1}{2}$ years
onwards become so excited in recounting what they have seen that
they stumble over themselves in a torrent of words and stuttering is
suspected by the mother.

Elsewhere Johnson[14,15] made the following comment:

"The mass of data collected indicated that stutterers are really
no different from non-stutterers and that their speech is initially
perceived and evaluated differently, usually by a parent. The negative
evaluations and misconceptions of the adults are communicated to the
children, who then view their own speech in the same anxious and
rejecting manner."

Most children pass through the stage of stuttering—rapid, confused
and jumbled speech. They can speak clearly if they try. As long as
nothing is done about it they nearly all grow out of it. Perhaps half the
children in nursery schools pass through a stuttering stage, which
lasts a few days.

Stutterers speak normally when alone, or singing, or when talking
to animals or to people whom they know well. There may be more
stuttering when speaking to one parent than to the other. An emotional
upset often acts as a trigger and starts an episode of stuttering.

There is a voluminous literature about stuttering, and there is
little doubt that the problem is a highly complex one. A study of the
previous development of stutterers shows that they have tended to be
later in learning to walk than controls, and later in beginning to speak.
There is often a family history of speech disorder, and apart from

the hereditary factor a child may readily stutter in imitation of another member of the family. It is more common in boys than girls.

It is probably not related to handedness. It is more a behaviour problem than a speech defect. Eisenson[9] in an excellent review of speech difficulties, quoted various studies to the effect that stutterers tend to come from a home in which there is excessive domination and discipline, overprotection and perfectionism.

Andrews and Harris[1] found that 1 in 100 school children stutter. They found no relationship between stuttering and handedness, change of handedness, crossed laterality and ambidexterity. Of 80 stutterers, 56 were right handed, 21 ambidextrous and 3 left handed. Of 80 controls, 52 were right handed, 23 ambidextrous and 5 left handed.

The essential part of treatment is the relief of parental anxiety. The parents must be reassured about their child's speech. They must stop trying to make him speak distinctly. His diction should be ignored.

If he is still stuttering when he reaches his fourth birthday, he should have speech therapy, because it is important that his speech should be normal by the time he reaches school. Some recommend earlier treatment. I would certainly not advise any treatment before 3 years.

Andrews and Harris[1] described their treatment of stuttering by "timed syllabic speech." They taught the children to separate syllables in speech equidistantly. Their results were good.

Tics

The term habit-spasm instead of tics, is not a good one, as tics are neither habits nor spasms. The common tics consist of blinking the eyes, wrinkling the forehead, rotating the head, or shrugging the shoulder, but a wide variety of other movements, some of them quite complex, may be seen. They are uncommon in the pre-school child. They disappear during sleep, and are increased by anxiety or tension. They are usually manifestations of insecurity. The peak age for their onset is 6 to 7 years.

Tics may lead to unpleasantness in the home, including conflict between parents, perfectionism with regard to their chldren, and quarrelling between parent and child. Mothers complain that they get on their nerves. Determined efforts by scolding and punishment are made to stop them, but they only aggravate matters and make them worse. They should be ignored completely. Any cause of insecurity should be removed. They tend to disappear when home conflicts resolve.[26]

It is wrong to say that all tics will disappear if ignored. They often do, but many tics last for years. Sometimes one tic disappears, only to be replaced by another.

Quarrelsomeness and Aggressiveness

All young children are aggresive, and no parent need be disturbed or surprised at games of killing and shooting. All young children are quarrelsome, though some are much more so, because of inherent personality, than others. Some bickering is inevitable in a family, however well the children are managed. Teasing and quarrelling are precipitated by fatigue, hunger (hypoglycæmia), and boredom.

The difficulty in management lies in deciding when to intervene in quarrels. On the one hand children have to learn to settle their own disputes. On the other hand good relationships with others are largely learnt in the home, and children have to learn in the home what is right and wrong. In general it is better to step in before quarrels develop rather than to wait till a quarrel occurs and try to stop it. One should anticipate by separating children when they are showing signs of having reached their limits of tolerance of each other, particularly if they are tired. The aim is to strike a happy mean between excessive interference and not interfering enough.

Excessive aggressiveness or quarrelsomeness is usually a sign of insecurity, and the cause must be looked for. It may, for instance, be due to overstrictness in the home, or to overindulgence. Determined efforts to stop a child hitting others are likely to lead to aggravation of the problem, for it will be continued as an attention-seeking device. A father told me that he had "tried everything" to stop his child hitting others. Although one cannot allow a child to injure others, the less that is done the better, because once the child recognizes the parental anxiety, he will enjoy the fuss and hit children all the more. It is better to treat the cause rather than the symptom, and the cause lies usually in one of the causes of insecurity. Douglas[7] wrote that even at the age of eight, children who are later going to get into trouble do badly in their work, and in particular score much lower than would be expected from their attainment and nonverbal intelligence. Teachers pick them out as being both nervous and aggressive.

It is worth remembering that undue fatigue, which leads, amongst other things, to excessive teasing and quarrelsomeness, may be due to a slight degree of anæmia. It may be due to inadequate sleep.

Stealing

As I have said in several places in this book, that which is normal at one age is not normal at another. Young children have a natural desire to take what they want, without distinguishing that which is theirs and that which is not. They have to learn, as they mature, to respect the property of others, and it is important that the parents should invariably set a good example of honesty. If a parent picks up coins at home when it is obvious that they do not belong to him, the child can be expected to do likewise. At all times, by act and in conversation, the parents should set the example of complete honesty.

One would not use the word "stealing" to describe the act of a pre-school child. In the case of a school age child, however, an act which is passed as normal and acceptable in the younger child, now becomes regarded as theft. The factors responsible for stealing are insecurity, bad example, revenge, self indulgence, or a feeling of inferiority when a child has no pocket money, or has less than others. It is apt to be a problem of overcrowding, when there is no one place for a child to keep his own property separate from that of others.

It is common to find that the stealing only occurs at home, and it is often confined to theft from the mother. This would immediately point to conflict between the child and his mother.

The treatment is that of the cause. It is useless to give the child a long sermon about honesty. Domestic conflict, particularly between parent and child, must be resolved. Wherever possible, the child should make restitution, restoring that which he has stolen, however embarrassing and difficult it is for him.

Lying

Lying is a similar problem. No one should expect the child of 2 or 3 to be truthful. The child of 5 or 6 may indulge in fantasy thinking, and make up the most remarkable stories, which he recounts in all seriousness to his parents. One has to distinguish this fantasy thinking from deliberate efforts to deceive. Once more, that which is normal at one age is not normal at another. Lies of exaggeration have to be distinguished from lies of deceit, and like fantasy thinking, do not justify a reprimand. Adults exaggerate so much in their conversation that it would not be surprising if their children had to do likewise; and they tell their children tall stories about Santa Claus at Christmas time. They may show tacit approval of the child's dishonesty and his evasion of trouble by deceit.

A child may lie to win praise, gain prestige, boost his ego, gain friends, or to escape punishment or the displeasure of his parents, particularly about school work. He should certainly be severely reprimanded for lying to get another child into trouble. It is commonly the result of lack of love and security at home, excessive religious strictness, domestic friction or a bad example set by the parents, who may condone and express pride at the child's dishonesty, on the ground that he is "clever." Moffatt[20] described it as the commonest juvenile crime.

The treatment, as usual, depends on the cause. Insecurity should be dealt with appropriately. It is unwise to insist on the child telling the truth when he is lying and will not retract what he has said. No child should be so afraid of the consequences that he lies to his parents. He should know that if what he did was an accident, they will not be in the least annoyed.

It is obvious that punishment for stealing or lying, when it is due to insecurity, will do nothing but harm.

Attention-seeking Devices

A very wide range of attention-seeking devices are adopted by children. Below is a collection of familiar ones. Most parents could add others. They are much more likely to be found in the insecure child than in the secure one, but it would be a mistake to think that they only occur in the absence of security. Any child likes power and attention, especially between the age of 1 and 3 years.

In connection with eating, the chief device is food refusal, sometimes refusal of a particular food which the mother has shown a special desire for the child to eat, particularly meat, milk, eggs and vegetables. The child may drop it on the floor or take it into the mouth, then spit it out or refuse to swallow it. Many mothers have thought that their child had some mechanical difficulty with swallowing, such as a disease of the œsophagus. Children may carry the meat around in the mouth for 2 or 3 hours. Others discover the trick of vomiting the food out. Some discover the particularly impressive trick of bringing it up over the tea-table.

Dirt eating (pica) is commonly a problem when the child discovers that it is a good way of drawing attention to himself, though psychologists have other explanations.

In connection with sleeping, screaming when put to bed and refusal to lie down are the chief devices used. One 18-month child was brought to me because it was feared that he had "gone wrong in the head." Every night when the mother put him to bed and left him he screamed, and as soon as she returned she found him standing on his head.

In connection with sphincter control refusal to sit on the pottie, withholding of urine or fæces, and the deliberate passage of a stool or urine on the carpet are the chief attention-seeking devices. Some discover that when they ask to be placed on the pottie the mother immediately jumps up and attends to them, and so they demand it every few minutes, having great fun as long as it lasts. Some boys refuse to pass urine standing up, simply because of the pressure which is brought on them by adults to do so. Stool smearing becomes an attention-seeking device if mismanaged.

Body manipulations—masturbation, sex play, head banging, head rolling, nose picking, tooth grinding, hair plucking, lip pulling and other manifestations are similar devices, or at least they become so if the initial manifestation is treated with anxiety and fuss.

Children may discover that they attract attention by abnormalities of speech, by facial distortion, by making certain noises, by coughing or gagging. One child achieves it by pulling up the best flowers in the garden; another by turning the gas tap on; another by banging the table; another by breath-holding attacks and tantrums; another by dawdling in dressing, tidying up or in other tasks; another by deliberate disobedience. One boy aged 3 greatly alarmed his mother, who feared that he was a sexual pervert, by frequently dashing up to ladies and lifting their skirts up. Another caused consternation in his mother's bridge parties by suddenly asking the ladies if they wanted to have a "wee-wee." Some children achieve their ends by feigning a pain or limp. A child may complain of pains in the legs when he does not want to go out for a walk, or abdominal pains at mealtimes when efforts are being made to compel him to take food. This is partly an attention-seeking device and partly a defence mechanism.

A successful device adopted by many children is frequently to ask the mother, "Do you love me?" This is highly successful when asked at the right time, just when the mother is showing signs of becoming angry. Another, when reprimanded, says "I'm sorry" with such feeling that the mother's heart melts and he gets his own way. The ingenuity of small children is remarkable and their powers of annoying considerable.

Any prank is likely to be repeated if the child discovers that it has attracted attention and put him in the centre of the picture. All too often parents describe his wrongdoing in his presence, for his pranks do supply a good topic of tea-time conversation. The inevitable result is that they are repeated. It is disastrous ever to let one's child know how much one secretly enjoys his wickedness. A child very readily becomes conscious of his parents' admiration of his tricks even though it has never been expressed in words.

The treatment of these problems is usually easy, but some of them tax the ingenuity to the utmost. Half the battle is won when the cause—the desire for attention, the development of the ego—is recognized. Not all of these tricks can be simply ignored. One cannot ignore the turning on of the gas taps or other dangerous tricks. Clearly the least possible anxiety should be shown. He should be distracted as soon as it is seen that he is about to repeat the trick. Distraction is much better than warnings or threats before the act or punishment after the act. Punishment may help towards the latter end of the third year, but it may make the behaviour worse. It is a matter of trial and error. It is preferable at this age to explain to the child that he is too old for that sort of behaviour. If such an appeal fails, stronger measures may have to be tried. For anything but dangerous tricks much the most effective method of dealing with them is to ignore them. That is the worst punishment that the child can have. When, in spite of the above treatment a child persists in turning the gas tap on, other measures must be tried. One would consist of fixing a toy tap for the child to operate, at a safe distance but near the gas stove, making it quite clear that that is his tap while the other one (the real one) is "Mummy's." This sort of method is more likely to succeed than punishment.

In all cases it is important to look behind the attention-seeking devices to the underlying cause. In simple cases the cause lies simply in the normal desire for attention which any child has and shows. In severe cases these tricks suggest that the child's basic needs are not being met, that in the normal course of events he is not being recognized sufficiently as a person, not being praised and loved sufficiently and not being given the responsibility which he wants. He then finds that the only way he has of attracting attention is being "naughty" and doing one of the tricks mentioned above.

Migraine and Periodic Syndrome

Recurrent headaches, vomiting and abdominal pain are common symptoms in children. They may occur singly or in association. Some children in addition have a rise of temperature in attacks. Others have some looseness of the stools, and the stools may be pale in attacks. There may be any combination of these symptoms. The term commonly applied to the condition is the "periodic syndrome." It used to be called "cyclical vomiting" or "acidosis attacks."

Apley[2] studied the incidence of some of these symptoms in an unselected group of school children, and found that 1 in 7 had headaches, and 1 in 9 had recurrent abdominal pains.

The syndrome is intimately related to migraine, and in 75 to 90 per cent. of cases there is a family history of that condition. Strictly speaking, the term migraine should only be applied to a unilateral headache, which is commonly associated with vomiting and sometimes with visual disturbance in the form of zigzag figures, or of blurring of vision. For a full description, readers are referred to the monograph by Bille.[5]

Before an attack begins, there may be an increase in weight with a reduction in the urinary output. The attack begins with pallor, sometimes with visual symptoms, and occasionally with difficulty in speaking or weakness or paræsthesiæ in an arm. The conjunctival vessels may be dilated. The symptoms are rapidly followed by vomiting and unilateral frontal headache. The child may go to sleep and awake normal, or the symptoms may persist for several hours or even a few days. Vomiting in rare cases is so severe that dehydration is marked. There is acetone in the breath and there are ketone bodies in the urine. In those who are not dehydrated the attack may be followed by an increased urinary output.

Attacks are often precipitated by emotional factors, including domestic quarrels and reprimands, or difficulties at school. They may also be precipitated by fatigue, bright lights, television viewing, a visit to the cinema, a loud noise, or a respiratory or other infection, a long car journey or hunger. It has nothing to do with errors of refraction. It is more common in rather nervous, sensitive children who are more liable than others to feel frustrated. It has been described, like innumerable other conditions, to allergy, but in the great majority of cases without any evidence to that effect. They have no connection with epilepsy. In some children, as in adults, migraine may be precipitated by foodstuffs containing tyramine,[11] of which the worst offenders are chocolate, cheese (especially cheddar and stilton), broad beans, Marmite and Bovril. Other foodstuffs which have been blamed include onions, tomatoes, cucumber and nuts.

It is said that affected children are more likely than others to have travel sickness. It is usually said that affected children are more likely to be intelligent than the reverse, but Bille did not confirm this. As compared with controls, there is more commonly a family history of peptic ulcer, headaches (not necessarily typically migrainous) and of nervous symptoms. The attacks may begin as early as 6 months of age—presenting with unexplained vomiting. Only later does the symptom of headache become obvious.

It has been shown that in the prodromal stage there is vasoconstriction of the cerebral vessels, accounting for the visual and neurological symptoms and signs, and that the headache is associated with vasodilatation of the cranial arteries, and the dilation of the scalp vessels in particular.

As there is commonly a psychological factor, it is important that little fuss and anxiety should be shown. Nothing should be said between the attacks about the episodes. The parents should avoid talking about their own symptoms. Where possible, sources of tension should be relieved.

In the attacks, the child will usually want to go to bed and that may be all that is necessary. An aspirin tablet or tab codein co. may be given if he is not vomiting. An ergotamine preparation (cafergot or ergotamine spray into the throat) may be tried, but success cannot be guaranteed.

It is quite useless to restrict the fat intake between attacks. This used to be done because it was thought that "acidosis" caused the attacks. The acidosis results from the attacks and does not cause them. But if any particular foodstuff (e.g. chocolate or cheese) is found to cause attacks, it should be avoided.

Other Headaches

Most children sooner or later have a headache. Headaches may be due to a febrile attack as the result of an infection. They may occur as a result of being in a stuffy room, or as a result of fatigue, dislike of a teacher, difficulty with a particular subject at school, or for other reasons. It is exceedingly unlikely that the headache will be due to eyestrain and it will not be due to an antrum infection unless there are obvious signs of such an infection such as a persistent nasal discharge.

Recurrent Abdominal Pain without Fever or Headache

Such pain is not necessarily related to migraine. Most children sooner or later have some abdominal pain. The reader is referred to the excellent book by Dr. John Apley on the subject.[2] In a statistical study of children with recurrent abdominal pain, he found that a history of similar pains in siblings or parents was six times more frequent than it was in controls. There was a higher incidence of migraine or bilious attacks, and of other emotional problems in the child and his family. In only 8 per cent. did full investigation reveal any organic cause. Kopel et al.[17] evaluated the rectosigmoid motility in 18 children with unexplained abdominal pain, and compared it with that of 18 normal children. Those with recurrent abdominal pain showed increased motility, and a heightened response to prostigmine. They regarded the recurrent abdominal pain as similar to the spastic colon variety of the irritable colon of adults.

Growing Pains

The term "growing pains" is a misnomer, because as far as we know these pains have nothing to do with growth. They certainly do not occur more often at the period of maximum growth. As Apley remarked, physical growth is not painful, but emotional growth may be. Naish and Apley[21] found that they occurred mainly between the ages of 8 and 12. Apley found that 1 in 25 unselected school children had them.

Elsewhere[3] he has related them to recurrent abdominal pains and headaches, in that children with limb pains are more likely than others to have these additional symptoms, and to have similar emotional factors. Winnicott described the pains as representing a "dramatization of persecution."

The pains are more common after fatigue and exertion. They are unrelated to infections, rheumatic fever or allergy. They are mainly confined to the lower limbs and to the calf and thigh muscles. The pains are non-articular. There is commonly a family history of non-specific rheumatic pains. They are not associated with organic disease.

The "Brain Injured" or "Brain Damaged" Child

This section is included, because children said to be "brain injured" may be normal, and show no evidence of disease.[6]

The terms "brain injured," "birth injured" and "brain damaged" are anathema to an increasing number of pædiatricians; they are certainly anathema to parents. Some psychologists refer to a child as being "brain injured"[22] if he is overactive, clumsy, impulsive, distractible, and has a short attention span, if he is destructive, excessively talkative, and shows scatter in his work, with a poor memory for some things, and a good one for others, and shows a discrepancy between verbal and performance tests (scoring well on verbal tests and poorly on performance). These children are apt to be called "bad mannered," "spoilt," or "badly brought up." Other children are apt to call them "queer," or "odd." As Birch[6] wrote in his book on the subject, much of the child's undesirable behaviour is the result of the attitudes of others, including their ridicule and unkindness. Reger[24] in his excellent review of the subject, wrote that some 43 symptoms have been ascribed to "Brain Injury" or "Birth Injury"—and added that probably all children in a class have some of them. The picture has been fully described in the two volume book by Strauss and Kephart.[25]

The terms "brain injury" and allied expressions are anathema to many pædiatricians for two main reasons. Firstly, there is no evidence that the symptoms are in any way related to birth injury; and secondly, it is most undesirable to suggest to parents that their child's annoying or even tragic symptoms are due to injury at birth, because this implies that the symptoms were preventable, and that someone, the obstetrician, the family doctor or the midwife, is to blame for what has happened. As it is quite impossible to prove that the symptoms are in fact due to birth injury, this is an altogether unwarranted aspersion. It gravely disturbs parents, for it is far better to feel that a child's difficulties were entirely unpreventable, than to feel that they could have been prevented by proper management. Even if a child with the symptoms described above suffered anoxia at birth, or was prematurely born, or had a difficult delivery, it is surely obvious that the symptoms may well have been due to something which caused the anoxia, the prematurity, or the difficult delivery. The use of the terms "brain injury" and "brain damage" imply that the cause of the symptoms is known—and that is not the case. The term "minimal cerebral dysfunction" is much more satisfactory.[4,12] Work and Haldane[30] used a similar term in their discussion.

Reger[24] wrote that "most of what is assumed to be known about the brain injured child is folk-lore. ... The fact that many children are distractible and hyperactive is no reason to assume that the concept of the brain-injured child is useful and worth retaining. ... There is no justification whatsoever to continue to call children 'brain injured' if there is no reason to assume that these children have injuries to the brain"—and he added that the only way the diagnosis can be made with certainty is at autopsy. There is certainly no psychological test which provides any evidence of brain injury. Reger added "The flippant way the label of brain injury is tagged on to children by persons, who, frankly, do not know what they are talking about, is hardly likely to further the cause of the profession."

As Reger wrote, almost all the 43 symptoms which are supposed to constitute the picture of brain injury occur in normal children, and some of them almost always occur in normal children at some stage. I have seen many children who were described as "brain injured" whose symptoms were obviously inherited from one of their parents. Many of the symptoms may be engendered by environment. For instance, a physically handicapped child may be over-protected, and deprived of environmental stimulation, and so develops symptoms ascribed to "brain injury." Admittedly, some use the term "brain damage" or "brain injury" in a broad sense, and mean to imply that the brain was damaged at any stage from conception onwards. Unfortunately parents will not interpret the term in this way. These expressions should not be used. Though the symptoms are frequent in abnormal children, they are also frequently found in normal children—and hence the inclusion of the subject in this book.

The Clumsy Child

In our book "*Lessons from Childhood*",[13] concerning the childhood of 450 famous men and women, we described several children who were clumsy in their movements. Napoleon could not throw a ball in the right direction. He was a poor shot, and not a good horseman. He was described as a boy who was not only awkward but who in many ways was helpless. Beethoven was a clumsy child. Henri Poincaré, famous

French mathematician, was clumsy with his hands and was ambidextrous. He had difficulties in spatial appreciation. Oscar Wilde and G. K. Chesterton were other clumsy children.

There is no precise definition of clumsiness. Some children and some adults are more adept with their hands than others. As I have stated elsewhere, there can never be an exact dividing line between the normal and the abnormal. Clumsy children tend to fall a great deal. They are awkward with their hands and write badly. They tend to hold the pencil in an odd way, to write with the whole body, often with the tongue protruding, and may place the paper at an unusual angle. They are awkward at tying shoe laces, and at buttoning their clothes. They may swing the arms in a strange manner. They tend to misjudge distances, as in steering an object (or themselves) through a doorway; they break objects more than others; they cannot thread a needle; they cannot throw a ball well; they cannot jump like a normal 3-year-old or hop like a 5-year-old; they are poor at dancing and physical training. They cannot stand on one foot as steadily as other children of the same age can; this is a useful test. The child of 3 can usually stand for a few seconds on one foot, and by the age of 4 he can stand steadily in this way. They tend to dislike physical training and organized games, because they are bad at them, and are apt to incur the ridicule of their fellows. This ridicule, and scolding by their parents and especially their teachers, who regard them as just naughty or careless, leads to a variety of manifestations of insecurity, such as truancy, poor school performance or bed wetting.

Mentally subnormal children tend to be "clumsy" as compared with intelligent children of the same age.

The clumsiness may be a normal variation. It may be inherited, and one must always ask for a family history of the same complaint. This is particularly important if the clumsiness is associated with difficulties of spatial appreciation, or with mirror movements (in which one hand "mimics" the other hand). It may be merely due to delayed maturation. All normal toddlers are clumsy, and if they are late in learning to walk, they are later than other children in walking and running steadily without falling. As they mature, the clumsiness becomes less obvious and may completely disappear.

Clumsiness may be largely of emotional origin. It is certain that clumsiness, of whatever the cause, is aggravated by scolding—and the repeated expression of opinion in front of him, that he is clumsy and awkward. He is expected to be clumsy, and he is.

The more carefully one examines clumsy children, the more likely one is to find abnormal neurological signs. These may point to mimimal cerebral palsy of the spastic, athetoid or ataxic types. The term "minimal cerebral dysfunction" can justifiably be applied to these children. In some of these children there is developmental apraxia and agnosia, and allied learning disorders.[28]

Organic causes of clumsiness include congenital myopathy, muscular dystrophy, chorea, cerebral tumours, familial dysautonomia, ataxia telangiectasia, and degenerative diseases of the nervous sytem.

A variety of drugs cause ataxia and clumsiness. They include anti-epileptic drugs, indomethacin, streptomycin and piperazine; and tranquillizing drugs, such as amitryptiline, chlordiazepoxide and meprobamate.

The treatment must begin with the treatment of the cause, if one can determine the cause, and if relevant treatment is available. Otherwise the main approach is that of making it clear to the parents and his teachers that the child is not just being naughty or lazy, and that he cannot help his clumsiness. Once teachers realize this, they are likely to be sympathetic and helpful, and to minimize their demands on the child. Physiotherapy or special exercises are unlikely to help.

Overactivity

Few features of the normal child disturb mothers so much as the constant fidgeting and restlessness of the overactive child. The fidgeting and restlessness are often coupled with a short attention span, distractibility, poor concentration, incessant activity, boundless energy and constant getting into danger. He exhausts his mother and teachers, but not apparently himself. The problem is nine times more common in boys than in girls.[29] Overactivity has been defined as a "chronic sustained excessive level of activity which is the cause of significant and continued complaint both at home and at school."[18]

In a study of 56 overactive children and 56 controls, the only significant difference was abnormally short or long labour followed by forceps delivery.[19]

All children from 5 to 7 or so are "constantly on the go," and never sit still. Many pre-school children behave in the same way. It is only occasionally that the distraught mother seeks expert help, because she cannot stand it any longer. The expert then has to decide whether the child's behaviour is normal or abnormal; and unfortunately it is never possible to draw the line between the two. Careful study of the overactive child shows that his movements are more purposeless than merely increased in quantity; it is not true that his overactivity is purely and simply an exaggeration of the activity of the more usual child. It is true to say that he may resemble the younger child, for what is normal at one age is not normal at another. Many an overactive child, with increasing maturity, comes to behave more like his peers.

It is fashionable in some quarters to refer to such a child as "brain damaged" or suffering from "brain injury." Knobloch and Pasa-manick[16] showed that there was some association between toxæmia, eclampsia, hypertension or other abnormalities of pregnancy and delivery, with overactivity in the child in later years. Drillien[8] showed that prematurely born children subsequently have more than their share of behaviour problems, notably defective concentration and overactivity, when at school age. These were not related to their intelligence. Prechtl and Stemmer[23] showed that there was some correlation between excessive drowsiness or irritability in the new-born and overactivity and poor concentration at school age. There is some evidence that anoxia suffered *in utero* or during delivery has a similar correlation. For instance Ucko[27] studied 29 boys who were asphyxiated at birth, comparing them with 29 boys without that history, and found notable overactivity, unusual sensitivity, and a tendency to perseveration—a dislike of changing from one task to another.

A common feature of mentally subnormal children is aimless overactivity and defective concentration. This is partly related to the delayed maturation of the mentally subnormal child. He is slower than others in growing out of the overactivity of earlier months.

Heredity is a most important and commonly forgotten factor in the causation of overactivity. I have repeatedly seen children described as "brain damaged" when it was obvious that the child merely took after his mother or father. I saw a highly intelligent grossly overactive child, who had been expelled from five schools because the teachers were quite unable to tolerate his presence in class. When he was taken for the first time to see his grandmother, who lived abroad, she remarked "Isn't it absolutely incredible? He is exactly like his mother was at that age!" In such a case the overactivity is largely a matter of inherited personality.

Overactivity and poor concentration may be one of the many manifestations of insecurity. They may also result from excessive restraint and limitation of freedom of movement.

The treatment is difficult. If there is an obvious cause of insecurity, it should be removed. Some workers have found that these children are helped by small doses of amphetamine, beginning with 2·5 to 5·0 mg per day, increasing, if necessary, to 20 mg per day. It must be remembered that amphetamine is a dangerous drug of addiction, but it can safely be used for the younger child, who has not yet grown out of his overactivity. Others have found that tranquillizing drugs may help, but I prefer not to use them because of their many side effects and the danger of addiction.

References

1. ANDREWS, G., HARRIS, M. (1964). "Syndrome of Stuttering." *Clinics in Develop. Medicine*, No. 17. London. Heinemann.
2. APLEY, J. (1959). *The Child with Abdominal Pain*. Oxford. Blackwell.
3. APLEY, J., MACKEITH, R. (1962). *The Child and His Symptoms*. Oxford. Blackwell.
4. BAX, M., MACKEITH, R. (1963). "Minimal Cerebral Dysfunction." *Little Club Clinics in Develop. Med.*, No. 10. London. Heinemann.
5. BILLE, B. (1962). "Migraine in School Children." *Acta Pædiat. Uppsala*, 51, Suppl. 136.
6. BIRCH, H. (1964). *Brain Damage in Children*. New York. Williams Wilkins.
7. DOUGLAS, J. W. B. (1966). "The School Progress of Nervous and Troublesome Children." *Brit. J. Psychiat.*, 112, 115.
8. DRILLIEN, C. M. (1964). *The Growth and Development of the Prematurely Born Infant*. Edinburgh. Livingstone.
9. EISENSON, J. (1956). In *Psychology of Exceptional Children and Youth*, by Cruickshank, W. M. London. Staples.
10. GESSELL, A. (1929). In *Foundations of Experimental Psychology*, by Murchison, C. Worcester. Clark Univ. Press.
11. HANINGTON E. (1969). in Smith R., *Background to Migraine*. London. Heinemann.
12. HATTON, J. E. (1966). "The Child with Minimal Cerebral Dysfunction." *Develop. Med. Child Neurol.*, 8, 71.
13. ILLINGWORTH, R. S., ILLINGWORTH, C. M. (1966). *Lessons from Childhood*. London. Livingstone.
14. JOHNSON, W. (1942). "Stuttering." *J. Speech Disorders*, 7, 251.
15. JOHNSON, W. (1959). *The Onset of Stuttering*. London. Oxford Univ. Press.
16. KNOBLOCH, H., PASAMANICK, B. (1959). "Syndrome of Minimal Cerebral Damage in Infancy." *J. Am. Med. Ass.*, 170, 1384.
17. KOPEL, F. B., KIM, I. C., BARBERO, C. J. (1967). "Comparison of Rectosigmoid Motility in Normal Children, Children with Recurrent Abdominal Pain, and Children with Ulcerative Colitis." *Pediatrics*, 39, 539.
18. LIVINGSTON, S. (1969). "Overactivity." *J. Am. Med. Ass.*, 268, 694.
19. MINDE, K., WEBB, G., SYKES, D. (1968). "*Studies on the Hyperactive Child.*" *Develop. Med. Child Neurol.*, 10, 355.
20. MOFFATT, J. (1969). "Stealing, a Pattern of Behaviour." *S. Australian Clinics*, 4, 235.
21. NAISH, J. M., APLEY, J. (1951). "Growing Pains—A Clinical Study of Nonarthritic Limb Pains in Children." *Arch. Dis. Child.*, 26, 134.
22. PINCUS, J. H., GLASER, G. H. (1966). "The Syndrome of Minimal Brain Damage in Childhood." *New Engl. J. Med.*, 275, 27.
23. PRECHTL, H. F. R., STEMMER, C. J. (1962). "The Choreiform Syndrome in Children." *Dev. Med. and Child Neurol.*, 4, 119.
24. REGER, R. (1965). *School Psychology*. Springfield. Charles Thomas.
25. STRAUSS, A. A., KEPHART, N. C. (1955). *Psychopathology and Education of the Brain Injured Child*. New York. Grune and Stratton.
26. TORUP, E. (1962). "A Follow Up Study of Children with Tics." *Acta Pædiat.*, Uppsala, 51, 261.
27. UCKO, L. E. (1965). "A Comparative Study of Asphyxiated and Non-asphyxiated Boys from Birth to 5 Years." *Develop. Med. Child Neurol.*, 7, 643.
28. WALTON, J. N., ELLIS, E., COURT, S. D. M. (1962). "Clumsy Children: Developmental Apraxia and Agnosia." *Brain*, 85, 603.
29. WERRY, J. S. (1968). "Developmental Hyperactivity." *Ped. Clin. N. Am.*, 15, 581.
30. WORK, H. H., HALDANE, J. E. (1966). "Cerebral Dysfunction in Children." *Am. J. Dis. Childh.*, 111, 573.
31. ZIMAN, E. (1950). *Jealousy in Children*. London. Gollancz.

CHAPTER 27

THE PREVENTION OF ACCIDENTS

In Canada, the United States, Holland and other countries, accidents are the chief cause of death in children of 1 year of age and over. They account for more deaths in children than the next six most common causes of death and more permanent crippling. They kill 15,000 children each year in the United States and cause permanent injury to some 50,000 children. About 15 million children seek medical attention each year on account of accidents.[12] Twenty-eight per cent. of all deaths of children aged 1 to 14 in England and Wales are due to accidents. In one year doctors and hospital departments treated about 15,000 severe burns or scalds, 16,000 bad cuts or bruises and 4,000 fractures among an estimated total of 1,740,000 children under 2 years of age in Britian in 1947. The accidents consisted chiefly of burns and scalds from radiators of fires or from boiling liquids; road accidents; falls from prams, chairs and stairs; suffocation; poisons; and electric shocks. Flammable cloths are a particular danger.

Eighty per cent. of scalds in children occur under the age of 4. About 10,000 children are admitted to hospitals in England and Wales every year on account of poisoning. In 1960 more children died from poisoning in New York City than the total dying from measles, rubella, poliomyelitis, tuberculosis, rheumatic fever, scarlet fever and other streptococcal conditions. Every year in the United States 600 children die from poisoning and 600,000 children recover from poisoning.[12] In a random sample of families in Syracuse, New York, a quarter of all families with five or more members had at least one case of child poisoning. It is estimated that about 6 per cent. of all children aged 1 to 4 take poison.

This may be due to a variety of factors[7]—attention seeking, insecurity, unconscious self injury as a result of guilt feelings, desire for independence, the avoidance of some unpleasant task, an attempt to seek sympathy, revenge, domestic conflict, broken homes, lack of discipline or excessive discipline, parental alcoholism, punitive or rejecting fathers, submissive or over-protective mothers, overcrowding or absence of adequate play space. Accidents are especially liable to happen when the mother is out at work, or is attending to someone who is ill, or is having a baby. Pavenstedt[13] noted the remarkable lack of motor caution displayed by slum children, their failure to learn from accidents, and their failure to adopt self-protective measures.

One study showed that there is a statistically significant correlation between a mother's menstruation and a child's admission to hospital for illness or accident.[4]

Carelessness and ignorance on the part of parents are important causes of accidents. Carelessness in the storage of poisons is a particularly important cause of poisoning in children. In a random selection of homes in a Swedish town with 1 to 2-year-old children in them, investigation[1] showed that chemicals were not accessible to children in 6·8 per cent. of homes; apart from cleaning agents, chemicals were safely stored in 3·4 per cent.; and chemicals were unsafely stored in 89·8 per cent.

In an Australian study[16] it was found that 50 per cent. of the scalds in children occurred at mealtimes. The kitchen was the most dangerous place with regard to burns and scalds. In 103 of 286 cases the accident occurred when the attention of the parents had been distracted. The parents had in general underestimated the abilities of the toddlers to get into trouble. MacLeod[11] estimated that 17 per cent. of accidents in the home were preventable.

Lambah[9] described 702 admissions of children with eye injuries to an eye hospital over a period of 10 years. Penetrating injuries were due to arrows, airguns, fireworks, chipping wood, thrown missiles or assaults.

The commonest poisons taken by children are aspirin and other salicylates, contraceptive pills, ferrous sulphate, barbiturates, cleaning agents, pesticides, disinfectants, deadly nightshade and berries, laxatives and petroleum derivatives. The number of children treated for poisoning has increased enormously over the last 20 years. There are at least 300,000 different noxious household products available to the child.[8] Pyman[14] wrote a useful review of 230 cases of inhaled foreign body. Two-thirds of the children were boys. Almost half the inhaled objects were nuts. Pyman recommended that children should not be given nuts either alone or in food in the first four years.

There is always a danger of a lilo floating out to sea. Water wings may spring a leak, or invert the child so that the head is under the water.

Factors concerned with accidents in children include hunger, fatigue, overactivity, illness at home, parental failure to understand what to expect of children at different ages, domestic friction, change of environment (e.g. a new house, holiday), imitation of the parents, anger directed against the parent, negativism, and emotional deprivation. Pica is an important factor in poisoning.

The Management of the Child

The proper management of the child is an essential step towards accident prevention. The child who has never had any sort of discipline, who is permitted by his parents to climb on to window sills, tables and other dangerous places and who is allowed to do exactly as he wants is particularly apt to become involved in accidents. The over-protected child is equally liable to become involved in accidents. The child who is constantly thwarted and prevented from any sort of ordinary activity because of some conceivable danger is apt to rebel and so get into difficulties.

An excellent discussion of the problem of accident prevention was given by Dietrich.[5,6] He wrote that safe behaviour, like any other form of behaviour, grows out of early parent-child relations. Accident prevention needs forethought, time and discipline: forethought—to think of and become sensitive to possible dangers to children; time— to watch them; and discipline—so that they learn how far they can go. "Mild, consistent, logical discipline is as necessary to a child's sense of security as it is to his life. It may be administered by a glance, a word, an act of deprivation, a tone of voice or the proper anatomic application of a dispassionate hand." In the first year there must be 100 per cent. protection, and any accident is entirely the fault of the custodians. If such absolute protection is maintained for a relatively few years the child becomes unusually vulnerable to accidents. Dietrich suggested that after 1 year, while one maintains protection against serious accidents, the child should be exposed to minor painful experiences for their educational value. He should at all times be protected from severe burns or scalds and from catching his clothes in an electric radiator, but he should be allowed to feel the heat of a coffee pot. "Instead of forbidding him to touch commonplace objects one should simply and objectively state: 'That is hot; if you touch it, it will burn you.' He does, it does, and a valuable lesson is learned." He must be prevented from reaching poisons, but a good lesson is learnt when a jar of vinegar or mustard is left in a place where the child cannot fail but discover it. He must not be allowed to fall from any dangerous height or on to a dangerous surface, but he may fall out of a low chair as long as he has not a dangerous implement in his hand. In other words, there must be a constant balance between protection and education, beginning with absolute protection at birth and finishing with almost complete independence by about 10 years of age. In these short intervening years the completely protected, totally dependent 1-year-old infant must be transposed into a secure, self-confident school child armed with safe behaviour.

I feel sure that the importance of wise loving discipline in accident prevention has not received sufficient emphasis. It is obvious that discipline will not prevent the young toddler from getting into trouble: but it can do much to prevent the older child from becoming involved in accidents. Overindulgence and lack of discipline on the one hand, and excessive strictness on the other hand, are both factors which lead to accidents. The child brought up without discipline is selfish and thoughtless, and disobeys. The child brought up with excessive discipline and overstrictness may rebel against restrictions and become involved in accidents.

Wise discipline includes the immediate stopping of all dangerous practices, such as door banging, throwing objects around the room, and playing on the stairs. It certainly does not include over-protection, which prevents the child from experiments, and which gives him an exaggerated and wrong idea of danger.

It is difficult when teaching caution to avoid implanting fear. The average child of 20 months can be taught some degree of caution. He can usually be trained to keep away from the kitchen stove or electrical connections. The ease with which forbidden acts are repeated as attention-seeking devices must also be remembered. The greatest ingenuity has to be used to stop such dangerous habits as turning the gas taps on and other acts which cannot be dealt with simply by ignoring them.

The child should be given positive instruction. He should be told the right and the wrong way of holding tools in woodwork, or of using any mechanical appliances. He should be taught water safety; he should be taught to swim as soon as he is old enough; to swim only in a safe place, and never alone; he should know of the danger of cramp, especially if he swims when tired; he should know about the undertow. He should be told about the danger of a current—and that if caught in one he should not swim against it, but with it, at an oblique angle, in order to get out of it. Parents and child should know about the dangers of inflated beach toys springing a leak, or being taken out with a current. Much can be done to prevent drowning accidents. Every year 1,100 drown around the coasts of Great Britain—a large proportion of them children.[2] They could largely be prevented if children were taught to swim, and if they were taught water safety as well as road safety. The use of life jackets in boats would save many child lives.

Children must be given positive instruction about road safety and hill safety. They should know the precautions which should be taken, and the reason. The older child should know about the folly of undertaking a dangerous ridge walk or climb if he is afraid of it. He should be taught that it requires more courage to refuse to tackle it than to try it—and run the risk of involving many others in trying to rescue him if he gets into difficulty. The older child should read and re-read the excellent booklet entitled *Safety on Mountains* published by the Central Council for Physical Recreation.[3] This gives valuable advice about clothing, equipment and instructions on hill walking and climbing.

Parents of small children must train themselves to anticipate danger, and to guess what the child can be expected to do in a particular situation. They must remove the hazard and teach him how to handle the situation. They must remember his climbing powers, his inquisitiveness, and his inability to anticipate the consequences of what he is doing. They know the personality of the child and they should allow for it. They should guess what toys are dangerous and they should know about the danger of such materials as bows and arrows and catapults. They should anticipate danger from electrical appliances in the kitchen. One paper[10] described 295 cases of washing machine accidents, causing mangling of arms.

The following is a summary of the steps required to prevent accidents in children, with many "Do's" and "Don'ts":

Specific Do's and Don'ts

Do set a good example.

Never stand on a rocking chair to fasten the curtains, or run across the road in front of traffic.

Burns

Never leave a small child alone in the house.

If there is an open fire, electric or gas fire, have an adequate fireguard, hooked in place so that it cannot be knocked or pulled out of place.

Don't allow the child to play with fire or matches.

Have the child in pyjamas, not a nightdress.

Remember the flammability of many clothes.

Don't let him climb into the fireplace to recover a toy.

Don't have a mirror above the fire, which will tempt the child to look at himself when his clothes are near the fire.

Don't leave a clothes horse in front of the fire; it may be knocked into the fire.

Remember the danger of portable stoves. They may be knocked over.

A Christmas tree is highly flammable; see that electric lights on it are properly wired by an expert.

Always see that there is a readily available fire extinguisher.

Be aware of the danger of fireworks.

Never let the child hold a firework.

Don't let him throw fireworks.

Don't let him bend over a firework to light one—or let him see you do it.

Don't let him put a rocket or other firework in a milk bottle to light it.

Never let him put a firework in the pocket.

Do not leave an electric iron where a child may come into contact with it.

Scalds

Don't leave a hot teapot or similar object near the edge of the table at mealtimes. The table cloth should not hang over the edge of the table.

Don't pass hot tea or other fluid in front of the small child. Never hold a baby on the knee when drinking hot liquid.

Always turn pan handles away from the front of the stove.

Never leave a hot bottle in the child's bed. It may burn by contact, or burst in the bed, scalding him.

Never leave the young child alone in the bath. The cold water should be run in before the hot.

Do not put hot water in the pottie before the child sits on it.

Electrocution

All electric points should be of the safe variety, so that the child cannot receive a shock by insertion of a lead pencil or other object through a hole.

Do not have an electric fire in the bathroom.

Keep all flex in good condition.

Always unplug electric equipment when it is out of use.

Do not fold electric blankets. See that they are regularly serviced. Don't let a child sleep on an electric blanket; he may receive a shock if he wets it.

Gas

Do not have a gas fire or gas water heater in the child's bedroom.

See that all gas taps are of the safety variety, so that if the tube is disconnected, no harm is done if the gas tap is turned on.

Drowning

See that all children learn to swim as soon as they are old enough.

Never allow children in a canoe, small boat or sailing boat without a life jacket on.

Do not allow an inflated lilo at the seaside if there is a possibility that it will be blown out to sea.

Remember that airwings may invert the child and keep him under the water; and air may escape so that they no longer support him.

Remember the danger that the child may get out of his depth. Remember the possibility of an undertow, or a current.

Never have a lily pond in the garden when there is a small child in the family.

Do not leave the baby or small child alone in the bath.

Never leave water on the floor in a bucket.

Poisons

Remember that the older child may pick up poisonous materials and give them to his young brother.

Wherever possible, cleaning agents, drugs and certainly pesticides should be locked in a cupboard and the key should be removed. The difficulty is that cleaning agents, such as detergents, are in such constant use that it is unreasonable to expect a mother to keep them always under lock and key.

The commonest drugs which poison children are aspirin and other salicylates, contraceptive pills, ferrous sulphate, barbiturates, laxatives, digitalis and strychnine. Keep them locked up.

Never leave medicines in the child's bedroom.

Destroy all discarded medicines.

Never take or give a medicine without first looking at it and reading the label.

Do not let the child see you take a medicine; he is liable to imitate.

Refer to the medicine as medicine, and not as sweets.

Never store inedible products on the food shelves.

Keep all poisons in their original containers, and not in fruit juice bottles.

Never let him see you hide a poison. It is a challenge to him to find it.

Don't leave toy fuel cubes or camphor balls about; they are poisonous.

Wax crayons are dangerous; they should not be given to a small child who is apt to eat them.

Don't have poisonous berries in the garden. Teach him that berries are for birds and not for people to eat.

Colours must be fast. Home decoration with lead paint must be avoided, for a child may bite the paintwork.

Mechanical Devices

The electric wringer has been responsible for innumerable grave accidents. It is safer not to have one if there is a small child in the house.

Electric mixers, electric fans and sewing machines are possible sources of serious injury to children; they should be kept out of reach when in use.

The rotary lawn mower has been responsible for the loss of hundreds of fingers and toes. It may hurl small stones at high speed into a child's eye. Keep him out of the way when using such a machine.

Bicycles

Children should be taught how a coat caught in the wheel will throw them.

Drain holes in the drive may cause accidents to children on bicycles or tricycles.

Road Safety

The danger of children running out into the street after a ball must be remembered, and the possibility or likelihood of the child doing it should be recognized.

The child may run behind a car when it is reversing into the street.

No child should be allowed to stand in the car when it is in motion—especially on the front seat or in front of the front seat.

The car door should have a door handle of the safety type which is locked, so that the door will not open when the car is in motion.

The car should be equipped with safety belts.

Eye Injuries

The common causes of eye injuries and loss of an eye are bows and arrows, catapults and airguns. Do not give them to small children. Splinters from wood chopping are another cause of eye injury. Do not allow a small child to play with sharp pointed objects.

Shotguns

The parent who supplies his child with a shotgun is guilty of culpable negligence.

Inhalation

Small detachable objects may be inhaled. Do not allow the child to throw peanuts into the air and catch them in the mouth. The baby may inhale the contents of a broken rattle. Never let a child run about with food in the mouth. Do not play with a child who is eating.

Falls

Have a safe high chair. Falls must be avoided by safe strapping. A bar between the legs prevents the baby sliding.

When he is old enough to climb out of the cot, he should be in a bed

The window of the child's bedroom must be safe, so that he cannot open it far enough to allow him to fall out. It is a mistake, however, to have all the upstairs windows so safe that no one can get out of them in case of fire.

The carpet or lino must not be torn or frayed.

If the floor is polished, the rug should have a non-skid device under it

Grease on the floor should be removed immediately.

Children should not be allowed to play on the stairs. When the child is just old enough to get up and down stairs alone, he should not be allowed to carry objects when going up and down.

The pram must not be overloaded, and it must be equipped with good brakes.

Do not let him remove the chair on which someone is about to sit.

Do not overload the pram; use struts to avoid tilting when the baby is in it.

Knocks

The danger of a swing is not the risk that the child will fall off; the danger is the possibility that a child will run behind the swing and receive concussion. The same applies to the "roundabout."

The practice of placing coins on the railway line is to be discouraged.

See that the street door is properly closed.

Trapped Fingers

The door banging game should always be inhibited. Parents should get into the way of opening and closing doors gently, and of looking to see where the child's hands are before closing a door.

The rocking chair and desk chair are common causes of minor injuries to the finger.

Cuts

Sharp objects, such as opened tins or scissors must not be left about.

No child should be allowed to run about with a plastic trumpet in the mouth. If he falls, it may break and perforate the palate.

He must not be allowed to place any sharp object in the mouth, and still less to run about with it there. He must not climb down from his stool with his fork in his hand to pick up dropped objects. Rusty nails should not be left in pieces of wood. Broken bottles must not be left about. Stone throwing must be discouraged.

Suffocation

The baby should never be taken into the parents' bed to sleep.

Children must always be forbidden to play with plastic bags over the head.

They must not play with elastic or a cord round the neck.

Elastic across the pram, with rattles or other objects on it, may strangulate the baby.

The safety harness in bed may strangulate.

The vertical cot bars must not be more than 3 inches apart; he may get his head stuck otherwise.

The parent should not play with the child who has food in the mouth.

The danger of the child shutting another (or himself) in the refrigerator must be remembered.

Conclusions

Parents must be aware of the possible dangers which their children face.

They must balance over-protection against carelessness.

They must allow the child to develop independence as soon as he is ready for it and take calculated risks.

The child must be taught firm loving discipline. Lack of discipline and excessive discipline may each lead to accident proneness.

Parents must set a good example.

Children must be given positive instruction in accident prevention—with regard, for instance, to water safety, road safety, safety on the mountains, and proper use of tools.

Having put together a long list of do's and don'ts with regard to the prevention of the common accidents in childhood, one is left with the thought that if our children do not have accidents, it is not just due to our own cleverness; we should regard ourselves as fortunate.

References

1. BERFENSTAM, R., BESKOW, J. (1962). "Storage of Poisons in the Homes of Families with Small Children." *Brit. J. prev. soc. Med.*, **16**, 123.
2. BOUCHER, C. A. (1962). "Drowning." *Monthly Bull. Minist. Lab. Hlth. Serv.*, **21**, 114.
3. Central Council for Physical Recreation (1965). *Safety on Mountains*. London.
4. DALTON, K. (1970) "Children's Hospital Admissions and Mother's Menstruation." *Brit. Med. J.*, **2**, 22.
5. DIETRICH, H. F. (1950). "Accidents, Childhood's Greatest Physical Threat, are Preventable." *J. Amer. med. Ass.*, **144**, 1175.
6. DIETRICH, H. (1965). "Accidents." *Clinical Pediatrics*, **4**, 1.
7. FABIAN, A. A., BENDER, L. (1947). "Head Injury in Children." *Amer. J. Orthoptychiat.*, **17**, 68.
8. JONES, J. G. (1969). "Preventing Poisoning Accidents in Children." *Clinical Pediatrics.*, **8**, 484.

9. LAMBAH, P. (1962). "Some Common Causes of Eye Injury in the Young." *Lancet*, **2**, 1351.

10. LUCK, J. W., MADDUX, R. (1955). "Washing Machine Accidents." *Gen. Pract.*, **12**, 87.

11. MacLEOD, D. A. (1962). "The Epidemiology of Children's Accidents." M.D. Thesis, Univ. of Manchester.

12. MEYER, R. J., KLEIN, D. (1969). "Childhood Injuries; Approaches and Perspectives." *Pediatrics*, **44**, Supplement, p. 791–896.

13. PAVENSTEDT, E. (1967). "The Drifters: Children of Disorganised Lower Class Families." London. Churchill.

14. PYMAN, C. (1971). Inhaled Foreign Bodies in Childhood." A review of 230 cases. *M. J. Australia*, **1**, 62.

15. SOBEL, R., MARGOLIS, J. A. (1965). "Repetitive Poisoning in Children." *Pediatrics*, **35**, 641.

16. WILLIAMS, H., BOWMAN, N., MALARE, G. (1958). "A Social Study of Burns and Scalds in Children." *Med. J. Aust.*, **2**, 599.

CHAPTER 28

TOYS AND PLAY—NURSERY SCHOOL

Play and play material is one of the basic needs for all children.

Play gives children emotional satisfaction. It keeps them occupied and prevents boredom. It can be difficult in wet weather or in winter to keep a young child occupied. It is important, for boredom rapidly leads to bad temper, irritability and destructiveness. A vicious circle is set up, for the child's behaviour annoys and tires the mother, and her irritability and loss of patience makes the child worse.

Play material may give a child a sense of achievement. It helps the child to sublimate his aggressiveness and primitive instincts. The hammer toy is a suitable weapon for a boy to use when he has pent up aggressive feelings. A girl may act out her aggressive feelings on her dolls. In hospitals toys help to keep a child happy and to reduce his anxieties.

Play is of intellectual value. It helps children to practise and develop their new skills. It teaches them to use their hands and to co-ordinate them with their eyes. To some extent all toys have educational value, but some have more value than others. Some toys, especially expensive mechanical toys, have little educational value and as a result they are unlikely to retain a child's interest for long. Toys which enable them to practise their new skills, to use their imagination and to experiment, are far more likely to hold their interest and to be used over and over again.

Play helps children to concentrate, to observe, to experiment. It teaches children how things work and how things are made. It helps to teach them to take care of their possessions.

Play helps children in their relationships with others. It helps them to co-operate with others, to learn to play the game, and to learn the consequences of cheating—isolation and loss of friendship. It teaches them to be honest. It helps them to learn to lose with equanimity. It teaches them the team spirit.

Out of door play gives healthy exercise in the fresh air and improves health and strength.

In any discussion of play material for children, one must consider the child's mental age as distinct from his actual age, together with his sex, personality, interests and aptitudes. Toys which will interest one child will not interest another. Some by the age of 3 can draw as well as the average 5-year-old. Some, of similar intelligence, are no good at all at drawing and have no interest in it. Even when a child's interests and capabilities are known, it is not usually possible to predict which toy will give the most lasting pleasure.

In all cases solitary play, though necessary part of the time, should be avoided in excess, but the child must learn to play without constant help from his mother. A mother makes the mistake of constantly interfering in play, so that he becomes utterly dependent on her and cannot entertain himself without her help. On the other hand, he should at frequent intervals visit the homes of others to play and to learn to give and take, and he should have friends into his house. All too often small children are denied the opportunity of mixing with others.

Apart from the out-of-door mechanical toys, there is no need to think that toys cost a great deal of money. It is by no means the most expensive ones which give the greatest pleasure. The costly hand-made doll will not necessarily please a little girl any more than a cheap doll with some hand-made rapidly-knitted garments so that the doll may be dressed and undressed by the child herself.

When in doubt about the suitability of a toy for a particular age, it is always wise to give one which is a little too difficult for him than one which is too simple. He will soon discard the one which is too easy for him. Wisely chosen toys are popular for many months. A good miscellaneous assortment of wood blocks, for instance, is enjoyed just as much by the 5-year-old as it is by the 1-year-old. The use to which the blocks are put is different, but in each case they teach the child to use his hands and brain. When a child gets bored with a toy and loses interest in it, it should be put away for a few weeks. It is likely to be thoroughly enjoyed as if it were a new toy when it reappears one wet afternoon a few months later. Children who are given an excess of toys are apt to become bored and destroy or waste them.

In the choice of toys it is always important to see that the toys themselves, or parts which can be detached, are not sharp enough to hurt the child; that the toys or detachable parts of the toys are not so small that they can be inhaled or swallowed, and that the paint does not come off when they are taken to the mouth.

A child should have a toy cupboard or a large box in which he keeps his assortment of odds and ends. A playroom is a luxury. It is of uncertain value in the first 3 years unless there are older children as well, for the child is likely to want to play near his mother, but it is of great value later, helping not only the mother, by allowing her to get on with her work away from the children, but helping the children by giving them a place of their own in which to play.

Between 3 and 6 months a wide-awake baby wants to see what is going on. He readily becomes bored if left in the pram all day with nothing but a view of a brick wall in front of him. Even when taken out for a walk he is apt to be kept lying down with the hood up and other obstacles to his vision, so that he cannot see anything. He should be propped up so that he can see what is happening. He may refuse to lie outside in a pram. In that case he should be wheeled into the kitchen, where he can watch his mother doing her household duties. At about 3 or 4 months he can hold objects if they are placed in his hand, though he cannot reach out for objects and get them. He should be given objects, therefore, such as plastic rattles or large curtain rings, which he can hold and play with. Highly-coloured objects will be more popular than dull colours. A toy may be tied on his pram so that it dangles in front of him. As long as this is a reasonable distance from his eyes it will not do them any harm.

He should begin to get used to seeing other children. It is a mistake to isolate a baby from other children. When eventually he sees them he is apt to be frightened and shy.

At 5 months the average baby can reach for an object and grasp it. From this time onwards he should be given an abundance of toys which will help him to learn to use his hands. A discarded tin with something inside, such as small pebbles or lentils, will be enjoyed. Bobbins, cubes, large beads on string, bricks (not paper covered), spoons and other large objects are suitable for him. He should be propped up in his high chair so that he can play with the toys on the tray in front of him.

From the age of 6 months onwards an ever-increasing range of objects interests the child. He is rapidly learning to use his hands, and he should be given a variety of toys to help him. Cubes, plastic rings on chains, bobbins and rattles continue to be favourites. Between 9 months and a year or so babies take a delight in placing objects in and out of containers, and baskets, boxes, tins and bricks of various shapes and sizes are particularly popular. Nesting boxes and barrels, nesting pyramids and interlocking building bricks will be enjoyed. Stiff books are likely to be enjoyed at about this age. They should be made of stout card, which is virtually untearable. Linen books are useful but not so satisfactory. The pages rapidly curl up. It is surprising how few mothers think of giving their children books at this age.

In the second year books become of increasing value. They should now be of two types, hard card books which the child can look at himself without risk of damage being done, and ordinary books which the mother will show him and read to him and then put away out of reach. The latter type includes nursery rhymes. Even before a year of age babies often show great pleasure in the rhythm of nursery rhymes and anticipate with appropriate bodily movement when a particular line is being approached. Picture books should preferably be simple, showing one object on a page. Many of the available books show pictures which are too complex and confusing to the child. When objects are pointed out to children in this way they learn a great deal and they can then themselves point out numerous objects long before they can say the appropriate word. This helps in the development of speech. Towards the latter part of the second year story books become popular. The Beatrix Potter books may become great favourites. Other books show coloured pictures of common objects. Scrapbooks composed of coloured pictures cut out of magazines and stuck into Press cutting books or albums will be enjoyed and instructive.

Boxes, tins and cubes continue to be useful. Sets of wood blocks of different shapes and sizes will occupy many hours. Toys which can be pushed and pulled, particularly if objects can be put into them, will be enjoyed. Children should be given opportunities to hear music on the wireless or gramophone. They enjoy drums, whistles and trumpets. Pile driving with wooden pegs which have to be hammered through holes is a satisfying pursuit.

Domestic mimicry is a characteristic feature of the $1\frac{1}{2}$–3-year-old child. Cookery sets, tea sets, doll's furniture, sweeping brushes and toy carpet sweepers will enable him to spend hours in this way. A doll and teddy bear enable him to use his imagination and he is likely to become attached to them.

Towards the latter half of the second year children are likely to be able to thread large beads (or cubes with holes through them). They often play with pencil and paper. At first it is a mere scribble, which the child may call a man or dog, but with practice the drawing rapidly improves. Lacing cards are useful. They consist of celluloid or similar material with holes punched through. Coloured laces are threaded through and through. Plasticine and modelling material will be used in this period. At about 2 children can pronate and supinate the wrists well enough to screw and unscrew jars. A sand-pit with simple wooden implements (rake, shovel, etc.) and tins will keep a child busy for hours. A bowl of water in the garden, with jugs and other containers, is always popular. Spinning tops, balls and trains have their uses. In my experience sets of farmyard animals have only temporary interests, in that they do not enable the child to think or use his imagination. There is nothing much to do with them.

In the third year books, building blocks, Plasticine, clay and other modelling materials find increasing use. Drawing books, paints, stencils, coloured shapes which can be stuck on to paper, bead threading, coloured pencils (with a pencil sharpener) all help to keep the child occupied. A blackboard and chalk can be provided. Domestic mimicry is now more advanced. Children delight in "helping" the mother to cook, and like to make pastries, shell peas, pick the tops off fruit and to set the table. "Cakes" made by the child have a specially delightful flavour for him. Home-made clothes or discarded baby clothes for the doll, with suitably large buttons, enable him to dress and undress the doll. A doll's cot and pram, with bits of rag to act as sheets, and doll's furniture, give him full scope for his imagination. A "Wendy" house can be constructed from clothes-horses if it cannot be made by the handyman; it, too, helps in developing the imagination. Scales and weights and a sweet shop are popular. Remnants from dressmaking find various uses if given to the child. There may be enough to enable her to dress up as a "nurse." The child should "wash up" his own cooking utensils. An hour or two may be spent in washing-up two or three cups. The doll's clothes may be washed and pegged out. He may play shops with the aid of his junk box.

Out of doors a small tricycle or pedal car will give great pleasure and provide him with exercise in the fresh air. A swing, rocking boat, wheelbarrow, balance bar, balls, sand-pit and bowls of water will keep him occupied for prolonged periods. A piece of rubber tubing is handy.

In the latter part of the third year simple jigsaws—beginning with those made of two or three pieces—may be given. Appreciation of size and shape is also learnt by peg boards and by a posting box with holes of various shapes carved in the side through which blocks of the appropriate size are "posted." There are simple form boards—pieces of wood with carved holes into which blocks of the right shape have to be fitted. Plastic mosaics serve the same purpose. Tracing books help in teaching finer manipulation. Other useful toys include the picture lotto, a magnet, magnetic shapes, construction kits, a gyroscope, animal templates, wood roadways.

Colour and picture matching is enjoyed. Sets of pictures of common objects have to be matched with corresponding pictures on a board; sets of five of each of a dozen or more pictures have to be put together in their proper pile. Assorted wools of various colours may be matched in the same way. Cut-out numerals which have to fit into a board, cardboard counters and cardboard coins and cut-out letters of the alphabet have a similar use.

Tile pictures can be made by shaped pieces of wood with holes in the middle which are hammered by means of nails on to a piece of beaverboard.

In the latter part of the third year the child is old enough to use blunt-ended scissors. Plastic scissors are available, but it is difficult to cut anything with them and they are of little use.

Gramophone records of children's stories, songs and other music may be purchased. On the wireless there are programmes of music which help to teach rhythm.

When the child is 3 or 4, many of the toys, such as building bricks, continue to be popular. Dinky cars and similar vehicles please the boy. Dolls, whose clothes can be put on and taken off, please the girl. Sets of paper dresses for dolls are useful. A shoe box can be made into a house or garage, doors and windows being made by scissors, the child being left to arrange the colour scheme. A child may be given a discarded pattern book, from which he can cut out the figures and dresses. A painting easel, finger paints, crayons and clay modelling are enjoyed. Stilts, a climbing frame with an old rubber car tyre, a rope ladder and slide are enjoyed. He may be allowed to colour pictures in old newspapers. Tracing and stencil books are popular. A dressing-up box, containing discarded clothes and pieces of material, provides endless pleasure.

The plastic building toy "Bildit" is a good toy for this and subsequent ages. The Raphael Tuck "Panorama Books" and the various Golden Play Books, published by Adprint, London, are much liked by boys.

Firms which specialize in educational toys include:

E. J. Arnold & Son, Butterly Street, Leeds, 10.
Wilkane Ltd., Eastbourne, Sussex.
Educational Supply Association Ltd., 181 High Holborn, London, W.C.1.
Galt Toy Shop, 30, Great Marlborough Street, London, W.1.
Paul and Marjorie Abbott, Wimpole Street, London, W.1.

These firms issue particularly good catalogues of the toys which they make.

The following books or series of books are recommended:

"Verses for Children." *Harry Golding.* Ward, Lock & Co., London.
"The Book of a Thousand Poems." *J. M. MacBain.* Evans Brothers Ltd., London.
The *Beatrix Potter* Series. F. Warne & Co. Ltd., London.
"Tirra Lirra." *Laura Richards.* George Harrap, London.
The Janet and John Books. *Mabel O'Donnell* and *Rona Munro.* James Nisbet & Co., London.
Gay Colour Books. *Alice Williamson.* E. J. Arnold & Son, Ltd., Leeds.
Colour Photo Books. E. J. Arnold & Son, Ltd., Leeds.
First Stories. *Margaret Barnes.* E. J. Arnold & Son Ltd., Leeds.
The Little Golden Books. *Various Authors.* Simon Schuster, New York.
"Tales to Read." *Mollie Clarke.* A. Wheaton & Co., Exeter.
Little Things Series. A. Wheaton & Co., Exeter.
My First Little Books Series. Evans Brothers Ltd., London.
Thomas the Tank Engine Series. *W. Awdry.* Edmund Ward, Leicester.
The March of Rhyme. Compiled by *Dorothy Green.* E. J. Arnold & Son Ltd., Leeds.
Listen with Mother Series. Juvenile Productions, London.
Blackberry Farm Books. *Jane Pilgrim.* Brockhampton Press Ltd., Leicester.

All children like to have pet animals. If the parents feel that they can tolerate the presence of a puppy in the house, his presence will be greatly appreciated by the children. They enjoy looking after and playing with animals. The medical man must be aware of the fact that animals may be responsible for the spread of any of a formidable list of diseases. They may harbour fleas or other insects which will cause urticaria in children who are sensitive to the bites. Cats may cause cat scratch fever. Dogs may carry lymphocytic choriomeningitis, toxoplasmosis or salmonella infections, and in countries abroad they may have rabies. They convey visceral larva migrans (toxocara canis) and other worms. Rabbits may carry tularæmia; guinea pigs may convey encephalomyelitis. Other diseases spread to humans by domestic pets include psittacosis, brucellosis, anthrax, leptospirosis, salmonella and fungus infections. Allergy to hair is of great importance to a child with asthma. The doctor must not exaggerate the risks, but he should be aware of them.

Nursery School

The question of whether or not to send a child to a nursery school sometimes arises towards the end of the third year. It is undesirable that he should be placed in a nursery earlier in order to enable the mother to work in industry or elsewhere. The child in his first two years needs his mother, and separation from her for the major part of each day is unsound psychologically and is apt to lead to insecurity and other behaviour problems.

In the latter part of the third year, however, it becomes increasingly difficult to keep the only child, if he is an active one, adequately occupied. The question hardly arises if there are siblings with whom he can play. The decision must be an individual matter. It depends largely on his personality, on his maturity, his ability to mix with other children and his readiness to be separated from home. The convenience of the mother, unless (as often happens) there is economic necessity, is a secondary matter; the essential factor to be considered is whether it will contribute to the child's happiness. It is valuable for him to play with other children. In general, I think that it is too early for most children to be separated from home. It is unfortunate that financial reasons compel many mothers to work in industry and so to leave their children in the charge of others.

CHAPTER 29

THE YOUNG SCHOOL CHILD

Bringing the best out of a child

In our book "Lessons from Childhood"[18] we described the childhood of 450 famous men and women of history, in order to learn about the indications or absence of early indications of mental superiority, the home environment, the parental attitudes, the personality of the children destined for fame, the opinions of parents and teachers about their children, the handicaps with which the children had to contend, and numerous other data. In the concluding chapter we put together the factors which seemed to have been at least partly responsible for the eminence which these children achieved. They included a reasonably good level of intelligence, ability to concentrate and work hard, persistence and determination, ambition, personality, the ability to learn from mistakes, an inquiring mind, creativity, opportunity, and a good home and good education. By no means all those destined for fame possessed these qualities; some may have achieved what they did because of adverse factors in the environment; but it would seem reasonable to suggest that the factors mention are desirable ones to bring the best out of a child.

I suggest that the first essential for a child to achieve his best is love and security—the satisfaction of his basic emotional needs. This means that the child must have affection, acceptance however meagre his performance and however difficult his personality may be; tolerance, sympathy and understanding for his developing mind; wise loving discipline in place of angry scolding; the gradual acquisition of independence and encouragement to acquire it as soon as the child is ready. He needs to have instilled into him good moral values, a sensible attitude to sex, thoughtfulness for others—features which depend largely on the atmosphere in the home and the example set by the parents. Insecurity is a major cause of backwardness at school. Children thrive on encouragement rather than discouragement, praise and rewards rather than punishment—though excessive praise should be avoided, for it could lead to an undesirable fear of failure. There must be an absolute avoidance of constant criticism, scolding, nagging, sarcasm, denigration, disparagement, favouritism, unnecessary prolonged separation of the child from his parents, constant friction with the child. The parents need ambition for their child, but not overambition, which demands more of him than his intellectual endowment will permit.

Secondly, suitable play material must be provided. In the previous chapter I discussed the importance of toys and play for a child's pleasure and intellectual development. The play material mentioned would provide the necessary visual, sensory, tactile, perceptual, kinæsthetic and intellectual stimulation which he needs. It would provide essential prereading matter. Good homes will have much of this material; the homes of the underprivileged and "disadvantaged" child will have virtually none of it.

Thirdly, bound up with the provision of suitable play material, he must be led to enjoy learning, to want to find out, to want to create. Dr. Kellmer Pringle,[26] in an address to the Royal Society of Medicine, said that "Learning to learn does not mean beginning to learn arithmetic or reading at the earliest possible time. It is far more basic and subtle, and includes motivating the child to find pleasure in learning to develop his ability to pay attention to others, to engage in purposeful activity, to delay gratification of his wishes, and to work for more distant rather than immediate rewards and goals. It also includes developing the child's view of adults as sources of information and ideas, as well as of approval and rewards. Through such learning the child develops his self-image, the standards he sets himself for achievement, and his attitudes towards others be they his contemporaries or adults. Evidence is accumulating to show that early failure to stimulate a child's desire to learn may result in a permanent impairment of learning ability or intelligence. The child should 'learn to learn' and decide whether learning is a pleasurable challenge or a disagreeable effort to be resisted as far as possible. The child must find very early that learning is pleasure."

The young baby should be given a chance to see things. The mother who leaves her baby outside in a pram all day, however much he cries, with nothing but a brick wall to see, cannot expect him to be as advanced as a baby who is played with, talked to, propped up in his pram to see what is happening, to watch the fascinating occupations of his mother in the kitchen.

Parents should read to their children. It is remarkable how many intelligent parents never think of reading to their child until he is four or five years old. The nine or ten month old baby enjoys sitting on his mother's knee as she reads to him, pointing out objects in the book; at first he understands little, but he soon learns to enjoy the rhythm of the nursery rhyme, and soon notices the omission of a word, and joins in the action as she reads to him.

Parents need to play with their child—but certainly not all his waking hours. It is important that he should learn to enjoy playing alone, planning his own games, planning his own constructions, seeking help when he needs it. Play should not be made too easy; he needs to acquire a sense of satisfaction when he has achieved something difficult; but failure should not be allowed. Josephine Klein in her "Samples from English Cultures" showed how "middle class parents provide a succession of problem solving tasks of gradually increasing difficulty for a child. The environment is manipulated so that success is nearly always achieved and confidence is built up, so that increasing degrees of uncertainty in the initial stages of a problem can be sustained".

It may be that there is a sensitive period for learning (Chapter 17). Madame Montessori many years ago taught that children should be given the opportunities to learn as soon as they are ready. They enjoy their new skills and should be given the chance to enjoy them. For instance, as soon as manipulative development will permit, the child is given beads to thread, building bricks and other suitable material. In our book "Lessons from Childhood" we described many examples of early learning made possible by the parents; but it is vital that the early learning should be enjoyed by the child.

A word of warning was given by Wolff and Feinbloom,[34] who pointed out that overanxious parents might create a harmful atmosphere of urgency about learning. They wrote that "There is no evidence at present to support the assertion that biologically fixed critical periods control the sequence of cognitive development, no evidence that scientifically designed toys are in any way superior to the usual household items available to most infants, no evidence that the systematic application of such toys accelerates intellectual development, and no persuasive evidence that acceleration of specific skills during the sensory motor phase of development even if possible, has any lasting effect on intellectual competence". Piaget wrote that what we want to know is when to teach the child and in what sequence to present the necessary materials.

The quality of conversation in the home is of importance to the child. The practice of keeping the children in another room when visitors are in the house is undesirable; it is a good thing for the child to hear intelligent adult conversation. The parents should avoid slovenly speech. In good homes there is much conversation between child and parent; the child constantly asks for explanations because he knows that he will be given them, or better still, given the means of finding out. The child should have stories told to him; he should hear conversation; he should be encouraged to join in leg-pulling if someone uses ambiguous words or expressions. Deutsch referred to "sustained, connected and relevant conversation with the child as participant" as being a feature of good homes as distinct from the homes of disadvantaged children.

Children, as soon as they are old enough, should be taught similarities, relationships, dissimilarities, cause and effect. They should be taught to think round a subject, particularly to look for other explanations, seek the evidence for what their parents say or what they read or what they see or hear on television; they should be encouraged to question the accuracy of what their parents say and ask the reasons for their statements.

They should be taught to argue, without being impolite. In all too many homes parents dislike having their authority questioned, and are intolerant of questioning—saying "Don't argue! I won't have another word from you."

Children need to learn persistence, accuracy, thoroughness; they should be encouraged to try, try and try again, being given judicious help so that failure is avoided and success achieved. They need to learn curiosity, originality, creativity—qualities which are implanted in the home.[1,15,16] They should be given freedom to explore, find out, make decisions as soon as they are ready—and to take the lead. The child should not be discouraged for untoward consequences of his curiosity. He will be introduced to the junior library and shown how to use it and the ordinary library and the reference section, and how to obtain help from the library staff.

Other important factors include interest in the child's education, the avoidance of unnecessary absence from school, and the wise choice of school. He should be provided if possible with a room of his own in which to work. Parents should establish and maintain contact with the teachers. They must themselves fully recognize the importance of education.

Attention to certain physical factors are important for a child's school achievement. The importance of proper nutrition in the early weeks was discussed in Chapter 3. Obesity must be prevented. Visual, auditory and speech defects should be diagnosed and treated.

Mental Superiority

The mentally superior child is much less likely to have troublesome behaviour problems at school than the child with a lower than average intellectual endowment.[10,29] He may become lazy, because he finds that the school work is too easy for him, and do badly as a result; he may become bored and become a daydreamer, and again do badly; he may be lonely at school, because he cannot find others of comparable interests; he may have difficulty with his teachers, because of his originality and creativity which make it difficult to accept rote learning, or because he has a special interest for which the school curriculum does not cater; he may show disdain to others who learn less quickly; and his physical and emotional development may lag behind his intellectual development, so that he does less well at sport than his older classmates and in addition is emotionally less mature.

The range of IQ levels is said to be as follows:

IQ	Incidence
over 180	1 in 1,000,000
170	100,000
160	10,000
150	1,000
140	170
136	100
125	17

The Backward Intelligent Child

We described elsewhere[18] numerous examples of backwardness in the early years of children who were destined for fame. For instance, Louis Pasteur was a mediocre pupil and a slow learner; Edison was always at the bottom of his class; Isaac Newton in the early years was bottom of his class but later improved; James Watt was regarded as dull and inept; the famous British Physician Dr. John Hunter was said to be impenetrable to anything in the way of book learning. Oliver Goldsmith was said to be a "stupid heavy blockhead, little better than a fool, whom everybody made fun of"; Sheridan was "by common consent of both parent and preceptor a most impenetrable dunce". Charles Darwin was regarded as dull, and said himself that he was a slow thinker. Leo Tolstoy was said to be both unable and unwilling to learn. Both Anthony Trollope and the Duke of Wellington had to be moved from school on account of their poor performance. Auguste Rodin was said to be the worst pupil in school. His father said "I had an idiot for a son." His uncle said that the boy was ineducable.

By far the commonest cause of backwardness at school is a level of intelligence which is low for the school in question. This section, however, is concerned with the "underachiever"—the child who is backward in relation to his level of intelligence. We are all conversant with the particularly futile and unconstructive comment so frequently seen in school reports, that "he could do better"—the implication being that the poor performance is inevitably the fault of the child. In fact when a child does badly at school (or later, at a University or Technical School), the cause may lie in the home, the school or the child. The trouble may well be caused by the teaching, the examination or grading system, or even the examiner. It is estimated that between 20 and 50 per cent. of all school children are "underachievers."[33]

Bartlett[1] investigated 715 children in their second year at Grammar or Technical schools who were doing so badly that a transfer to a less exacting type of education was planned. He found that 70 had an IQ score of 120 to 135, 65 had a score of 135 to 140, and 73 a score of over 140.

The home. It is a regrettable fact that children born in the lowest social class achieve less at school than these of the same level of intelligence born into the upper social class. The factors involved are complex and not fully known. Bloom attempted to enumerate, for statistical purposes, the various factors which he thought were chiefly responsible. It is obvious that the factors must include the interests of the home; the parents' recognition of the importance of education; the opportunity which they give the child to enlarge his vocabulary and to acquire knowledge and experience outside the home and school; the opportunity and facilities which they give him to do his homework; their expectations of achievement, the stimulation which they provide, and the reward for good work. A home with no books and no opportunity for the child to learn, with interests confined to dog racing, football and pop singers, is hardly conducive to achievement at school. Many parents have little appreciation of the value of education; they may not only fail to encourage the child to do his homework but may actually discourage it. They encourage him to take spare time work, such as newspaper rounds; they fail to provide him with any room in which to work—away from the television. The parents do not hesitate to keep him away from school to help in the home; they let him stay at home for a prolonged period for no good medical reason at all— after a trivial cold or cough. Burt[7] showed that serious non-attendance at school is three times more common in the case of backward children than of controls. He found that barely 1 per cent. of children from a socially "good" neighbourhood in London were underachievers, as compared with 20 per cent. from a poor neighbourhood. Poverty, he wrote, "impairs health, and it limits general knowledge. By weakening the child's physical vitality it lowers his capacity to learn; and by narrowing his mental range it deprives him of that elementary fund of worldly knowledge and experience that most schools take for granted." He ascribed 11 per cent. of backwardness purely and simply to poor attendance at school.

Poor attendance may be due to illness, but at least 20 per cent. of school absence is unrelated to illness.[6] Bransby,[4] in a study of 9,444 children, showed that non-medical causes of absence increase with age—over 30 per cent. of 12-year-old girls being absent without any medical justification. "Medical" causes for absence were much more common in the case of the only child. Most of the "medical" conditions were diagnosed by the parents alone, and consisted largely of coughs, colds, abdominal pain and headache. Absence from school correlated strongly with poor parental care and lack of appreciation of the importance of education. A follow up study showed that absence from school correlated with poor performance in army selection tests in adolescence, with poor army conduct record, and with a poor civil employment record.

Those interested in the subject of school backwardness in children of normal intelligence should read the books by Dale and Griffith[8] and Kornrich.[22] Dale and Griffith studied 39 children whose work at a Grammar school deteriorated. Only one of 78 parents of the deteriorators had been to Grammar school, as compared with 83·4 per cent. of the controls. In the case of 62 per cent. of children in the A stream, both parents had attended a Grammar school, as compared with 6 per cent. of those in the C stream. A quarter of the deteriorators came from a home in which there was domestic turmoil. Fifty per cent. had no room in which to work at home. Thirty-seven out of 39 of the deteriorators came from social classes 5 to 7; all 36 of the "improvers" came from social classes 2 to 5. Various studies comparing the performance of negro and white children in America[19] have shown that there is no difference in the preschool period, but that thereafter the coloured children drop behind the white ones, the gap rapidly increasing with age. It is presumed that the main factor is the quality of the home.[16]

The child may be an underachiever because his parents want him to leave school in order to earn money, despite the fact that his intellectual ability is adequate to enable him to achieve a brilliant University career; they give him no opportunity to widen his knowledge of the world outside his home and school; and they express no interest in his achievement at school. They expect little of him, and he achieves little. Douglas[9a] showed that children from a low social class home or neighbourhood tend to be sent to a school of which little is expected, and at which little is achieved. The children of manual workers tend to be placed in a lower school stream or group—and their work deteriorates.

The school. When a pupil does poor work at school (or University),[17] the cause may be any of the reasons mentioned earlier or in the degree of motivation, or interaction between the personalities of the child and his teacher. Kornrich[24] remarked "the underlying notion is that pupils could do better but won't, so we interpret this as a kind of delinquency on their part, forgetting that it may be as much our fault for putting them in the wrong environment, or teaching them badly, or expecting them to fulfil our needs rather than their own. Moreover, the underachiever has not, in fact, failed to learn, but he has learnt hostility, inattentiveness, getting by with as little as possible, or perhaps success in athletics or social popularity, instead of what we wanted."

The child tends to be assessed entirely on his performance in the school curriculum, no attention being paid to the possibility that some children are never going to be good at some subjects, their interests and aptitudes being elsewhere; and the child with originality and creativity may be condemned because of his poor performance in the subjects of the curriculum. It is unlikely that children will achieve their best if they are bored, because of poor teaching and lack of motivation, or if they dislike the teacher. All teachers have behaviour problems, like all children, and it is easy to understand how a teacher who has to deal with difficult parents may come to dislike the child— and the feeling becomes mutual, with the result that the child does badly. Some teachers, furthermore, use the method of threats, ridicule, sarcasm and discouragement in their teaching, instead of encouragement—with bad results in the work done.

It stands to reason that the cause of poor performance in examinations may lie in the inadequacy of the examination. I know of no evidence at all that once a person qualifies as a teacher, he is automatically able to examine.

The child. Many factors may retard the progress of an intelligent child. Emotional problems are of particular importance. The child who is unhappy is liable to do badly at school. Douglas[9a] showed that children who bite their nails, have recurrent abdominal pain, repeated nightmares or enuresis, do less well at school than other children; and the more behaviour problems they had, the worse their performance.

Laziness is another important cause of poor performance at school. It may be a personality problem, or due to lack of interest in the subjects of the curriculum. A child may be lazy because he finds the work too easy. The problem may be the result of gang influence, or of lack of stimulation at home.

Some are slow thinkers, and develop an emotional block when the teacher tries to hurry them; some are unable to express themselves well, though they think well; some, like Honoré de Balzac, and Hans Christian Andersen, are daydreamers; some are so devoted to sport that they neglect their work; some have sensory defects, poor eyesight or poor hearing, which are unrecognized by the teacher; some have other physical handicaps, which make learning difficult; some suffer from overactivity and poor concentration, and do badly as a result; some suffer from overdosage of antiepileptic drugs, which impair concentration.

14

Many other reasons for poor performance could be cited; but enough has been said to indicate that backwardness at school in relation to intelligence is an important problem of multiple ætiology— many factors often operating in one child. Their elucidation is a matter of much difficulty, and a problem for the expert. It is clear that it is futile merely to blame the child, and to think that one has uttered words of wisdom when one has said that "he could do better"— and one has then done nothing about determining the reason why.

Reading difficulty. Many young children lag a long way behind their fellows in learning to read. By far the most common cause is an intellectual deficit, and hence it is essential, before diagnosing a specific reading disability, to have the child's intelligence quotient assessed by a competent psychologist, who will also relate his IQ score to his reading ability. Reading difficulties are more common in large families and in poor homes. There is commonly a history of lateness in speaking. Spelling is commonly a later problem. Various factors often act in combination.

The reason for delayed reading may lie in poor teaching, or in prolonged absence from school. Emotional difficulties are an important cause of delayed reading. Worries about home and school, and unhappiness for any reason, may be the reason for the difficulty. Worry and embarrassment about reading difficulties may further retard his progress, setting up a vicious circle. Defective eyesight or hearing may delay a child in his learning to read. Delayed maturation may explain the problem in some children. Just as some children are late in learning to sit, walk, talk, or acquire control of the bladder and bowel, so others are late in learning to read. It may be a familial pattern.

There remains the so-called "specific dyslexia," or "specific reading disability." Those interested should read the excellent articles by Ingram and Mason of Edinburgh,[20,21,25] and the book by Hermann of Copenhagen. Specific dyslexia is usually familial. It is commonly associated with dysgraphia (difficulty in writing) and spelling difficulties. It commonly follows lateness in learning to speak. Many affected children are also clumsy, and have difficulty in establishing handedness, or in differentiating right from left. They are frequently ambidextrous or left handed. They tend to write slowly and hesitantly, wriggling as they write, and contorting the face, with tongue protusion. In writing they tend to leave two small or too large a space between letters and to write at an acute angle. They frequently reverse letters, interpreting p for b, and confusing letters of similar shape. They may read from right to left, and interpret, for example, *was* for *saw*, *but* for *tub*, transposing whole letters or syllables. There may be mirror writing. I saw a whole page of an exercise book of a highly intelligent boy with calculations like the following:

$$16 + 1 = 71$$
$$14 + 1 = 51.$$

Ingram and Mason[20,21,25] broke down the difficulty into visuospatial (e.g. transposition of letters) and audiophonic (poor auditory discrimination of speech sounds, interpreting, for instance, *but* as *bud*, though the hearing is normal). These children fail to synthesize into their correct words letters sounded correctly individually—pronouncing C-L-O-C-K as COCK. They may be able to speak a word correctly, but prove unable to write it. Ingram and Mason have found that in younger patients, dyslexia always includes one or more visuospatial difficulties, poorly established laterality, clumsiness or poor writing, but that those disappear as the child gets older, leaving behind "pure" dyslexia.

Dyslexia commonly presents as a variety of behaviour problems, such as truancy and other manifestations of insecurity. It causes the child considerable anxiety and embarrassment.

Treatment is difficult. Some lose their disability altogether as they mature. Others never lose it completely. It is uncertain how much remedial teaching really helps. It is essential that the teachers should be aware of the problem, and not merely accuse the child of being lazy, stupid or naughty. Remedial teaching consists of combining the visual, kinæsthetic and auditory senses—the child looking at the letters and words, at the same time feeling the cut-out plastic letters, while the word is pronounced slowly and clearly, so that he hears what he sees and feels.

Dislike of School. School Phobia and Truancy

Children may express their distaste for school by a variety of means. They may include tears, particularly on starting at school, frank and unequivocal views on school, somatic symptoms, such as headache, abdominal pain or vomiting, any of the signs of insecurity, already mentioned, or frank school refusal (true school phobia). Other children play truant.

Tears on starting school are nothing unusual or abnormal. In some ways they are more likely if there has never been separation from the parents before, the parents never having been away even for a week-end without the child. They are more likely if the parents have been unwise in their remarks about school—suggesting, quite unintentionally, but plainly enough to the child, that he will not like it. If the mother attempts to encourage the child by saying, "You will be all right, it's not so bad as all that," or similar comment, it will suggest to the child that there is something unpleasant about school. It is far better to cause the child really to look forward to starting school, by suggesting to him in many different ways that he will thoroughly enjoy it, making new friends, playing games, and so forth. An unwise parental attitude, interacting with the child's personality, is the main reason for serious difficulties on starting school.

The child's frank disapproval of school should not be taken seriously, but somatic symptoms before going to school in the morning can be troublesome. The parent has to decide whether his complaints of headache or abdominal pain are genuine or not. He can only be guided by what he knows of the child's personality, by his appearance and by his temperature. If he looks well, he is unlikely to have a severe headache. When in doubt, it is always as well to take his temperature.

School phobia is the term used by many for school refusal. The child absolutely refuses to go to school. The problem has been admirably reviewed by Kahn and Nursten.[23] Other good reviews are those by Hersov,[14] and Tyerman.[30] It is a complex subject, but it is now commonly accepted that the problem is more one of anxiety about separation from the mother than fear of going to school. There is commonly an excessively close tie between the mother and child, the parents letting it be known in subtle ways that they doubt whether the child will like school, and they would not object seriously if he stayed at home—though he really ought to go to school. They insist on his going to school but fail to convince him that they mean what they say. It would not be reasonable to say that factors in the school are irrelevant. There may be some bullying or teasing at school. The refusal to go to school is commonly precipitated by a change from one school to another, or by an illness, or by absence from school for other reasons, or even by some punishment. The child's personality is also of great importance; the common characteristics include immaturity, timidity and dislike of games. The usual intellectual level is average or above average, and progress at school is entirely satisfactory; yet he is apt to feel unable to live up to the high aspirations of his teachers or parents, and he may feel that he cannot compete with his siblings. Various studies have indicated that the mother is commonly a domineering type, though overprotective and overindulgent, while the father is ineffective and disinterested.

Treatment is difficult, especially in the case of older children. Parent and child should be weaned from each other, but forceful methods will fail. The help of a child psychiatrist, working in conjunction with the teachers, should be enlisted. In general, the longer the child is away from school, the more difficult it becomes to get him back; yet actual compulsion will almost certainly fail, and may do more harm than good. A change from one school to another is rarely successful. One should do one's best not to make the parents feel guilty on account of the problem.

Whereas the child with school phobia usually has an average or an above average level of intelligence, with good school work, the truant may be a poor attender, whose work is below average. The truant tends to come from a large family, and a home with little discipline, while the child with school phobia is more liable to be an only child from a good home. The truant has commonly experienced more than average separation from his parents when he was young, while the child with school phobia has commonly had fewer separations than usual.

Bullying and Teasing

If a child is a bully, it is likely that he is being bullied by other boys, or by his siblings, or by his parents or by a teacher. It is a reaction to insecurity at home or school, and may arise from lack of discipline or excessive discipline with corporal punishment. The treatment must consist of a search for the cause; punishment of the bully, and particularly corporal punishment, is futile and will do far more harm than good.

A child is liable to be bullied if he fails to stand up for himself, is timid, subsides into tears, and is poor in sport. The child who is tall for his age but who is not proportionately more mature is liable to be bullied. At home his parents may have stepped in to stop every dispute between the children, instead of letting them settle their own arguments; or the child may be an only child, who has been seriously overprotected. Treatment is not easy, but the essential thing is to encourage the child to stand up for himself. It is usually possible to arrange classes in Judo, wrestling, boxing or Karate, particularly Judo. This will build up his self confidence and enable him to deal effectively with a bully.

Teasing at school is invariable, but sometimes it is excessive and causes unhappiness. Children may be teased because of their accent, their social class, their manner of speech, and particularly because of obesity, clumsiness or deafness; they are liable to be teased and taunted if they have a short temper, or if they tale tales, show off, try to boss others, are poor in sport, prudish, "know alls", and court favours from the teacher. The less bright children may tease the brighter more successful ones, partly because of envy. Children are unlikely to be teased on account of dwarfism, or handicaps such as cerebral palsy, a weak leg (such as that due to poliomyelitis), or defective vision.

The treatment must be that of the cause. The cause is likely to lie at home, in overprotection, inhibition of normal aggressiveness, and perhaps the absence of siblings.

Solvent Sniffing

In some areas solvent sniffing is a serious problem. In two years 130 "glue sniffers" were arrested in Denver, Colorado, and their average age was thirteen.[11] In some schools two to five per cent of pupils are solvent sniffers.[10] It is associated with delinquency, and is much more common in the lower social classes.

The solvents sniffed are varied; they include glues, nail polish removers, spot or stain removers, petrol, lighter fluid, plastic cements in building kits, aeroplane glues, lacquers, aerosols, enamels, paint thinners. They may squeeze some glue onto a hankerchief and smell it, or add nail polish remover to Coca-cola and drink it.[10] The solvents contain a variety of poisons, such as carbon tetrachloride which is hepatotoxic; benzene which is toxic to the bone marrow; toluene in cleaning agents (hepatotoxic, renal-toxic); naphtha which may cause hæmolysis or cardiac arrest; petrol which may cause hepatitis or lead encephalopathy; various central nervous system depressants which may cause intoxication, ataxia, coma or sudden death.[4] One result of the practice is deterioration in school work.

Smoking

Smoking is an important problem of the school child. Its causes are varied[27]; the example set by the parents, siblings and teachers is particularly important. Smoking may be a status symbol; the result of a challenge by others (when smoking is forbidden); a desire to be regarded as tougher or older than they really are; a reaction to stress—arising from examinations, insecurity at home or school; boredom; curiosity; a desire for conformity—the child smoking because others do; or an attention seeking device—perhaps just because the parents object to it. Numerous studies[24] have shown that regular smokers of both sexes have lower average grades at school, and a higher school absence and illness rate. There is more smoking in the C stream at school than the A stream. There is more smoking in children of lower social classes—partly because the children have more pocket money than those of upper classes.

Prevention is difficult. The setting of the example of not smoking has been shown repeatedly to be important. Parents can do much by encouraging independence of thought, leadership and a willingness not always to conform if conformity is undesirable. Children should learn by precept and example to think for themselves. The use of fear for prevention is useless; no child knows what it is like to die of cancer of the lung or bladder. If he has a cough due to smoking, he may understand the cause and effect. If he is interested in sport, he may be persuaded that smoking is spoiling his athletic performance.

Delinquency

There is a vast literature on delinquency; the subject is mentioned briefly because all are potential delinquents, and there is no hard and fast dividing line between those who get into trouble and those who do not. In one year a million juveniles (1 in 43 of the age group) were taken to court in the United States, but only one in four of those coming to the notice of the police were taken to court. It seems reasonable to mention the problem in a book about the normal child. The following is a summary of many articles and books.

Delinquency is five times more common in boys than girls. Twenty per cent. have a delinquent brother or sister, and 40 per cent. a father with a criminal record. Their intelligence is about average. Delinquents tend to have a poor record at school, with more frequent absences than others; they are more likely to get into trouble at school, to be unpopular, poor at sport, to play truant, to be hostile and defiant, with little respect for authority, and to be immature. Truancy is a common problem. They tend to be selfish, to lack a conscience, to show little respect for the property of others, and to show little affection. The father is commonly weak, alcoholic, punitive, and hated by his children; he is especially liable to have suffered himself from an unhappy childhood. Insecurity is an important feature in the life of a delinquent; he has little love at home and seeks security in a gang.

Delinquents tend to come from lower social classes and a poor neighbourhood where there is overcrowding, large families, unemployment and a poor educational standard, with parental ignorance and broken homes. The parents are likely to set a bad example, and to show pride in their child's dishonesty. Lack of discipline is the rule, but sometimes there has been excessively strict discipline with much corporal punishment. Prolonged separation of the child from his mother in the first five years, and from his father after five years, is a common finding. Delinquency has been described as the culmination of many years of unsatisfactory home life.

The subsequent history of juvenile delinquents is unsatisfactory. Robins[23] studied the adult status of 524 child guidance clinic patients and compared them with 100 others of comparable age, sex, race, intelligence and neighbourhood who had not attended such clinics. He found that antisocial boys had a 71 per cent. risk of future arrest, and a 50 per cent. risk of divorce—while the girls had a 70 per cent. risk of divorce. Antisocial children were more often arrested or imprisoned as adults, had more marital difficulties, poor occupational, social and army records, more alcoholism, more physical disease and more hysteria or schizophrenia.

References

1. ARASTEH, J. D. (1968). "Creativity and Related Processes in the Young Child; A Review of the Literature." *J. Genet. Psychol.*, **112**, 77.
2. BARTLETT, E. M. (1965). In Howells, J. G., *Modern Perspectives in Child Psychiatry*. London Oliver and Boyd.
3. BLOOM, B. J. (1964). *Stability and Change in Human Characteristics*. New York. Wiley.
4. BRANSBY, E. R. (1951). "Absence from School." *Medical Officer*, **86**, 223, 237.
5. *British Medical Journal* (1971). "Sniffing Syndrome." Leading article, **2**, 183.
6. BURN, J. L. (1956) in *Report of Chief Medical Officer*. Minister of Education for years 1954 and 1955. London. H.M.S.O.
7. BURT, C. (1953). *The Causes and Treatment of Backwardness*. London. University of London Press.
8. DALE, R. R., GRIFFITH, S. (1965). *Downstream*. London. Routledge and Kegan Paul.
9. DEUTSCH, M. (1967). *The Disadvantaged Child*. New York. Basic Books Inc.
9a. DOUGLAS, J. W. B. (1964). *The Home and The School*. MacGibbon and Kee.
10. FREEHILL, M. F. (1961). *Gifted Children: Their Psychology and Education*. New York. MacMillan.
11. Gellman V. (1968). "Glue Sniffing Among Winnipeg School Children." *Can., Med. Ass. J.*, **98**, 411.
12. GLASER, H. H., MASSENGALE, O. N. (1962). "Glue-sniffing in Children." *J. Am. Med. Ass.*, **181**, 300.
13. HERMANN, K. (1959). *Reading Disability*. Copenhagen. Munksgaard.
14. HERSOV, L. A. (1960). "Persistent Non-attendance at School." *J. Child Psychol. and Psychiat.*, **1**, 130.
15. HUDSON, L. (1967). *Contrary Imaginations: A Psychological Study of the English Schoolboy*. London. Penguin.
16. HUDSON, L. (1970). *The Ecology of Human Intelligence*. London. Penguin.
17. ILLINGWORTH, R. S. (1964). *The Normal School Child; His Problems Physical and Emotional*. London. Heinemann.
18. ILLINGWORTH, R. S., ILLINGWORTH, C. M. (1966). *Lessons from Childhood: Some Aspects of the Early Life of Unusual Men and Women*. Edinburgh. Livingstone.
19. ILLINGWORTH, R. S. (1968). "How to Help a Child to Achieve His Best." *J. Pediat.*, **73**, 61.
20. INGRAM, T. T. S. (1963). "Delayed Development of Speech with Special Reference to Dyslexia." *Proc. Roy. Soc. Med.*, **56**, 199.
21. INGRAM, T. T. S., MASON, A. W. (1965). "Reading and Writing Difficulties in Childhood." *Brit. med. J.*, **2**, 463.
22. JAHODA, M., WARREN, N. (1968). "Intelligence, Nature and Nurture." *New Scientist*, **39**, 188.
23. KAHN, J. H., NURSTEN, J. P. (1968). *Unwillingly to School*. London. Pergamon.
24. KORNRICH, M. (1965). *Underachievement*. Springfield. Charles Thomas.
25. MASON, A. W. (1967). "Specific (Developmental) Dyslexia." *Develop. Med. Child Neurol.*, **9**, 183.

25a. MICHAL-SMITH, H. (1957). *Management of the Handicapped Child.* New York. Grune and Stratton.
26. PRINGLE, M. L. K. (1967). "Speech learning and Child Health." *Proc. Roy. Soc. Med.*, **60,** 885.
27. ROBINS, L. N. (1966). *Deviant Children Grown Up.* Baltimore. Williams Wilkins.
28. ROGERS, K. D., REESE, G. (1964). "Smoking and High School Performance." *Am. J. Dis. Child.*, **108, 117.**
29. TERMAN, L. M., ODEN, M. H. (1926 to 1959; 5 volumes). *Genetic Studies of Genius.* Stanford. Stanford University Press.
30. TYERMAN, M. J. (1958). "A Research into Truancy." *B. J. Educ. Psychol.*, **28, 217.**
31. VERNON, P. E. (1969). *Intelligence and Cultural Environment.* London. Methuen.
32. WEHRLE, P. F., BRENT, R. L., DOYLE, J. L., FARR, L. E., FAGAN, E. L., FINBERG, L., NAHMIAS, A. J., PICKERING, D. E., YAMAZAKI, J. N., HORTON, J. R. M. (1969). "Smoking and Children; a Pediatric Viewpoint." *Pediatrics,* **44,** 757.
33. WIMBERGER, H. C. (1966). "Conceptual System for Classification of Phychogenic Underachievement." *J. Pediat.*, **69,** 1092.
34. WOLFF, P. H., FEINBLOOM, R. I. (1969). "Critical Periods and Cognitive Development in the First Two Years." *Pediatrics,* **44,** 999.

CHAPTER 30

THE SICK CHILD

A child wants to be loved at all times, but at no time does he want love more than when he is feeling poorly. It is unfortunate that just at that very time some children have to be sent into hospital.

When the sick child is at home, discipline must be relaxed. One cannot teach discipline when a child is poorly. There must be no fear of spoiling him if the illness is only a short one. It is essential, however, that as soon as he is convalescent, normal discipline should be exerted.

Many children learn bad habits during an illness as a result of some indulgence, and the habit proves difficult to break. The mother may sleep in the child's room or the child in the parent's room, or a warm drink is taken to him every time he cries out at night, and instead of reverting to the normal practice immediately after the acute illness (which in most cases is only 1 or 2 days) the parents make the mistake of continuing the indulgence too long.

Food forcing should always be avoided. It is wrong to attempt to persuade a feverish child to eat. He should be given what he wants, and no more. Not all children when feverish take enough fluid if left to regulate their fluid intake merely by their thirst. It may be necessary to persuade a child gently to drink more, and to make him want to drink more by supplying palatable fluids. Severe dehydration may occur in a toddler who acquires a simple upper respiratory tract infection, and is not given sufficient fluid. Babies and toddlers do not usually demand sufficient fluid for their needs when suffering from infections with fever.

Medicine forcing should be avoided. If a child is forced to take medicine once, he is almost certain to resist next time. There is always a risk that if there is a struggle, some of the dose will be lost, and that some will go down the wrong way. It is far better to get the medicine down by guile than by force. Syrup preparations of medicine may be strongly disliked by children. A tablet is often more likely to be preferred, provided that it is crushed up and given in jam. Under the age of 5, few children will swallow the average sized tablet intact.

The role of suggestion must always be remembered. Parents make the mistake of repeatedly asking a child if he is going to be sick again, or if he still has a pain or headache, with the result that the symptom is suggested. It is far better to make light of his symptoms and distract his attention to other things.

When a child who has recently acquired sphincter control becomes ill, "accidents" are apt to occur. The parents should be warned of this and told not to make any fuss about it and not to scold the child.

It is always difficult to keep a poorly child occupied in bed. The book by Cornelia Stratton Parker entitled *Your Child can be Happy in Bed* (New York, Thomas Crowell) gives useful ideas in this respect. She suggested that periods of illness should be anticipated, books and suitable toys, along with such materials as Christmas calendars, sea shells, and pictures to colour or cut out, should be kept in a box, to be used only when the child is ill.

On Keeping the Child in Bed

I am convinced that children are kept in bed during the day far more than they need be. I have reviewed this matter in detail elsewhere.[1]

I agree with Browse, who in his excellent book on bed rest, wrote that "the bed is often a sign of our therapeutic inadequacy rather than a therapeutic measure deserving of praise. The bed is *the* non specific treatment of our time, *the* great placebo."

It is a common practice to put a child to bed for almost any symptom, such as abdominal discomfort, a cold or diarrhœa. If a child wants to be up and about, it is difficult to see the rationale of putting him to bed. It is thought that in the preparalytic stage of poliomyelitis, complete rest reduces the spread of paralysis. There is evidence that infective hepatitis clears up more quickly with rest. It is customary to keep a child in bed in the acute stage of rheumatic fever with carditis, but the duration of bed rest in this condition has been greatly reduced. Otherwise it is difficult to think of medical conditions for which bed rest is essential when the child is well enough and anxious to get up.

I find it difficult to understand why it should be thought better to keep a child with a sore throat, even if his temperature is raised, sitting restlessly in bed playing, than to allow him to be up and play in his room or sit in a chair reading. A restless child exerts himself more when in bed than he would do if allowed up in his room; and in any case there is no evidence in the vast majority of conditions that trivial exertion will in any way harm him even if his temperature is 100°F.

Confinement to bed bores a child: it makes sleep at night more difficult; it is less easy for him to play games; it tends to isolate him from his siblings. I firmly believe that before we confine a child to bed we should think about the disadvantages of so doing, and we should think about the possible disadvantages and the obvious advantages of allowing him up. If we do that, we shall be much less likely to bore children by unnecessary confinement to bed.

The Child in Hospital

It cannot be doubted that some young children suffer an emotional disturbance when admitted to hospital. This has been exaggerated by some and minimized by others. The extent of emotional trauma, if any, is governed by a variety of factors, especially the age and especially the developmental age of the child; his personality; the parent child relationships at home; his psychological preparation for admission to hospital; the duration of hospital stay; the experiences in hospital; and the attitudes of the parents when he returns home. The nature of the illness itself may be relevant.

As for the age, it seems likely that the most vulnerable age is 6 months to 2 or 3 years.[3] It is uncertain whether a baby in his first 6 months suffers psychological harm by being separated from his mother, though it has been suggested that some of the behaviour characteristics of children who were prematurely born may be related to the prolonged separation of the baby from the mother in the new-born period. There is abundant experimental evidence that animals are affected by separation from their mothers at birth, and there is some evidence that the damage is caused by the lack of the normal tactile stimulation which the young receive from their mothers. The developmental age, as distinct from the chronological age, is important.

The personality of the child has a considerable bearing on the emotional effect of admission to hospital. Some children readily adapt themselves to the new circumstances. Some are firmly attached to their mothers and are severely disturbed when separated from them.

The quality of the parent child relationship is important. It would be wrong, however, to suggest that a 3-year-old who is exceedingly upset at being separated from the mother has been in any way mismanaged at home.

Where possible the child should be prepared psychologically for admission to hospital. This is impossible in the case of the young child. The older one, such as the 3-year-old, can be shown into the ward beforehand, and told a little about the experiences which he is likely to have in hospital. The worst thing which parents can do is to threaten the child that if he does not do what he is told he will no longer be loved, or he will be changed for another child, or will be taken to the doctor, or worse still taken to a hospital and left there. Such a child will inevitably regard his admission to hospital as a punishment.

As for the experiences in hospital, there is no country in which more has been done for children than this one: yet there is still more to be done. I have discussed these in detail elsewhere.[3] The problems are reviewed in the book by Vernon and colleagues.[6] When a child is admitted, he should be taken up to the ward by his mother, who should see him into bed, if he has to go to bed, and stay with him for a time until he has settled down. There is nothing to be said for the old idea of separating child from parent in the casualty department, stripping the child and bathing him, removing all his clothes, and then putting him to bed—however necessary it is that he should go to bed.[6] We should try to imagine the feelings of the small child when he is admitted to hospital.

If he is an infant he is likely to be placed in a cubicle because of the risk of cross-infection. He is visited occasionally by someone in a white coat and mask, someone he has never seen before. No one picks him up, however much he cries. He is left crying longer than he has ever been left before. He is thought to be "spoilt." No one realizes that this is a normal reaction for a child of his age who has the firm attachment to his mother he ought to have.

Meals come round at fixed intervals to which he is not accustomed, and he cries from hunger long before these times. They contain items of diet which he has never tasted before, or which he does not like. No one knows anything about his likes or dislikes. His favourite cup and dish are missing. He wants a drink. His mother would know perfectly well, but the nurse does not realize that this is the reason for his fussing.

He has no toys, or perhaps a single teddy, but it is not his favourite one. He is given no chance of practising his newly-learned skills. His personality and individuality are not recognized. He is just left to cry.

A doctor comes in at intervals, and he is held down by a nurse while needles are pushed unexpectedly into his back, neck or thigh, causing great pain. This happens at intervals throughout the day. He is carried away to another room, and there a dark thing is held over his nose and mouth. There is a nasty smell in it and it hurts his nose and throat. He screams in terror, but is held down firmly by two nurses until he goes to sleep.

The type and design of hospital is relevant to the problem. If a child has to be admitted to hospital, the best place for him is a Children's Hospital, where everyone is used to dealing with children, and the next best place is a large Children's Unit in a General Hospital. The worst place for him is an adult ward, and after that a private ward or a nursing home, in either of which he will be alone, and isolated from other children. A child is far happier in the presence of other children. Even if he is in bed himself, ambulant children can come and talk to him and play with him. For this reason cubicles should be kept to a minimum.

It is now widely accepted that regular visiting is essential, where possible. Parents should be allowed to visit at times convenient to them. The old idea of an hour's visiting in the evening should be a thing of the past. It is true that small children cry when their parents leave.[2] It is far better that they should see their parents daily, even though they know that they will have to go, than they should be allowed to become more and more convinced that they have been deserted by their parents.

Every Children's Hospital and large Children's Unit should have accommodation for mothers to share a room with their child. When it is obvious that a child is going to be disturbed at being separated from his mother, and that the mother is going to be disturbed at being separated from her child, it is desirable that the two should be given a room together. The mother then looks after her own child and takes her part in bringing about his recovery. If she has other small children at home she is unlikely to be able to come in with her child. In that case she can usually arrange to spend the day with him. Some Infectious Disease Hospitals still have antiquated ideas about visiting— making it impossible for the parents to do more than look at the child through a window.

Much can be done to make the child's stay in hospital a happy one. A little foresight will reduce venipunctures and pricks to a minimum—a battery of tests being carried out on a single specimen. The use of ultramicro-methods, which make venipunctures unnecessary, helps to reduce discomfort. Rectal temperature taking should be avoided. Every effort should be made to attend to the child's toilet needs. Much distress can be caused by failure to attend to them. The child should be kept occupied by a liberal supply of toys and books suitable for his age group, with the help of an occupational therapist and voluntary workers. Food at mealtimes should be food liked by children. All unpleasant procedures should be carried out in a treatment room out of sight of other children. No one should tell lies to a child—saying that a prick will not hurt, and that parents are about to visit when they are not.

Children should not be kept in bed during the day unless it is absolutely necessary. They are far happier if allowed to walk round the ward, and to sit at the table to play or have meals. The duration of stay in hospital should be kept to a minimum. For instance, in the case of an operation for an inguinal hernia, there is no need for the child to be detained for more than one day.

Before his discharge the management of the child should be discussed with his parents. They should know about possible behaviour problems which may arise when he gets home.

The reaction of small children when admitted to hospital has been described by many writers. The sequence is commonly an initial protest (crying), followed by a stage of negativism, and thereafter a stage of withdrawal, in which the child is quiet and subdued. In this stage he is apt to be subdued and quiet until an attendant or the parent approaches the bed, when he cries. Many babies fail to gain weight when separated from their mothers. This may be due partly to excessive use of energy and fluid loss in crying.

On discharge from hospital children may revert to infantile habits. Common problems are night terrors, bed wetting, fear of strangers and clinging to the mother. Parents are apt to spoil children who have been seriously ill and add to the problems. The child may feel insecure, however, and the parents have to make every effort to restore his feeling of security.

Levy[5] and others have written about the psychological trauma of operations, particularly tonsillectomy. He described children who as a result of such operations in the first 3 years had developed night terrors, negativism, dependency reactions, causing the child to cling to the mother, and various fears—fears of the dark and of strange men. He thought that they were due chiefly to the removal from the mother just at the time when the child most needed her and to painful experiences such as an anæsthetic.

There are other ways in which a period in hospital disturbs a child. It upsets his whole rhythm and he is liable to develop sleep and sphincter disturbances on his return home, fears of the dark, fears of strange people and negativism.

Parental Attitudes

A person's whole attitude to illness is likely to be implanted by the parents in his childhood. The child will be greatly influenced by his parent's attitude to their own symptoms. If they constantly complain about their gastric or other symptoms in the child's presence, constantly express anxiety about their own symptoms, real or imaginary, and are always worried about illness, exaggerate every complaint and have fetishes about good health, then they are setting their child on the way to neurosis and hypochondriasis. If in addition they make a fuss about every symptom of which the child complains, express anxiety about it, put him to bed, give him medicine, keep him indoors, get him excused from gym, or keep him off school totally unnecessarily, they are doing great harm to the child. Leo Kanner remarked that 53 per cent. of 145 hypochondriacal children seen by him had parents who were hypochondriacs. When a boy falls and grazes his knee, the wise parents, having seen at a glance that he has not broken his leg, virtually ignores the injury—except that he may clean the leg up on return home; whereas the unwise parent shows great anxiety, picks the child up and pets and comforts him, gives him a sweet—and makes a fool of him. Parents have to strike a difficult balance between hardness and lack of sympathy, and excessive sympathy and fussing. They must not allow their child to use his symptoms to get his own way—or worse still, to make use of a simple knock in play, by screaming, to get his siblings into trouble.

References

1. BROWSE, N. L. (1965). *The Physiology and Pathology of Bed Rest.* Springfield. Charles Thomas.
2. ILLINGWORTH, R. S., HOLT, K. S. (1955). "Children in Hospital." Some observations on their reactions with special reference to daily visiting. *Lancet,* 2, 1257.
3. ILLINGWORTH, R. S. (1958). "Children in Hospital." *Lancet,* 2, 165.
4. ILLINGWORTH, R. S. (1963). "Why Put Him to Bed?" *Clin. Pediatrics,* 2, 108.
5. LEVY, D. M. (1945). "Physic Trauma of Operations in Childhood." *Amer. J. Dis. Child.,* 69, 7.
6. VERNON, D. T. A., FOLEY, J. M., SIPOWICZ, R., SCHULMAN, J. L. (1965). *The Psychological Response of Children to Hospitalization and Illness.* Springfield. Charles Thomas.

CHAPTER 31

THE WHOLE CHILD

There have been so many recent advances in knowledge that it is no longer possible for a pædiatrician to be an expert in all aspects of pædiatrics. No doctor can be an expert in congenital heart disease, electroencephalography, electromyography, neonatology, respiratory function, the orthopædic surgery of infancy and childhood, the radiology of childhood, air encephalography, genetics and chromosomes, biochemistry, hæmatology and endocrinology of childhood—and all the other branches of pædiatrics. The tendency now is for a pædiatrician to become an expert in one particular field—and fellow pædiatricians, who are experts in other subjects, refer children to him if they present problems in his field. This is inevitable, but the great danger is the likelihood that no one will view, assess and treat the child as a whole—and where relevant, as it so often is, view, assess and treat the family as a whole.

It is with this in mind that I thought it desirable, after discussing infant feeding, various features of mental and physical development, and numerous behaviour problems, that I should conclude with this brief chapter on the Whole Child.

The History

No examination of a child is complete without a good history. This includes not only the history of the main complaints, but a history concerning all other systems of the body. For instance, when a child is referred to one on account of a cough, one must ask the history of symptoms referable to the ear, nose, throat, appetite, bowels, urinary system, the amount of energy or lassitude which he has, and the presence or absence of pains. The family history, including that of tuberculosis, is always investigated. If the child is referred for a feeding problem, a detailed history of the method of feeding must be obtained.

In the case of a behaviour problem, and in the case of many diseases, one has to enquire in detail about the whole environment. It is important to know about the father's alcoholism, ineffectiveness and disinterestedness in the children, or his excessive strictness and his punitive attitudes. It is important to know about the housing conditions, which may be highly relevant to the child's behaviour. For instance, an infant's sleeping problems may be due to the unkindness of the mother-in-law, who owns the house, and who complains as soon as the baby cries—so that the mother has to try to make him go to sleep. Friction between the mother and her mother-in-law may be an important factor in the ætiology of behaviour problems in the child.

Inadequate sanitation, with the absence of an indoor lavatory, may be at the root of a problem of enuresis. A boy's bad behaviour may be due to boredom, and the lack of suitable playing space outside the house.

The services of the medical social worker may be essential in this connection. She may visit the home, and interview both parents there. In the case of the school child, she will contact the teachers concerned—and obtain a completely new and important view of the child's problems.

Insecurity may be due to a wide variety of causes, and one has to determine why the child feels insecure. For this reason one has to know much about the home environment. It might well be important to know about prolonged absences of the father, or about the mother being out at work. In the case of the school child, who is doing badly at school, the parents' attitude to his homework, and to his whole education, must be determined.

Remembering that a child's behaviour problems are due to a conflict between his developing personality and the personality and attitudes of his parents, one has to determine not just what the parents' attitudes are, but why they have them. It is not enough to know that the conflict between the child and his mother is due to the mother's bad temper; one has to know the reason why she loses her temper, why she beats the child, or why she over-protects him. She may be anæmic without knowing it, or have an unrecognized thyrotoxicosis—which could be remedied.

There are many problems which are partly somatic and partly psychological in origin. The family background of the child with asthma is of great importance. Overprotection or rejection, or a combination of both, may be vital factors in the child's asthma. A child may have somatic symptoms because of psychological factors, or have psychological problems as a result of organic disease. He may respond to specific dyslexia, at school age, by playing truant; he may wheeze because of worries at home. He may have abdominal pain, not because of a peptic ulcer, but because his father has a peptic ulcer—and constantly impresses the children with the abdominal discomfort which he experiences—making them fear that they may suffer in the same way.

Many a mother takes her child to the doctor with a complaint of symptoms which bear little relation to her real fears. She may fear that the child has leukæmia, a cerebral tumour, tuberculosis, asthma, or early insanity—because a relative of hers experienced one of these conditions. Yet she tells the doctor about a variety of symptoms, none of them pointing directly to her inner fears. The sensitive pædiatrician, in taking the history, assesses the mother and realizing that there is something behind what she has said, determines what it is that she really fears.

The Examination

It is bad pædiatric medicine to treat a child's cough and ignore the much more important behaviour problems, which, untreated, may have a permanent effect on his emotional development, and affect his whole adult life—and the life of the next generation, because of his attitude to his own children. It is not enough to look at a baby's nævus and ignore the fact that he is starving; to treat a child's tics and ignore the need for orthodontic treatment to prevent an unfortunate facial appearance which would be with him for life. It is poor medicine to examine a baby for an umbilical hernia, and to ignore the squint which if untreated will cause blindness in one eye. It is poor work to investigate a baby's feeding problem, and to fail to realize that the baby is deaf—a failure due to the fact that a hearing test was not a routine part of the examination.

It would be inadequate to allay the mother's anxiety that the baby had a squint, by telling her that the eyes were normal, while the congenital dermal sinus in the lumbar region, which would lead to pyogenic meningitis, was not seen, because only a small part of the child was examined.

A rapid screening developmental examination must be part of the routine examination of any baby. It would be inadequate, when a mother suspected that the child was not responding well to sound, to inform her that the child's ears and hearing were normal, without having assessed the child's development, in order to determine whether the poor response to sound was merely part of general mental retardation.

One must add that in some cases, such as thyroid deficiency, the mental retardation is reversible, if proper treatment is promptly instituted, and for this reason alone, early diagnosis is important.

The examination of any baby, in a baby clinic, private house, in-patient or out-patient department of a hospital, must include a rough developmental assessment, the measurement of the maximum head circumference (and its relation to the weight), an inspection of the back for a congenital dermal sinus, examination of the hip for congenital subluxation, and of the genitalia. The eyes are always examined for nystagmus, cataract or other abnormalities. After 3 or 4 months, one always tests the hearing. The urine is examined for phenylpyruvic acid. The developmental examination is a rapid one, unless an abnormality is suspected. It includes motor development and an assessment of muscle tone in all cases. It includes an assessment of the child's alertness and responsiveness to his mother—and of her response to him.

Perhaps the most common abnormal feature to be ignored in the child after infancy is obesity. It is wrong to ignore early obesity, because it is so much easier to treat in the early stages than later, when the child is seriously overweight.

I constantly tell my students that if they fail to notice things when they don't matter, they won't notice things when they do matter. They are taught to notice every patch of pigmentation, every bruise and scar, and every abnormal mark on the child. One must always be concerned with the whole child, and not just a little bit of him.

Much more could be said about the inspection and examination of the child. I have not touched on the examination of the heart, chest, abdomen and lymph node areas, or on the features commonly found in children with chromosome abnormalities (e.g. low set ears). Enough has been said, however, to indicate that it is altogether wrong to confine one's history or examination to that part of the anatomy which seems to be relevant to the symptoms for which the mother refers the child. In pædiatrics one is concerned not just with treatment but with prevention. We are concerned with the whole child—and therefore, very often, with his family.

SOME RECOMMENDED READING

APLEY, J., MACKEITH, R. (1967). *The Child and His Symptoms*. Oxford. Blackwell.

AUSUBEL, D. P., SULLIVAN, E. V. (1970). *Theory and Problems of Child Development*. New York. Grune and Stratton.

BAKWIN, H., BAKWIN, R. M. (1966). *Behavior Disorders in Children*. Philadelphia. Saunders.

BOWLBY, J. (1961). *Child Care and the Growth of Love*. London. Pelican.

BRECKENRIDGE, M. E., VINCENT, E. L. (1965). *Child Development*. Philadelphia. Saunders.

BURTON, L. (1968). *Vulnerable Children*. London. Routledge and Kegan Paul.

CAPLAN, G. (1961). *Prevention of Mental Disorders in Children*. London. Tavistock Publications.

CARMICHAEL, L. (1967). *Manual of Child Psychology*. New York. Wiley.

FALKNER, F. (1966). *Human Development*. Philadelphia. Saunders.

FOSS, B. M. (1961, 1963, 1965, 3 vols.). *Determinants of Infant Behaviour*. London. Methuen.

GESELL, A., AMATRUDA, C. S. (1947). *Developmental Diagnosis*. New York. Hoeber.

GESELL, A., HALVERSON, H. M., THOMPSON, H., ILG, F. L., CASTNER, B. M., AMES, L. B., AMATRUDA, C. S. (1940). *The First Five Years of Life*. London. Harper.

GESELL, A., ILG, F. L. (1943). *Infant and Child in the Culture of Today*. New York. Harper and Row.

HADFIELD, J. A. (1962). *Childhood and Adolescence*. London. Pelican.

HARPER, P. A. (1962). *Preventive Pediatrics*. New York. Appleton Century Crofts.

HOWELLS, J. G. (1965). *Modern Perspectives in Child Psychiatry*. Edinburgh. Oliver and Boyd.

HURLOCK, E. B. (1964). *Child Development*. New York. McGraw-Hill.

HYMES, J. L. (1961). *The Child Under Six*. New Jersey. Prentice Hall.

ILLINGWORTH, R. S., ILLINGWORTH, C. M. (1966). *Lessons from Childhood*. Edinburgh. Churchill Livingstone.

ILLINGWORTH, R. S. (1964). *The Normal School Child: His Problems Physical and Emotional*. London. Heinemann.

ILLINGWORTH, R. S. (1972). *Development of the Infant and Young Child, Normal and Abnormal*. 5th ed. Edinburgh. Churchill Livingstone.

ILLINGWORTH, R. S. (1971). *Treatment of the Child at Home. A Guide for Family Doctors*. Oxford. Blackwell.

ILLINGWORTH, R. S. (1971). *Common Symptoms of Disease in Children*. 3rd ed. Oxford. Blackwell.

JENSEN, G. D. (1962). *The Well Child's Problems*. Chicago. New York Medical Publishers.

JONES, P. G. (1970). *Clinical Paediatric Surgery, Diagnosis and Management*. Bristol. John Wright.

KAHN, J. H. (1965). *Human Growth and the Development of Personality*. London. Pergamon Press.

MITCHELL, ROSS G. (1970). *Child Life and Health*. London. Churchill. Livingstone.

MUSSEN, P. H., CONGER, J. J., KAGAN, J. (1963). *Child Development and Personality*. New York. Harper and Row.

NEWSON, J., NEWSON, E. (1963). *Infant Care in an Urban Community*. London. Allen and Unwin.

PARKHURST, H. (1951). *Exploring the Child's World*. New York. Appleton Century Crofts.

SMART, M. S. (1967). *Children, Development and Relationships*. New York. Macmillan.
STUART, H. C., PRUGH, D. G. (1960). *The Healthy Child*. Cambridge, Mass. Harvard Univ. Press.
VERVILLE, E. (1967). *Behaviour Problems of Children*. Philadelphia. Saunders.
WATSON, E. H., LOWREY, G. H. (1967). *Growth and Development of Children*. Chicago. Year Book Publishers.

INDEX